PRINCIPLES OF BIOMECHANICS & MOTION ANALYSIS

PRINCIPLES OF BIOMECHANICS & MOTION ANALYSIS

Iwan W. Griffiths, BSc, PhD (Wales)

Department of Sport Science
University of Wales Swansea

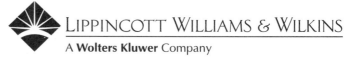

LIPPINCOTT WILLIAMS & WILKINS
A **Wolters Kluwer** Company

Philadelphia • Baltimore • New York • London
Buenos Aires • Hong Kong • Sydney • Tokyo

Acquisitions Editor: Emily Lupash
Managing Editor: Karen Ruppert
Marketing Manager: Christen Murphy
Production Editor: Jennifer Ajello
Designer: Doug Smock
Compositor: Maryland Composition
Printer: Quebecor World-Dubuque

Library of Congress Cataloging-in-Publication Data

Griffiths, Iwan W.
   [Principles of motion analysis and mechanics]
   Principles of motion analysis & mechanics: a handbook for sports science students/Ivan W. Griffiths.
       p. cm.
   ISBN 0-7817-5231-0
    1. Kinesiology—Handbooks, manuals, etc. 2. Human mechanics—Handbooks, manuals, etc. I. Title.

QP303.G75 2005
612.7′6—dc22

                                                                    2005051188

To purchase additional copies of this book, call our customer service department at **(800) 638-3030** or fax orders to **(301) 824-7390**. International customers should call **(301) 714-2324**.

Visit Lippincott Williams & Wilkins on the Internet: http://www.LWW.com. Lippincott Williams & Wilkins customer service representatives are available from 8:30 am to 6:00 pm, EST.

05 06 07 08 09
1 2 3 4 5 6 7 8 9 10

PREFACE

Motion analysis is a fascinating subject that is intricately linked with the field of measurement. *Principles of Motion Analysis and Mechanics: A Handbook for Sports Science Students* has been written for all students of human movement who require an introduction to mechanics of human movement, the instrumentation used for motion and force measurement, signal processing and manipulation using software packages, mathematics, human anatomy, and fundamental statistics. The study of motion analysis is relevant to biomechanics and motor control, sports engineering, sports medicine, various types of therapy, sports science, and kinesiology.

The main thrust of the book is to introduce mechanical concepts using examples drawn from human movement and often using real data collected at the Motion Analysis Laboratory, University of Wales Swansea. Real data often introduce problems and questions whereas hypothetical or idealized data do not. For example, distances might appear in non-standard units such as millimeters or screen pixels, data on moving objects do not obey a simple model of their movement due to frictional effects or instrumental factors becoming apparent, or the data might require processing before any conclusions can be drawn from it. These problems and questions, however, often bring new insight and deeper understanding of the subject. Therefore, the problems introduced by real data are not ignored or bypassed in this book; rather, they are confronted head on and used to aid the teaching and understanding of the principles.

Pedagogical Features

New students of motion analysis and mechanics often find the mathematics difficult which slows down their progress in the subject. The following features help the students understand and retain the material:

Several examples and their solutions are given in the text to aid the understanding of the relevant mathematical principles.

New physical principles are explained thoroughly as they are introduced and any new mathematics are summarized in Appendix 1 "Units and Mathematics."

The headings in the book are numbered so that students and instructors can more easily see the hierarchy of the material. Main sections are double-numbered with the chapter and section number. Second-level heads are triple-numbered, and so on.

Case Studies are used to illustrate some important applications of the principles being taught; the case studies are drawn either from the literature or from real motion capture data collected at Swansea.

Each chapter begins with Objectives and Outcomes to guide the reader through the chapter.

Each chapter concludes with a Chapter Summary; key concepts are highlighted as they are introduced and defined.

Most chapters have Study Questions that are based on application of the concepts covered.

Answers to the Study Questions are included at the end of the book.

Organization and Structure

Chapter 1 provides an overview of the subject and should interest anyone who is new to the field. The optical methods of motion capture are outlined and all types of modern camera systems are covered. Some of the systems available for force measurement are also introduced including force platforms and insole pressure sensors. The chapter concludes with three case studies summarizing some of the important applications of mechanics and motion analysis to studies of human movement.

Chapters 2 through 8 introduce the mechanical principles required for the study of kinematics and kinetics and cover all aspects ranging from vectors, through linear and angular motion to mechanical analyses of human movement. Real data are introduced at all stages to maintain interest and to demonstrate how to use calculations in practical situations. The mathematics required for these chapters is summarized in Appendix I.

Chapters 9 and 10 discuss manipulation and analysis of data in spreadsheet form. An important attribute of modern motion capture systems is the quantity of data they produce. Data streams of positional and force information can often flow into files of hundreds of megabytes or even gigabytes in size. Software packages are essential for handling data in this form and this book shows how to do fundamental calculations for kinematic and kinetic quantities using computer-based techniques.

Chapter 11 examines the forces and resulting motion of balls in flight including the effects of dynamic fluid forces. Study Questions for Chapters 9, 10, and 11 require the use of electronic data files available on both the Instructor's Resource CD and on the book's Connection website, http://connection.lww.com/go/griffiths.

Chapter 12 discusses gait analysis. The preceding chapters can be viewed as essential reading before reading this chapter. This chapter explains gait analysis and how segmental positions can be calculated from three-dimensional marker positions. Some kinematic and kinetic data are presented as examples of the data that can be obtained by using modern motion capture methods. The anatomy of the lower leg and foot required for this chapter is summarized in Appendix 2.

REVIEWERS

Neil Fowler, PhD
Undergraduate Program Coordinator
Department of Exercise and Sport Science
Manchester Metropolitan University
Alsager, United Kingdom

Peter Walder, BEd(Hons)MA
Senior Lecturer in Sport and Exercise Science
School of Sport and Leisure Management
Sheffield Hallam University
Sheffield, United Kingdom

Jonathan Wheat, BSc. (Hons)
Sport, with Coaching and Exercise Science
School of Sport and Leisure Management
Sheffield Hallam University
Sheffield, United Kingdom

Peter Sinclair, PhD
Lecturer
School of Exercise and Sport Science
The University of Sydney
Lidcombe, Australia

Randall Jensen, PhD
Professor
Department of HPER
Northern Michigan University
Marquette, Michigan

David Pearsall, PhD
Associate Professor
Department of Kinesiology & Physical Education
McGill University
Montréal, Canada

ACKNOWLEDGMENTS

I would like to thank Gretchen Miller and Rebecca Keifer at LWW together with their colleagues Emily Lupash, Acquisitions Editor, and Christen Murphy, Marketing Manager, who made preparing the book a rewarding and almost pain-free experience. I thank the reviewers of the text, who made many wonderful suggestions: Neil Fowler; Manchester Metropolitan University, Peter Walder; Sheffield Hallam University, Jonathan Wheat; Sheffield Hallam University, Peter Sinclair; The University of Sydney, Randall Jensen; Northern Michigan University, David Pearsall; McGill University.

I would also like to thank my co-workers at Swansea — Colin Evans, Jim Watkins, Paul Schembri, Neil Griffiths, Dave Sharpe and Gerwyn Hughes — for discussions and practical help when required. My thanks also to the University of Wales Swansea for the use of experimental facilities and time to devote to the project.

And finally, thanks also to my family, Esme, Caryl, Owain, Seth and Dafydd for their forbearance while the work was done.

Iwan W. Griffiths
Department of Sports Science
University of Wales Swansea
UK

BRIEF CONTENTS

CONTENTS

CHAPTER *three*

CHAPTER *four*

CHAPTER one

INTRODUCTION TO MOTION ANALYSIS

CHAPTER *objectives*

To give an explanation of what motion analysis is and how it can be applied to kinematic and kinetic studies. The chapter emphasizes the instrumentation and methods available in modern motion analysis laboratories.

CHAPTER *outcomes*

After reading this chapter, the reader will be able to:

- Describe the camera systems available for two-dimensional (2D) and three-dimensional (3D) kinematic analyses.
- Differentiate between motion analysis systems that have 2D and 3D capabilities.
- Compare several different force systems for measuring foot pressure and ground reaction forces.
- Appreciate the three main areas for application of this technology, which are in the design of equipment, improvement of sports techniques, and injury prevention and rehabilitation.

1.1   Introduction to Motion Analysis

Motion analysis is the science of comparing sequential still images captured from photographing a body in motion in order to study the **kinematics** (i.e., the motions themselves) and the **kinetics** (i.e., the external and internal forces) involved. Motion analysis can be used not only to develop more efficient training programs for athletes but also to evaluate physical educational programs for cerebral palsy patients, test the action of prosthetic devices, and determine the evolution of patterns of locomotion.

I

1.2 Two-dimensional (2D) Motion Analysis

Recording of images may take place using a variety of possible methods. For example, **digital video cameras** (camcorders) with digital video tape (DVT), digital video disk (DVD), or hard disk drives (HDD) are cheap and convenient devices for capturing visual images of relatively large objects, such as the human body, in movement. Almost all analysis is now done with the use of computers and software to analyze the recorded images separately or in sequence or to compare them with other single images or sequences in order to detect patterns and make predictions. Digital video cameras, as illustrated in Figure 1.1, produce **two-dimensional (2D;** i.e., flat) images at a frame rate of 50 or 60 Hz and are easily transferred in digital form to computers for processing.

Digitization of visual images (i.e., conversion of parts of an image to numerical position data) may be either manual or automatic. In manual digitization, the operator displays a single image on a video screen, moves a cursor (usually an arrow) in turn to the various points of interest (e.g., ankle, knee, hip joints), and clicks a key or mouse to define a data point. For automatic analysis, the body is fitted with small reflective markers before image capture at strategic points (e.g., on the outer joint surfaces of the hip, knee, and ankle), usually using an adhesive sticker of some sort.

Digitizing software (which is included with basic motion analysis system packages) detects each reflective spot in the captured frame, calculates the center of each marker, and transforms its relative position into a data point, represented in either tabular or graphical form for analysis. In this 2D case, the marker positions, whether obtained by manual or automatic means, are of the form

$$(x_1, y_1),\ (x_2, y_2),\ (x_3, y_3), \ldots \ldots \ldots \ldots \ldots (x_n, y_n),$$

where (x_1, y_1) is the coordinate pair for the first marker etc. and (x_n, y_n) is the coordinate pair for the nth and final marker. Here x is used to stand for distance measured along an axis pointing along the horizontal direction in the captured frame, and y stands for distance measured along an axis pointing vertically up. The use of the symbols x and y is conventional but not compulsory. Indeed, some manufacturers of motion analysis systems specify the vertical direction using the symbol z so that coordinate pairs would then appear perhaps as (x_j, z_j). It is also worth bearing in mind that n coordinate pairs will be produced for each video frame that is captured. Thus, if M frames are digitized, there will be nM coordinate pairs of positional data. For example, using a video camera with a frame speed of

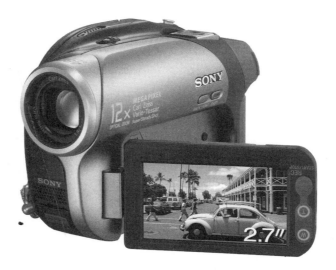

Figure 1.1 A modern digital video camera with a DVD facility. (Courtesy of Sony Corporation.)

50 Hz, if 15 markers are digitized for a clip lasting 1 second, the number of coordinate pairs is $15 \times 50 = 750$.

1.3   Three-dimensional (3D) Motion Analysis

To produce video-based **three-dimensional (3D)** motion capture, a number of cameras need to be used so that "depth" data can be obtained as well as the planar information obtainable from a single camera. One good technique for doing this is the **direct linear transform (DLT)** method using two or more video cameras. This technique relies on a mathematical transformation between raw 2D camera data (u,v) and the actual 3D coordinates (X,Y,Z) of a point. The basis of the transformation is the idea that the views from each camera are governed by the laws of perspective so that apparent distances and orientations in the image are determined by the position and orientation of the camera and the transform itself is characterized by 11 constants (i.e., camera parameters). An example of the effects of perspective from the points of view of two cameras is shown in Figure 1.2.

The DLT equations are:

$$u = \frac{aX + bY + cZ + d}{iX + jY + kZ + 1}$$

and

$$v = \frac{eX + fY + gZ + h}{iX + jY + kZ + 1}$$

If you have six or more calibration points with known (X,Y,Z) and corresponding raw camera coordinates (u,v), the camera parameters $a, b, c \ldots \ldots, k$ can be calculated because you have 12 or more equations (two for each calibration landmark) with 11 unknowns. This is done for each camera. When the camera parameters are known, the unknown (X,Y,Z) coordinates of other landmarks can be obtained from the (u,v) data of two or more cameras because there are four or more equations for the three unknowns (X,Y,Z). Some modern automated systems for optical 3D motion capture use reflective markers (usually partly or completely spherical) to

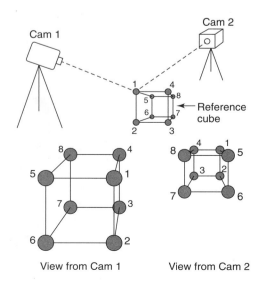

Figure 1.2 The views from two separate cameras of a cube with markers at each corner.

identify joint locations. Figure 1.3 shows an experimental subject with reflective markers in a 3D motion analysis laboratory.

The cameras emit visible or infrared light that is reflected back by the retro-reflective markers. Often the analysis system measures only the 3D coordinates of the markers, and subsequent kinematic analysis is based purely on these data. Analyses can be done in two or three dimensions (requiring separate software modules) and can produce 2D or 3D graphics of the motion paths of selected points, such as the path of the ankle in a person running or the flexion of an elbow during a baseball pitch.

Basic statistical routines to determine standard deviation and significance of variation in data are usually part of the software. In the case of 3D motion capture, the data returned will be in the form:

$$(x_1, y_1, z_1), (x_2, y_2, z_2),\dots\dots\dots\dots, (x_n, y_n, z_n),$$

where x and y are distances measured along two horizontal axes and z is the distance along a vertical axis. The orientations of x and y are sometimes aligned along convenient directions, for example, x to coincide with the direction of someone walking (anterior–posterior) so that y would be the medial–lateral axis. Again, some manufacturers define symbols differently, so that the y axis may be vertical, x is anterior–posterior, and z is medial–lateral. In this book, when dealing with xyz axes, the z axis is taken as a vertical axis unless stated otherwise. However, in 2D axes, x and y are usually used with y vertical.

Most optical motion analysis systems have similar hardware components, but they may vary in flexibility or capacity or in the analytical capabilities of the software component. A typical camera used in an optical motion analysis system is shown in Figure 1.4. It is normal to have between six and 12 cameras in use simultaneously with each camera trained on the moving object. It is also possible to use other types of motion analysis systems; for example:

Magnetic systems: Sensors are linked by cables to a computer.

Electromagnetic: The subject wears a body suit.

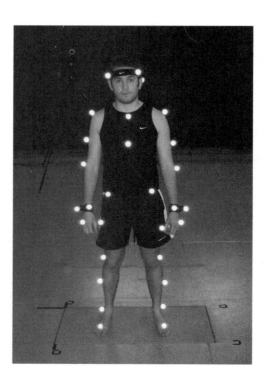

Figure 1.3 A subject marked up with reflective markers in a laboratory setting surrounded by a three-dimensional motion analysis system. *(Courtesy of University of Wales Swansea.)*

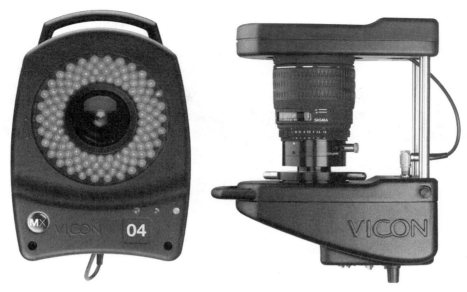

Figure 1.4 A digital video camera fitted with visible red light–emitting diodes used for three-dimensional motion capture. *(Courtesy of Vicon Peak Limited.)*

A typical digital video camera with DVD storage available at the time of writing uses a 1.0-megapixel charge-coupled device (CCD) imager that delivers high-quality video images. This means that the image is composed of 1 million picture elements laid out in a rectangular array. The DVD recording format delivers digital picture and sound quality comparable to that of Mini-iDV tape but on a DVD, the disc plays back in compatible DVD players or computers. When used in video mode, the camera has 690 K of effective pixels and provides 520 lines of resolution. With a maximum resolution of 1152 × 864, it is possible to capture more than 6000 still images on a single disc.

10× optical/120× digital zoom: The optical zoom helps to bring the action up close from far away. The digital zoom interpolation means that extreme digital zooming is clearer, with low distortion.

Burst mode: Captures up to four images in 1152 × 864 or 12 images at 640 × 480 consecutively for capturing fast action.

Picture stabilization system: Controls a large range of shake and vibration frequencies to achieve a high level of smoothness without degradation of video quality.

USB 2.02 interface: Provides an easy way to connect the DVD camcorder to computers for fast transfer of video and still images to a computer for editing and analysis. The camcorder can also be used as an external DVD burner, which is convenient for copying DVDs and edited movies.

Recording capacity of one disc: 20 minutes at high-quality setting; 30 minutes at standard-quality setting; 60 minutes at low-quality setting.

Shutter speed: 1/4 to 1/4000 s. The shutter speed is important if fast movements are to be captured without loss of detail. The faster the shutter speed, the sharper moving objects will appear on playback.

Four frames from a typical recording are shown in Figure 1.5. The toe end of the bat in this figure takes a complicated trajectory (i.e., path through space) during the execution of the stroke. We can differentiate between the overall distance traveled by the toe end of the bat (the overall length of the trajectory) and its displacement (the difference between its end point and starting point). The displacement of the toe end of the bat is clearly much smaller than the total distance traveled and, moreover, the displacement needs to be specified by both its magnitude (in meters) and its angle relative to the starting point. The distance traveled by the toe end of the bat is also measured in meters but is much larger in magnitude. The distance does not have a direction, so it is known as a scalar quantity. The displacement, on the other hand, is known as a vector quantity. Both displacement and distance traveled can be calculated after the analysis system has been calibrated. This is a recurring theme in kinematics, and the distinction between vectors and scalars is re-emphasized in Chapter 1.

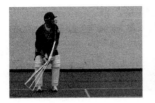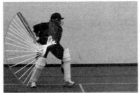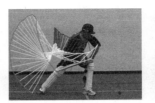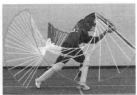

Figure 1.5 Four still frames taken from a video recording of a batsman playing a shot.

Optoelectronic: The subject wears light-emitting diodes.

Acoustic systems: Sonar uses reflected sound waves.

Non-invasive: Uses a high-speed video camera or cameras.

But in all cases, the objective is the same: to determine the coordinates of the marked points as a function of time. In this introduction for kinesiology and sport science students, we restrict our attention to the commonly used methods of 2D video analysis and 3D optical motion analysis systems.

1.4 Calibration of Motion Analysis Systems

1.4.1 Video-Based Two-Dimensional Systems

The screen displays available for video and still image playback come in various resolutions (i.e., the level of detail discernible on the screen). Commonly available resolutions are 640 × 480 pixels and 800 × 600 pixels. This means that the image can be thought of as a pattern of small dots on the screen distributed regularly on a rectangular array. Commonly available software packages for viewing and analyzing video images make use of the pixel information to furnish information on the kinematics of the marked points, provided a suitable calibration is available. A typical video screen is shown in Figure 1.6 together with the location of the origin of horizontal and vertical coordinates and a marker point.

The location of the origin is purely arbitrary but in most cases is defined by the manufacturer of the analysis software as being in a definite location on screen; here, for example, it is at the top left. **Calibration** of a 2D video analysis system is usually achieved by using a reference object of known size placed in the field of

Figure 1.6 A typical video screen together with an indication of the pixel coordinates used for analysis.

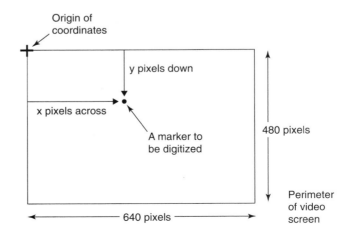

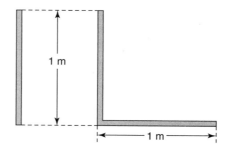

Figure 1.7 Two possible reference objects for two-dimensional video calibration.

view at approximately the same distance from the camera as the markers. Figure 1.7 shows two typical calibration objects for video-based analysis systems.

The reference object may be a one-dimensional object (*left panel* of Fig. 1.7) placed in a given orientation within the field of view, or it may be a 2D object (*right panel* of Fig. 1.7) so that it can be oriented along two mutually perpendicular directions. Note that the reference object can be any desired size or shape provided it is accurately known. The length of the reference object is usually measured within the analysis software in terms of pixels. The calibration of the system is then inferred from this result. For example, a 1-m reference length might correspond to 150 pixels on the video screen. This implies that each screen pixel corresponds to a real separation of $\frac{1}{150} = 0.00666$ m. This result can only be expected to be accurate for subjects observed at one distance from the camera and even then does not take into account possible distortions in the image caused by optical limitations, for example, at the edges of the screen view. Also, it is expected that, even under ideal focusing and illumination conditions, the reference object can only be measured to ± 1 pixel. Thus, the calibration quoted in the example above might be in error by as much as $\pm 0.7\%$.

1.4.2 THREE-DIMENSIONAL OPTICAL MOTION CAPTURE SYSTEMS

These systems are calibrated using reference objects of known dimensions and usually incorporating reflective markers at known separations, with some using a static calibration (stationary reference object or objects or a dynamic calibration [moving reference object or objects]). Figure 1.8 shows a typical pair of calibration objects for a 3D motion analysis system calibration.

The L frame (*left panel* of Fig. 1.8) is positioned at a fixed point in the laboratory and defines the directions of the coordinate axes while the wand (*right panel* of Fig. 1.8) is waved around within a predetermined capture volume. This process ensures

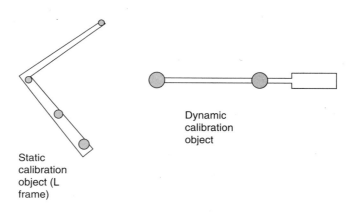

Figure 1.8 A static and a dynamic reference object for three-dimensional motion capture calibration.

Static calibration object (L frame)

Dynamic calibration object

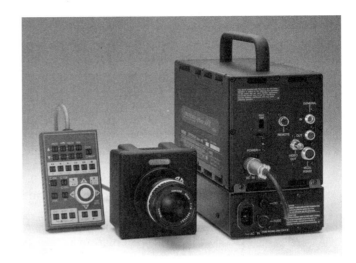

Figure 1.9 A high-speed video camera capable of up to 1000 frames per second. *(Courtesy of Photo-Sonics International Ltd, United Kingdom.)*

that the locations and orientations of the cameras are known so that overall calibration is as accurate as possible.

1.5 High-speed Videography

It is possible to obtain special high-speed cameras for capturing images of very fast movements such as the swing of a golf driver, the impact of a bat on a baseball, or the motion of a runner's foot during stance. A typical high-speed camera can be used with an aperture speed of from 10 microseconds upward so that rapid movements can be captured without blurring. (A microsecond is one millionth of a second.) The high frame rates (picture speeds) from 100 per second to 10,000 per second mean that quickly moving objects can be captured fully before the motion has finished. The camera shown in Figure 1.9 has a 512 × 512 pixel sensor. This camera can operate up to 1000 pictures per second using all sensor pixels but can achieve picture speeds as high as 32,000 per second by reducing the number of pixels used.

Figure 1.10 shows some still pictures of a golf swing captured by a high-speed video camera at a picture speed of 350 pps (pictures per second) in daylight. The head of the golf club is moving at over 50m.s^{-1} in this sequence of pictures. Clearly, an ordinary video camera operating at 50 Hz would be inadequate to capture this movement. Illumination of the subject often becomes an important issue when operating at high picture speeds because of the limited amount of light available during the exposure time. Very high picture speeds are only obtainable by reducing the resolution of the picture; this means selecting fewer of the sensor pixels. Illumi-

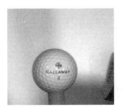 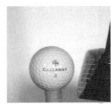 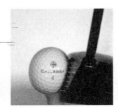 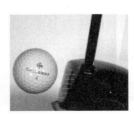 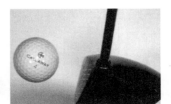

Figure 1.10 A golf shot captured by a high-speed video camera at 350 pictures per second.

Table 1.1	The picture speed as a function of the horizontal and vertical resolution available from a typical digital video camera		
		Horizontal Resolution	
	512	**256**	**128**
512	1000	1908	3132
256	2115	3731	6038
Vertical Resolution **128**	4125	7142	11261
64	7861	13157	19841
32	14367	22727	32051

nation by lamps is sometimes required to increase the available light to acceptable levels. Therefore, there is a tradeoff between resolution and picture speed. Table 1.1 shows how resolution can be traded for picture speed in a typical system.

1.6   Two- and Three-dimensional Kinematics

A typical 2D video screen view ready for analysis is shown in Figure 1.11. This shot was captured using a long focal length lens; the camera was placed about 35 m from the soccer player. This soccer player's knee is marked by a circular marker and is measured as 315,465 pixels with respect to the origin at the top left corner of the screen. The ankle and toe points are also marked. In such cases, it is not

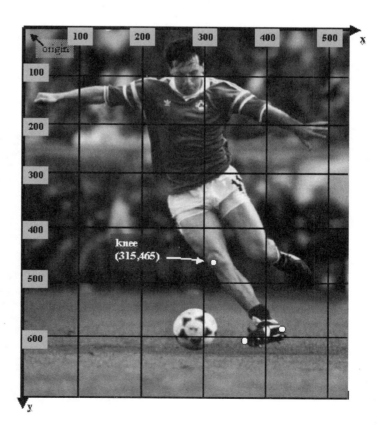

Figure 1.11   A soccer player captured in action. The pixel coordinates and origin are shown.

BOX 1-2

Automated Multi-camera Systems with Light Emitting Diode (LED) Strobes and Retro-reflective Markers

Modern 3D automated multi-camera analysis systems can be used with retro-reflective markers to provide unprecedented speed and accuracy in a laboratory setting. The markers can be as small as 2 or 3 mm in diameter. A typical camera at the time of writing has a 4.1-MPixel CMOS sensor and a maximum frame rate of 160 Hz at full sensor resolution. By appropriate use of windows, the sensor frame rate can be increased to a maximum of 10,000 Hz. The strobe can be specified as a visible, infrared, or near-infrared ring light; a typical system can be configured easily within working volumes as small as 0.2 m^3 (linear dimension 0.5 m) up to 275 m^3 (linear dimension 16.5 m). Positional accuracy is routinely 1 mm or better. A typical result, shown in Figure 1.12, is a rendered skeleton based on the 3D coordinates of the marker positions.

always possible to include a reference object in the camera shot, but an alternative in this case is to use the diameter of the ball as a calibrating object.

In 2D kinematics, it is necessary to compute:

■ Displacement (vector) or distance moved (scalar) in meters (m)
■ Velocity (vector) or speed (scalar) in meters per second (m/s or ms^{-1})
■ Acceleration (vector or scalar) in meters per second squared (m/s^2 or ms^2)

Also of interest are:

■ Angular displacement and distance (in degrees or radians)
■ Angular velocities and speeds (in degrees per second or radians per second)
■ Angular accelerations (in degrees per second squared or radians per second squared)

In the case of 2D analyses, the above kinematic quantities can be calculated only in the plane of the video recording, and kinematic components perpendicular to this plane will be missed. This limitation of 2D systems can often be overcome by careful alignment of the video camera to record action in the most meaningful way. For example, if an athlete is running on a straight track, most of the action occurs in the sagittal plane, so the camera could be set up at the side of the track to record movements in this plane.

The kinematic information available from a 3D analysis is itself 3D in nature.

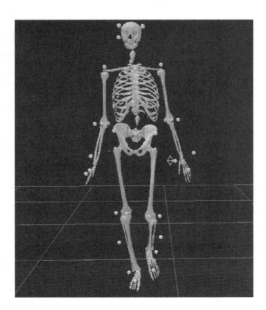

Figure 1.12 A rendered skeleton based on the marker information obtained from three-dimensional motion capture.

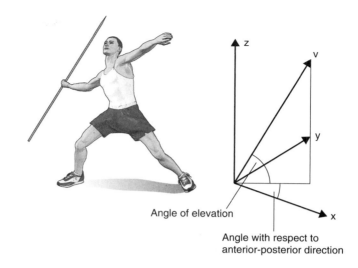

Figure 1.13 A javelin being thrown. The velocity of the javelin is shown together with the angles of projection.

For example, displacements, velocities, and accelerations can now be quoted as their components along the x, y, and z axes. An alternative is to specify the magnitude of the 3D vector together with at least two angles to specify its direction. In Figure 1.13, the velocity of the javelin can be specified as 25 ms^{-1} with angle of elevation 48° and angle with respect to posterior–anterior 20°.

The alternative is to say: $v_x = 15.72$, $v_y = 5.72$ and $v_z = 18.58$ ms^{-1}. More information on resolution of vectors into components is given in Chapter 2.

With 3D analysis, it is also possible to give information on body rotation angles. For example, Figure 1.14 shows the shoulder joint can give rise to three separate movements: flexion/extension, abduction/adduction, and internal/external rotation. Applications of these ideas are extended in Chapter 12.

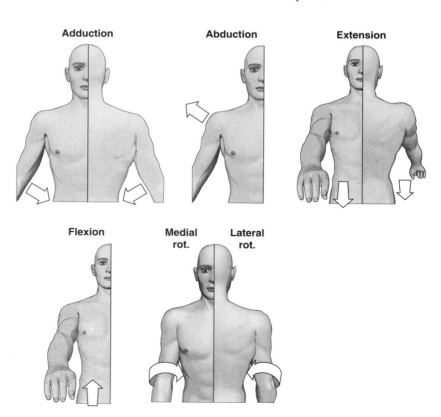

Figure 1.14 The three-dimensional joint motions possible at the shoulder joint.

1.7   Instrumentation for Measurement of Force and Pressure

1.7.1 INTRODUCTION TO FORCE TRANSDUCERS

To take into account the effects of external forces on bodies, it is essential to have some instrumentation to measure these forces and the moments produced by them. In general, these devices are known as **force transducers** and **force plates**. A force transducer gives an electrical signal (voltage or current) proportional to the applied force (e.g., if the force doubles, the electrical signal doubles). There are many kinds available relying on different principles:

Strain gauge: A metal plate undergoes a very small change in one of its dimensions (strain), altering the resistance of a semiconductor or metallic sensor.

Capacitive: A separation between two electrode plates changes and alters the ability to store charge.

Piezoelectric: Very small deformations of crystalline materials change the electrical characteristics such that a potential difference is generated between the faces of the crystal.

Piezoresistive: The atomic structure of a crystal is altered in such a way as to change its electrical resistance.

For the interested reader, more information about instrumentation is contained in a book by Regtien (2004).

1.7.2 FORCE PLATES

Ground reaction forces (GRFs) are the most common forces that act on the human body. These forces act at the feet during walking, running, and jumping. The GRF can be represented as a 3D vector consisting of a vertical component and two shear components acting in the ground plane. This force can be measured with a force plate, illustrated in Figure 1.15. Typically, an instrumented force plate produces electrical signals corresponding to forces F_x, F_y, F_z and moment outputs M_x, M_y, and M_z. Some characteristics of a typical strain gauge force plate are shown in Table 1.2.

Specific uses of such plates include gait analysis; stability analysis; athletic performance; and force, power, and work studies. Some force plates are waterproofed with pressure compensation, so they can be used under water. Some important features are high sensitivity (how many volts for every Newton applied), low crosstalk (does not indicate horizontal force if a vertical force is applied), repeatability (gives similar results over and over again under the same load), and stability (properties do not drift much with time or temperature). Most commercially available force plates have been engineered to be good in all these respects. Strain gauge–based

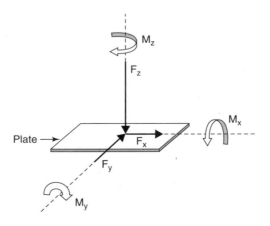

Figure 1.15 A typical force plate produces outputs corresponding to three-dimensional force and moment inputs.

Table 1.2   Some typical characteristics of a strain gauge force plate

Typical Strain Gauge Force Plate Specifications

F_x, F_y capacity	4450
F_z, capacity	8900
M_x, M_y capacity (Nm)	2300
M_z capacity (Nm)	1100
F_x, F_y sensitivity μV/[VN]	0.34
F_z, sensitivity μV/[VN]	0.08
M_x, M_y sensitivity μV/[VNm]	0.79
M_z, sensitivity, μV/[VNm]	1.69
F_x, F_y natural frequency (Hz)	370
F_z, natural frequency (Hz)	530
Weight (kg)	45
Height (mm)	82.50
Top plate	Aluminum 463 × 508 mm

force plates require bridge excitation (power supply) and signal amplification (boosting the voltages to convenient sizes), and these are normally supplied via a combined power supply and amplifier unit. Piezoelectric force plates are also available with the advantage of requiring no power supply. Force plates come with their own software for automated data collection and reduction; typical modules feature hardware setup, data logging, and analysis. See Regtien (2004) for further information on sensor characteristics.

1.7.3 PLANTAR PRESSURE DISTRIBUTION MEASUREMENT

Insole devices incorporate a large number of individual pressure sensor elements arranged over the area of the insole so that plantar pressure distribution can be mapped. The location of the center of pressure can be calculated by a weighted average of the matrix of sensors. It is important to note that these devices record only the vertical component of the applied force and that shear forces are ignored. These devices can also display the averaged plantar pressure, the instantaneous plantar pressure, and any obvious high-pressure points, as shown in Figure 1.16.

Some typical characteristics of a capacitive sensor–based insole system are given in Table 1.3. This system features a power supply/data acquisition box normally worn on a waist belt by the subject and connected to the insoles by cables.

Insole systems are accurate and reliable for the measurement of pressure distribution and monitoring local loads between the foot and the shoe. Some systems can be tethered to a personal computer (PC) with a fiberoptic USB cable, and they can sometimes function in a mobile capacity with built-in state-of-the-art Bluetooth® technology that is able to communicate with Bluetooth-compatible pocket computers, notebook computers, or standard PCs. Another alternative is a system with a built-in flash memory storage that allows data to be collected anywhere and later downloaded into a computer. All of these features make insole systems extremely mobile and flexible to meet virtually all testing needs such as walking, running, climbing stairs, carrying loads, playing soccer, and even riding a bicycle.

A console containing the power supply and electronics usually connects to highly conforming elastic sensor insoles that cover the whole plantar surface of the foot or sensor pads for the dorsal, medial, or lateral areas of the foot. Many systems allow multiple synchronization options to use with electromyography (EMG) and video systems for gait analysis.

Insole systems may function with wireless telemetry functions (e.g., Bluetooth).

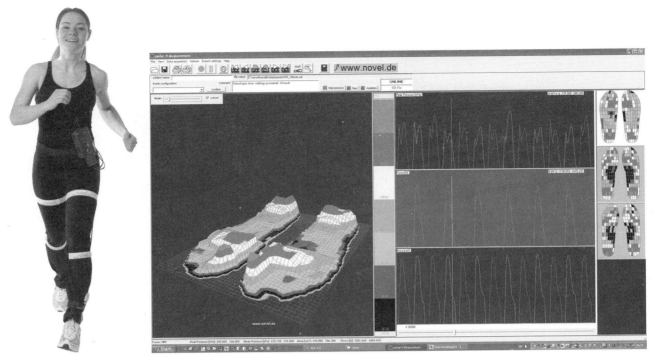

Figure 1.16   An insole pressure measurement system based on capacitive sensors. *(Courtesy of Novel Gmbh.)*

The telemetry allows the user to watch the subject while at the same time fully controlling the testing from a PC. Then the dynamic pressure data can be viewed online and the subject advised how to perform. Such systems are ideal for teaching and for biofeedback testing.

Personal digital assistants (PDAs) can be used in conjunction with insole pressure measurement systems for data collection and presentation. A PDA is a Windows-based handheld pocket PC. Additional functions such as sensor calibration and data analysis are usually completed on a PC. The PDA transfers the data to a notebook or desktop computer. Typical applications of insole plantar pressure measurement systems include:

■ Shoe research and design
■ Aid in orthotic design

Table 1.3   Some typical attributes for a capacitive sensor insole system for plantar pressure

Pressure Measurement	Measurement
Box dimensions (mm)	150 × 100 × 40
Box weight (g)	400
Number of sensors (max)	256 (1024)
Measurement frequency	20,000 sensors/s
Storage type	8-MB internal flash
Computer interface	Fiberoptic/USB and Bluetooth
Operating system	Windows
Power supply	Li-Ion battery
Insole sizes	22 to 49 (European)

- Rehabilitation assessment
- Kinetic analysis of free gait
- Long-term load monitoring
- Sport biomechanics
- Biofeedback

Many insole pressure measurement systems are tested by inserting the insoles between the upper and lower surfaces of a calibration device operated by compressed air or able to apply a known load with fixed weights. Some useful features of insole plantar pressure measurement systems are:

- Individual sensor selection
- Online and offline modes
- Online 2D or 3D display
- Isobar display (lines connecting points of equal pressure)
- Numeric display
- Animation of foot contact phases
- Maximum pressure picture (MPP)
- Step selection
- Step timing analysis
- Averaged and individual gait lines

CASE *Study 1.1*   Application of Motion Analysis to Design of Sports Equipment

Many sports involve dynamic mechanical loads on athletes' feet. Sports shoes are very important to improve sports performance and give the feet good grip and protection from injury. The forefoot and rearfoot experience different forces, so it is often beneficial to make the sole of a sports shoe from a complex combination of different materials to give the response required for each part of the foot. Testing the elasticity and damping characteristics of a sports shoe under realistic conditions is an essential part of research and development for major manufacturers. For example, Adidas-Salomon AG has a test center dedicated to the investigation of new materials and designs.

Sports shoes are demanding in terms of their design requirements. During running, for example, the heel of the foot contacts the ground first with up to two or three times the bodyweight applied rapidly to the heel. The energy resulting from this impact must be absorbed by the heel material in order to protect the foot and the heel from the large impact force. This requires viscous (energy absorbing similar to the dampers on a car's suspension) and elastic (springiness) properties in the material making up the heel of the shoe. During the contact or "stance" phase, the foot unrolls and then pushes off from the ground through the forefoot. During this propulsive phase, very little energy should be absorbed in the sole material, so that its springiness gives the athlete assistance to move forward and upward. This is shown in Figure 1.17 for running at medium speed where the stress in the sole material is shown shaded and with arrows.

Figure 1.17 The stress developed in the sole material of a running shoe at three separate instants of stance.

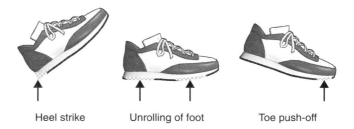

Heel strike   Unrolling of foot   Toe push-off

Figure 1.18 The forces acting on the heel and forefoot for a 70-kg runner.

$$1 \text{ msec} = 1 \text{ ms} = \frac{1}{100}\text{th sec}$$

1 kN = 1000 N
(Courtesy of Adidas Salomon.)

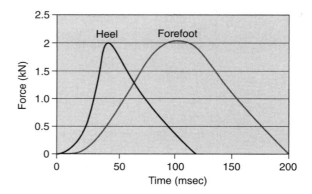

Enhanced performance can be delivered by shoe structures that incorporate viscous and elastic foam materials such as ethylene vinyl acetate (EVA) and polyurethane (PU). Viscous plastics in the heel provide cushioning during initial foot contact, and elastic plastics in the forefoot area minimize energy losses. In all circumstances, it is important to keep the shoe from "bottoming out," that is, the sole material being compressed down to very thin dimensions and the loading forces building up to unacceptable levels.

The forces acting on different parts of a shoe during running can be shown on a force–time graph. The graph in Figure 1.18 shows the forces acting on the heel and forefoot for a 70-kg runner. The force on the heel reaches a maximum of 2000 N about 30 to 40 ms after first contact. On the forefoot, a similar force is reached at a time of about 100 ms. This information helps to determine the deformation properties of the sole of the shoe.

The materials for shoe soles should have force deformation curves that are not linear (like a spring) but progressive in different grades so that the more they are compressed, the stiffer they get. It is important to carry out mechanical testing of the plastic materials to check on their suitability as shoe materials. To simulate real running conditions, the testing machine must be capable of compressing samples with a thickness of up to 20 mm in a time interval of 30 ms. In this extremely short time, the testing force must increase from 0 to 3000 N maximum with a force application speed of 0.0 to 1.6 m.s^{-1}. Adidas uses an Instron testing machine to test the damping properties of existing shoe soles and to investigate and optimize new materials.

Using testing machines like the one shown in Figure 1.19, new shoe designs can be

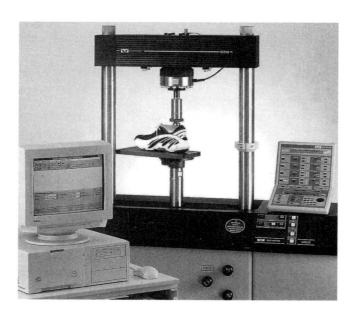

Figure 1.19 An Instron testing machine applying known loads and stresses to new materials. *(Courtesy of Adidas Salomon.)*

developed and testing methods developed. Running movements are often recorded using 2D and 3D cameras to investigate the effect of the shoes on gait and non-neutral foot behavior. Laser scanning can produce a 3D foot profile of an athlete in a few seconds.

CASE *Study 1.2* **Application of Motion Analysis for Improving Sports Techniques**

Kinematic and kinetic analyses can often inform coaches and instructors on the best ways to improve athletes' performance. Some sports consisting of simple movements involve reasonably straightforward analysis, but other sports that include more complex movements require full biomechanical treatment for full understanding. An example in the latter category is the discus throw, one of the four throwing events in track and field. The complex movements in the discus throw take place at high speed and within a small volume. One attempt at full analysis was made at the Atlanta Olympics in 1996, where three video cameras were used with a DLT procedure to investigate the release velocities, the heights of release, and the projection angles (Ariel et al., 1997). This investigation was used to provide biomechanical data on the Internet for analysis at remote sites.

Three-dimensional videographic and force plate data (Yu et al., 2002) have been used to investigate the relationships between official distance and selected ground reaction measures during the throw and the relationship between GRF and lower extremity joint kinetics

Figure 1.20 shows a discus throw at six critical instants: maximum back swing, right foot takeoff, left foot takeoff, right foot touchdown, left foot touchdown, and release. These six instants divide the throw into five critical phases: initial double support, first single support, flight, second single support, and delivery.

The experimental setup of force plates (FPs) and cameras used in this investigation is shown in Figure 1.21. FP-1 was used to record the GRF at the left foot for the first double support of the throw, and FP-2 and FP-3 were used to record the GRFs at the second single support and at delivery. A DLT procedure was used to collect 3D coordinates of 21 body landmarks and the center of the discus for each subject in a series of trials. Three time-synchronized S-VHS video cameras were used to record a control object and the performances of the subjects at a frame rate of 60 frames per second.

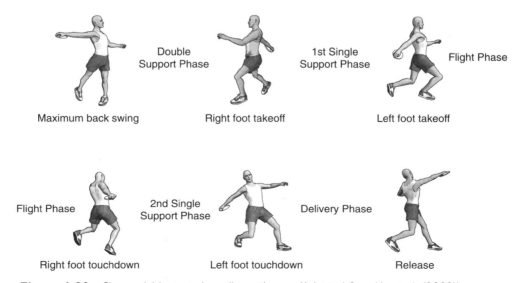

Figure 1.20 Six crucial instants in a discus throw. *(Adapted from Yu et al. (2002))*

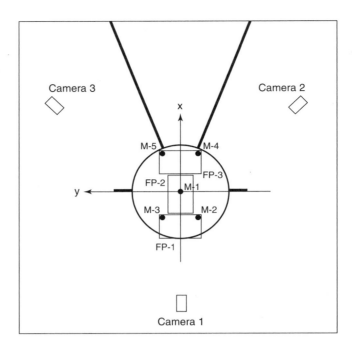

Figure 1.21 Experimental setup of force plates in an investigation of the discus throw. *(Courtesy of Yu et al. (2002)*

The results from an investigation such as this can be divided into two categories:

1. The effects of GRFs on performance:

   As an example of the results produced in this category, consider the normalized forward–backward driving impulse on the right foot during the second single-support and delivery phases and its relationship with the official distance shown in Figure 1.22.

   In this example, the driving impulse is the area under the force–time graph (see Chapter 6) and is normalized by dividing by the bodyweight. The official distance is said to be *significantly correlated* with the impulse. The precise meaning of this term has to be understood in terms of basic statistics, but this book will not dwell on an explanation of this subject. Suffice to say that correlation is a method for looking for a linear relationship between two variables, as, for example, in this graph, where the straight line drawn implies a relationship between the official distance and the driving impulse.

2. The effects of lower extremity joint resultant moments on GRFs:

   Joint resultant moments at the knees and hips during the first single-support, second

Figure 1.22 The normalized forward-backward driving impulse on the right foot during the second single-support and delivery phases of a discus throw and its relationship with the official distance. *(Courtesy of Yu et al. (2002))*

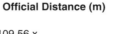

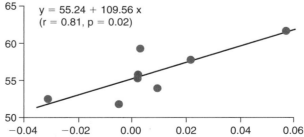

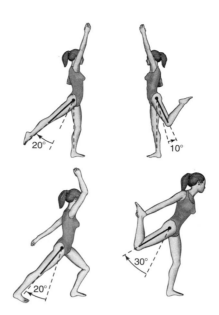

Figure 1.23 Flexion at the hip in a number of different movements.

single-support, and delivery phases were estimated using an inverse dynamic procedure (see Chapter 10). The component of a joint resultant moment vector perpendicular to the plane defined by the thigh and lower leg was referred to as the flexion–extension moment. The component of a joint resultant moment vector parallel to the thigh or lower leg was referred to as the internal–external rotation moment. The component of a joint resultant moment vector perpendicular to both the flexion–extension and internal–external rotation moment vectors was referred to as the abduction–adduction vector. To take one example, consider flexion at the hip shown in Figure 1.23.

The hip flexion moment is a measure of the strength of the turning effect at the hip joint. The idea of a turning moment is further explored in Chapter 10, but for this specific case, it can be thought of in terms of flexing the hip against no resistance, or against a weight attached at the ankle.

The hip flexion moment (Fig. 1.24) has to be higher in the weighted case because the weight attached now adds to the weight of the leg itself and because the attached weight is at a large distance from the hip joint. As an example of the results found by Yu et al. (2002), consider the graph of Figure 1.25, where official distance is plotted against normalized right hip peak extension moment during the second single-support and delivery phases.

Although a linear relationship can be claimed from these data, it is clear that the data have a large amount of scatter. In this graph, the data are normalized for bodyweight and

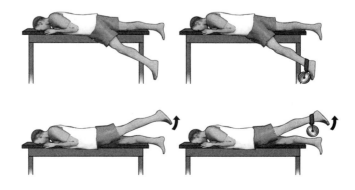

Figure 1.24 Left: Easy—lower hip flexion moment. Right: Hard—higher hip flexion moment.

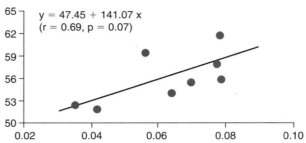

Figure 1.25 The official distance in a discus throw plotted against normalized right hip peak extension moment during the second single-support and delivery phases.

height—that is, the moments are divided by weight and height. The hip extension data was also examined to see if there was a correlation between right hip peak extension moments with the normalized forward impulse on the right foot during the second single-support and delivery phases. The impulse of a temporary or transient force is basically force × time, or area under a force–time graph. The concept of impulse is discussed further in Chapter 6. In the graph of Figure 1.26, the impulse is normalized by dividing by the bodyweight (Yu et al., 2002).

This study included many more variables, and the main conclusions were:

1. Discus throwers should drive their bodies plus the discus system forward as vigorously as possible toward the throwing direction during the first single-support phase.

2. Throwers should also generate vertical thrust during the first single-support phase to increase the height of flight.

3. A hard right foot landing after the flight may assist discus throwers to generate ground reaction impulses on the right foot during the second single-support phase and delivery phase for long official distance.

4. Throwers should drive their right legs forward and to the right during the second single-support phase and delivery phase for long official distance.

5. Discus athletes should drive their left legs upward and backward as vigorously as possible to obtain maximal vertical thrust for long official distance. The knee and hip extension strengths are critical for a vigorous left leg drive during the delivery phase.

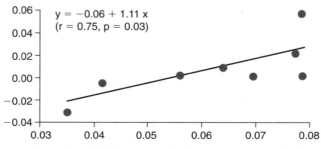

Figure 1.26 The normalized forward *impulse* on the right foot during the second single-support and delivery plotted against right hip peak extension moments. Discus throw. *(Courtesy of Yu et al. (2002.))*

CASE *Study 1.3*   **Application of Motion Analysis to Injury Prevention and Rehabilitation**

Field event coaches focus on the main tasks of directing a training program that ensures progression of athletes in their events while avoiding injury. Burnett (2001b) has produced a nice summary of the causes of injury in jumping events (Fig. 1.27).

High GRFs are high in jumping activities, particularly those done on artificial surfaces. Excessive loads may then be borne by fascia, ligaments, tendons, and bones. Injuries may occur if large numbers of jumps are performed, especially on hard surfaces; after how long this happens is determined by the athlete's resilience against injury. Forces can be measured by force plates, instrumented insoles, or other force sensors and, as we have seen, this leads to important conclusions about the type of shoes to wear while jumping.

Overuse means that the same jumping movement is performed over and over again; for example, in the high jump, a high-intensity activity is repeated and judged by the measuring tape.

Poor physical preparation means that an athlete has not undergone an adequate amount of physical training to sustain high–intensity, high-volume training.

In general, landing on a flat foot is a good way to avoid injury in most jumping activities. Landing on the ball of the foot may give a shorter contact time but can lead to injury. Landing on the side of the foot can lead to sprains.

Some jumpers may have an anatomical structure, inflexibility, or a muscle imbalance that may leave them liable to injuries. Many lower limb injuries are caused by excessive pronation, excessive pelvic drop, Achilles tendon problems, or leg-length discrepancy.

Pronation (Fig. 1.28), a normal part of human gait, is a movement at the ankle joint after foot strike. When a foot pronates, it rolls outward (**eversion**), the lower leg moves forward over the foot (**dorsiflexion**), and the foot moves away from the midline (**abduction**). **Supination** occurs after pronation and consists of the opposite movements: the foot rolls inward (inversion), the ankle joint extends (plantarflexion), and the foot moves toward the midline (**adduction**). Such movements of the foot and lower leg can be seen in detail by using a camera mounted behind the runner to take still photographs or video pictures.

Pronation is thought to be linked to a variety of common injuries to the foot, ankle, knee, and invertebrae of the back and can be corrected by orthotics.

Another example in which video recording may be beneficial is that of pelvic drop during single-limb stance. Pelvic drop can occur in running and jumping when all the weight of the body is supported on a single leg. If the middle gluteal muscles (underneath the buttocks) are weak or lack control, a large drop will occur in the pelvis on the side opposite to the weight-bearing leg (Fig. 1.29). This problem often occurs after lower limb injuries and usually requires a physiotherapist to supervise the rehabilitation. Burnett (2001a) has advocated the

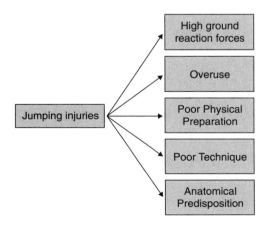

Figure 1.27 A summary of the causes of injury in jumping events. *(Courtesy of Burnett. (2001b.))*

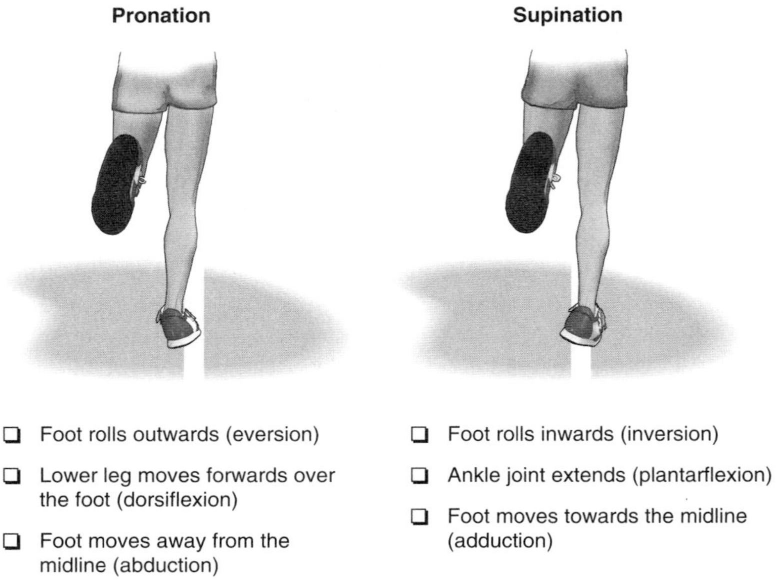

Pronation

Supination

❏ Foot rolls outwards (eversion)

❏ Lower leg moves forwards over the foot (dorsiflexion)

❏ Foot moves away from the midline (abduction)

❏ Foot rolls inwards (inversion)

❏ Ankle joint extends (plantarflexion)

❏ Foot moves towards the midline (adduction)

Figure 1.28 Pronation and supination, both normal movements in human gait. *(Adapted from Burnett (2001b.))*

following exercises for the lower limb as part of a regular training program to delay or prevent injury. The same exercises can also be used as part of a rehabilitation program.

Feet: To maintain the structural integrity of the foot: towel scrunches, barefoot running, and picking up objects with the toes

Ankle: To strengthen the lower limb: using theratubing to perform ankle inversion, eversion, and dorsiflexion exercises; using an ankle board to perform various exercises; walking sideways across a hill; walking on the toes, heels, and inside and outside of the feet. The still photographs shown in Figure 1.30, which were extracted from a video, show ankle inversion being performed with a theratube (i.e., resistance tube used for therapy).

Knee: To strengthen the joint and prevent injury: squats. By controlling the downward (eccentric) phase of the squat, the patella tendon is strengthened.

It is also possible to devise exercises for the rest of the body, including the back, hips, and so on, but these are not presented here. This book mainly focuses on the mechanical principles and the application of motion analysis to human movement and sports.

The remainder of the book begins with a chapter on basic vector analysis and then proceeds to develop linear and angular kinematics and kinetics with many examples and case studies that are relevant to human movement or sports. The book has been written for students of human movement, kinesiology, or biomechanics who require a good working

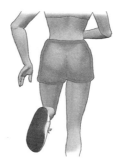

Figure 1.29 A drop in the pelvis on one side opposite to the weight-bearing leg may occur after a leg injury.

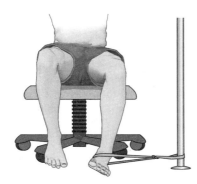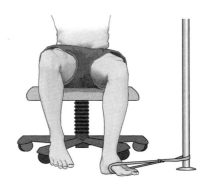

Figure 1.30 An ankle inversion exercise being performed with a theratube while being recorded using a video camera. *(Adapted from Burnett (2001 b.))*

knowledge of mechanics and want to apply motion analysis to their subjects. The subjects are introduced assuming no prior knowledge of mechanics. A little knowledge of mathematics is assumed, but the methods used are introduced in the text the first time they are used and with a full explanation.

SUMMARY

This introductory chapter has reviewed some of the modern methods and instrumentation available for motion analysis. The main objectives of kinematic and kinetic analysis are outlined, and three case studies are presented illustrating the three main reasons for doing such analyses: application to design of sports equipment, improvement in sports techniques, and prevention of and rehabilitation from injuries.

REFERENCES

Ariel GB, Finch A, Penny MA: Biomechanical analysis of discus-throwing at the 1996 Atlanta Olympic games. Presented at the XV International Symposium in Sports. Texas Women's University. Denton, TX; June 20–28, 1997.

Burnett A: Biomechanics of jumping: The relevance to field event athletes. *Modern Athlete and Coach* 39:3–8. 2001a.

Burnett A: Jumping injuries: Their cause, possible prevention and rehabilitation. *Modern Athlete and Coach* 39:3–6. 2001b.

Yu Bing, Broker J, Silvester LJ: A kinetic analysis of discus-throwing techniques. *Sports Biomechanics*, 1(1):25–46, 2002.

SUGGESTED READINGS

Abdel-Aziz YI, Karara HM: Direct linear transformation from comparator coordinates into object-space coordinates. In Proceedings ASP/UI Symposium on Close-Range Photogrammetry. Falls Church, VA; American Society of Photogrammetry; 1971:1–18.

Burnett A: Coach Information Service. Available at http://www.coachesinfo.com/articles/50/

Regtien PPL: *Electronic Instrumentation*. Delft, The Netherlands: Delft University Press; 2004.

Dengler K, Lang A: Material requirements of sport shoes. *Materials World* 7:739–740, 1999.

Woltring HJ, Huiskes R: Stereophotogrammetry. In *Biomechanics of Human Movement.* Edited by Berme N, Capozzo A. Worthington, OH: Bertec Corporation; 1990: 108–127.

Wood GA, Marshall RN: The accuracy of DLT extrapolation in three-dimensional film analysis. *J Biomech* 19:781–785. 1986.

CHAPTER two

SCALAR QUANTITIES AND VECTOR QUANTITIES IN MECHANICS AND MOTION ANALYSIS

CHAPTER *objectives*

To give students a good basic understanding of vectors and scalars and their application to mechanics.

CHAPTER *outcomes*

After reading this chapter, the student will be able to:

- Distinguish between vectors and scalars.
- Add and subtract vectors by the tip-to-tail method.
- Add and subtract vectors using unit vectors or vector components.
- Resolve a vector into components along orthogonal axes.
- Use the Pythagorean theorem to add two orthogonal vectors.
- Use the cosine rule to add two non-orthogonal vectors.
- Use the scalar or "dot" product of two vectors to evaluate work done by a force.
- Use the vector or cross"product of two vectors to evaluate turning moments or torques.

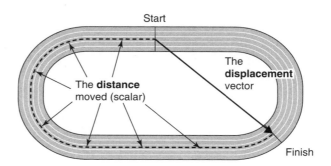

Figure 2.1 Distinguishing between a distance moved (a scalar) and a displacement (a vector).

2.1 Addition and Subtraction of Vectors

The study of **mechanics** involves the measurement of physical quantities such as position, mass, velocity, acceleration, force, moment of inertia, time, and angular speed. Some of these quantities are called **scalar** quantities because they can be described completely by single numerical values and are nondirected quantities; mass, time, angular speed, and moment of inertia are all scalar quantities. **Vector** quantities, on the other hand, are completely described by a magnitude and a direction. Displacement, velocity, acceleration, and force are all vector quantities. With vector quantities, the size or magnitude of the quantity must be specified along with the direction.

The difference between a vector and a scalar can be most successfully demonstrated by comparing a displacement and a distance moved. A **displacement** is a vector movement joining the initial position to the final position by a straight line. The **distance**, on the other hand, is a scalar quantity indicating the total distance moved, including any diversions from a straight path. For example, Figure 2.1 shows a runner running three quarters of the way round a 400-m oval track in a time of 40 s. In this example, the displacement, *d*, is a vector approximately 130 m long pointing in the direction shown, but the distance s moved is 300 m measured all the way along the track. Likewise, we can distinguish between velocity (vector **v**) and speed: the velocity is displacement divided by time taken and so is a vector in the same direction as **d**. The speed is the distance traveled divided by the time taken and is a scalar. Therefore, in this example, velocity = 3.25 m/s and speed = 7.5 m/s.

2.1.1 Addition of Scalars

Scalars can be added by simple addition. Two masses of 50 kg each would make a total of 100 kg. In general, if S_1, S_2, S_3, ..., S_n are scalars to be added together, then the sum of all of them is:

$$S = S_1 + S_2 + S_3 + \ldots\ldots\ldots\ldots\ldots + S_n$$

BOX 2-1   **Examples of Scalar Quantities**

A mass of 80 kg
A moment of inertia of 0.2 kg/m² $\quad$ A time of 55 s
$\qquad\qquad\qquad\qquad\qquad\qquad\qquad\quad$ An angular speed of 10 rad/s (radians per second)

BOX 2-2 | Examples of Vector Quantities

A velocity of 12 m/s directed due east
A force of 20 N acting vertically upward

An acceleration of 5 ms^2 from left to right
A displacement of 5 m along the line joining A and B

Sometimes this is written in textbooks or scientific publications as:

$$S = \sum_{i=1}^{n} S_i$$

where the symbol Σ stands for summation or "the sum of." The "dummy" index or subscript i is used to show that there are n terms to the summation with i taking on all the whole-number values from 1 to n.

2.1.2 ADDITION OF VECTORS

Vectors add together by simple addition provided that they are both pointing along the same straight line. A displacement of 100 m due south followed by a further displacement of 200 m due south gives a total displacement of 300 m due south. However, vector addition does not proceed so simply if there is an arbitrary angle between the two vectors. We adopt the convention in this book that vectors are represented by bold, italicized capital letters in the text. Two or more such vectors can then be added by the "tip-to-tail" approach. Let's take two vectors, *A* (a displacement of 50 m due north) and *B* (a displacement of 75 m due northeast) and try to add them using the "tip-to-tail" method (Fig. 2.2).

Starting from point P, a person (or any other object) undergoing these two displacements, say *A* first and then *B*, the person or object would move first to point Q and then to point R. The overall displacement is clearly a vector pointing from P (the starting point) to R (the finishing point). Also, the result would still be the same if *B* was executed first and then *A*. We can summarize this as follows:

If the addition of the two vectors is represented by *C*, then:

$$C = A + B$$

BOX 2-3 | Examples of Scalar Addition

25, 30, and 45 kg add to give 100 kg.
Times of 20, 10, and 15 s add to give 45 s.
Moments of inertia 0.2 and 0.1 kg/m^2 add to give 0.3 kg/m^2.
Angular speeds of 5 and 2.5 rad/s add to give 7.5 rad/s.

CAUTION:

The values of moments of inertia depend on what axis is taken, so that it may not make physical sense to simply add moments of inertia as we have done here. Also, angular speeds, which, although in principle, can be added together simply like this, in practice, other physical laws may be at work, meaning that addition of angular speeds proceeds according to different rules. (See Chapters 6 and 7, which deal with angular kinetics and dynamics.)

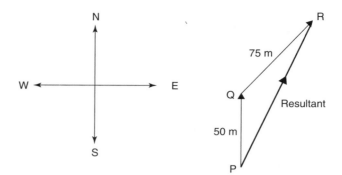

Figure 2.2 Addition of two vector quantities by the tip-to-tail method.

(i.e., resultant displacement PR = displacement PQ + displacement QR) and

A + **B** = **B** + **A** (The order in which the displacements are done is unimportant.)

The result in the above example is 115.88 m at an angle of 27.2° to PQ, but this will not be proved here. This can be shown approximately by a graphical method. Take a piece of graph paper with 1-cm squares, preferably also with 1-mm small squares, and draw the vectors starting from a point near the center of the graph paper, which we will call the origin (0,0). It always makes sense to choose the vertical and horizontal scales according to a "simple-to-use" rule. For example, if we choose each centimeter on the graph paper to represent 10 m, it is easy to draw vectors such as 50 m north because it would be 5 cm on the graph paper and pointing straight up. Also, if we wish to be able to measure angles on the graph paper, then it is essential to make the scales on the horizontal (x) and vertical (y) axes the same. If we wish to draw a vector at some other direction (e.g., for a vector northeast), we would draw it at an angle of 45° using a protractor and pointing in the positive x, positive y direction. Figure 2.3 shows the two vectors, **A** and **B**, and their resultant; in this case, it can be measured with a ruler as being 11.6 cm long and with a protractor as being 27° with respect to **A**.

The magnitude of 11.6 cm translates to a displacement of 116 m and is only as accurate as the length measurement in percentage terms. In this case, the result-

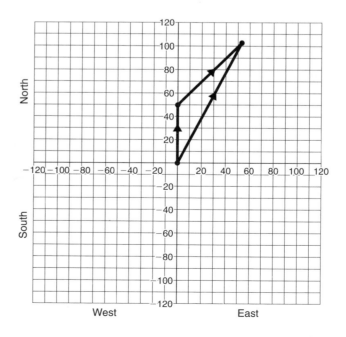

Figure 2.3 Addition of two displacements **A** and **B** using a graphical method.

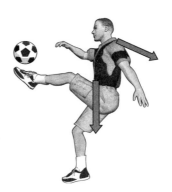

Figure 2.4 A football player subject to two forces: his weight acting vertically down from his center of mass and a force exerted by another player on his shirt acting down at an angle of 25° below the horizontal.

ant can only be measured with a ruler to ±0.1 cm, so the displacement can only be quoted to ±1 m, or about ±1%.

It is not always clear how two or more vectors can be added using the tip-to-tail method when the vectors themselves do not appear, at first glance, to be in a tip-to-tail position. Consider the example of the football player shown in Figure 2.4 subject to some shirt tugging. In this unbalanced position, he is likely to fall down and injure himself because of the combined effect of his weight and the force exerted by the other player tugging his shirt. In this case, one or both forces can be translated in the plane of the figure so that they meet tip to tail. The result of this is shown in Figure 2.5 together with the resultant of the vectors **W** and **F**.

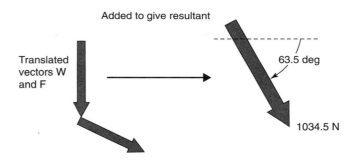

Figure 2.5 The two vectors *W* and *F* shown translated, without rotating either of them, and then added to form the resultant using the tip-to-tail method.

Here are some arbitrary vectors **A** and **B** and their resultant **C**:

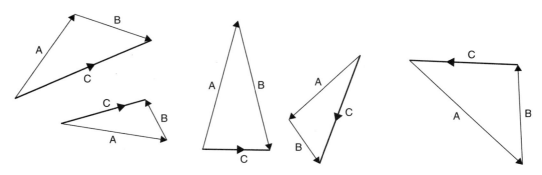

It also follows that any number of vectors **A, B, C, D, ... ,M, N** can be added by placing them tip to tail and producing a polygon of vectors (Fig. 2.6), the resultant **R** being found by completing the polygon to make a closed figure.

The order in which the vectors are added is not important. Again, the vectors can be translated in the plane of the figure to get them to be in the tip-to-tail position.

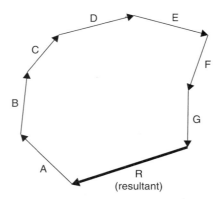

Figure 2.6 Polygon of vectors.

Subtraction of vectors, as in $A - B$, can be achieved by adding A and (B multiplied by scalar -1). This has the effect of changing the direction of the B vector by 180° (Fig. 2.7).

■ **EXAMPLE 2.1**

A man throws a baseball with a velocity of 20 m/s at an angle of 30° with respect to the horizontal. Then he does the same throw, but this time he is running with a velocity of 5 m/s in the same direction as the throw. What is the resultant velocity of the ball?

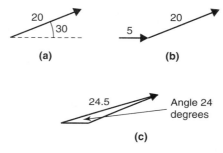

(a) shows the velocity achieved in a normal throw
(b) shows the velocities caused by running and throwing respectively
(c) shows the formation of the resultant by the tip-to-tail method

The resultant velocity with which the ball can be thrown is 24.5 m/s at an angle of 24° with respect to the horizontal, as calculated using the tip-to-tail method on graph paper. (Accurate values for these answers are 24.46 m/s and an angle 24.13°; see section 2.1.4 for the method.)

2.1.3 ADDING TWO VECTORS AT RIGHT ANGLES

When two vectors act at right angles, the resultant can be easily found by adding the vectors using any of the techniques discussed so far. The result can also be

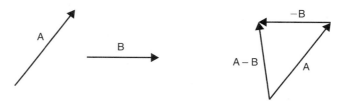

Figure 2.7 Subtraction of two vectors, **A** − **B**.

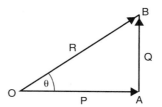

Figure 2.8 Addition of two vectors, **P** and **Q**, which are perpendicular to each other.

accurately found by using the **Pythagorean theorem** to find the diagonal in the rectangle formed.

Consider a vector **P** represented by OA and a vector **Q** at right angles to **P** represented by AB (Fig. 2.8). The resultant **R** is represented by OB on Figure 2.8. The Pythagorean theorem gives this length as:

$$(OB)^2 = (OA)^2 + (AB)^2$$

or

$$R^2 = P^2 + Q^2$$

giving

$$R = \sqrt{P^2 + Q^2}$$

If the angle θ is required, it is given by:

$$\tan \theta = OA/AB = P/Q$$
$$\theta = \tan^{-1} (P/Q)$$

■ **EXAMPLE 2.2**

An ice skater is propelling herself along a level horizontal ice field with a posterior force of 50 N and a lateral force of 40 N. What is the resultant force of propulsion?

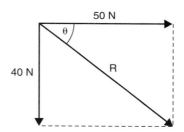

The resultant **R** can be evaluated in terms of magnitude and direction:

Magnitude $R = \sqrt{(50)^2 + (40)^2} = \sqrt{2500 + 1600} = \sqrt{4100} = 64.03N$

Direction $\tan\theta = 40/50 = 0.8$

Therefore, $\theta = \tan^{-1}(0.8) = 38.66°$ or 0.6747 radians

Appendix 1 on Units and Mathematics gives further information on the Pythagorean theorem and trigonometry.

CASE *Study 2.1*   **Magnitude and Direction of Force Vectors During Walking**

An AMTI force plate is used to measure the ground reaction force (GRF) of someone walking across the plate. For this particular force plate, the z axis is vertically up, and the x and y axes are in the horizontal plane. The following diagram shows the force plate and its relationship with the rectangular coordinate axes. The person walks across the plate in the positive x direction.

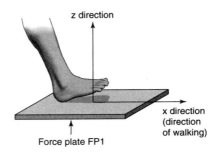

The plate produces voltage outputs corresponding to the x, y, and z components of the GRF as a function of time. The graph shows the components of primary interest, namely the x and z components of the GRF, using a data collection frequency of 600 Hz for all force components.

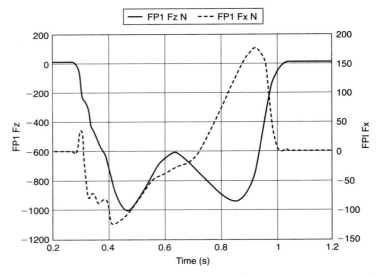

The graph shows the force components F_x and F_x of a normal walking gait. The vertical component F_z is shown as a solid line and has two minima at approximately 0.47 s and 0.86 s. The horizontal component F_x is shown as a dashed line and commences with a mainly negative section before changing to a positive value at approximately 0.72 s. The significance of the positive and negative signs of the force components in this example is clarified by considering the forces acting on the person's foot during the push-off phase.

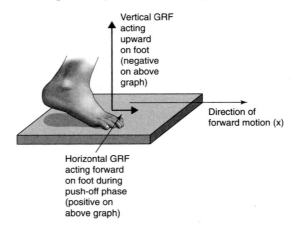

	Table 2.1	z- and x-force components at five selected times		
Time t (s)	**z-Component of Force (N)**	**x-Component of Force (N)**	**Comment**	
0.3583	−501.585	−87.3915	50% of F_z min	
0.47	−990.525	−102.3729	Local minimum in F_z	
0.64	−605.555	−26.0391	Local minimum in F_z	
0.86	−937.135	134.1192	Local minimum in F_z	
0.9533	−469.27	159.8016	50% of F_z min	

The picture shows the foot in contact with the force plate during the push-off phase showing the x and z force components acting on the foot. Table 2.1 shows the values of F_x and F_z at five selected times.

Using these force components, we can calculate the angle θ and the magnitude of the force **F** at these times. The angle θ at time t = 0.3583 s can be calculated from:

$$\tan \theta = \frac{87.3915}{501.585} = 0.1742$$

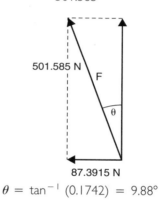

$$\theta = \tan^{-1}(0.1742) = 9.88°$$

Let us call this a positive angle, although such a distinction is arbitrary, with the benefit that if the x component becomes positive, the angle will become negative. The magnitude of the GRF acting on the foot is:

$$F = \sqrt{(501.585)^2 + (87.3915)^2} = 509.14N$$

Likewise, the angles and magnitudes of the force acting on the foot can be calculated at the other times, so giving a table of force magnitudes and angles (Table 2.2). The vector diagram shows the force vector F and its angle of lean roughly to scale.

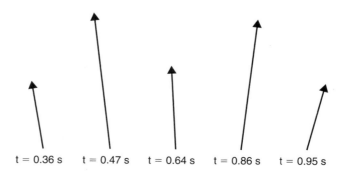

t = 0.36 s   t = 0.47 s   t = 0.64 s   t = 0.86 s   t = 0.95 s

Table 2.2	Magnitude and angle of the resultant force vector at five selected times	
Time (s)	**Magnitude of GRF (N)**	**Angle θ(deg)**
0.3583	509.14	9.88
0.47	995.80	5.90
0.64	606.11	2.46
0.86	946.68	−8.14
0.9533	495.73	−18.8

GRF = ground reaction force.

2.1.4 PARALLELOGRAM RULE

If OA and AD (Fig. 2.9A) represent two vectors P and Q making an angle ϕ with one another, then the resultant R can be calculated using the cosine formula:

$$OD^2 = OA^2 + AD^2 - 2OA.AD \cos(180 - \phi)$$

or, using R, P, and Q to stand for the magnitudes OD, OA, and AD, respectively:

$$R^2 = P^2 + Q^2 - 2P.Q \cos(180 - \phi)$$
$$\text{or } R^2 = P^2 + Q^2 + 2P.Q \cos\phi$$

The angle θ between R and P is given by

$$\tan \theta = \frac{DE}{OE} = \frac{Q \sin\phi}{P + Q \cos\phi}$$

The angle ϕ between P and Q appears as an exterior angle in the triangle. For this reason and another reason discussed later, it is often considered best to draw OB = AD to represent Q (Fig. 2.9B) so that a completed parallelogram is formed, of which the diagonal through O represents R. Thus, if OA and OB represent the size and direction of two vectors P and Q, their resultant R is represented in size and direction by the diagonal OD of the parallelogram OADB.

When dealing with the **cosine rule**, it is essential to label the angles and lengths of the sides of the triangle with a logical system of symbols and to be able to link them with the appropriate formulae. To give an example, let us consider a sprinter on the starting blocks before the starting pistol has been fired. The forces acting on the sprinter are his weight acting vertically down, the reaction force at the blocks,

Figure 2.9 (**A**) and (**B**)
The parallelogram rule.

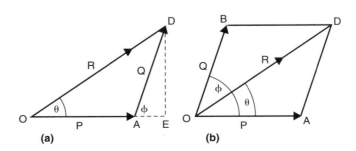

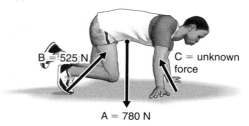

Figure 2.10 The sprinter in the starting blocks experiences three forces: the weight, **A**, acting at the center of mass; the reaction force, **B**, at the blocks acting on his body of magnitude 525 N and at an angle of 70° with respect to the horizontal; and **C**, an unknown force acting at an unknown angle and with an unknown magnitude. The mass of the sprinter is 78 kg, and the magnitude of **A** is, therefore, approximately 780 N. The blocks are instrumented with strain gauges and give an accurate measure of the force **B**.

and the reaction force that the ground exerts on his hands. This example is shown in Figure 2.10, in which **A** represents the weight of the sprinter, **B** represents the reaction force exerted by the blocks on the feet (sum of the left and right feet), and **C** represents the total reaction force exerted by the ground on the hands.

If the sprinter is not moving and not accelerating, the three forces, **A**, **B**, and **C**, will be in equilibrium (see Chapter 3) and will form a closed triangle of forces; there is 0 overall resultant. This fact together with the cosine rule can enable us to find the unknown force **C**.

The forces **A**, **B**, and **C** can be shown on a vector diagram (Fig. 2.11A). Figure 2.11B shows the preferred general labeling of any triangle for application of the cosine rule. Based on Figure 2.11B, the formulas for the cosine rule can be written as:

$$A^2 = B^2 + C^2 - 2BC\cos\alpha$$
$$B^2 = A^2 + C^2 - 2AC\cos\beta$$
$$C^2 = A^2 + B^2 - 2AB\cos\gamma$$

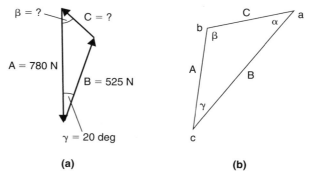

(a)   **(b)**

Figure 2.11 (A) The forces **A**, **B**, and **C** exerted on the body of the sprinter with a resultant of 0. The force **C** is unknown and can be calculated from the cosine rule. This is true provided the sprinter is stationary and not accelerating. (B) The general labeling of a triangle before application of the cosine rule. The lengths of the sides of the triangle are allocated symbols A, B, and C on an arbitrary basis. The angle opposite the A side is labeled α, the angle opposite the B side is labeled β, and the angle opposite the C side is labeled γ. This should be adhered to carefully so that the cosine rule formulae can be applied correctly. If the angles α and β are interchanged, for example, errors may occur in calculation of lengths and angles. If desired, the three apexes can be labeled *a*, *b*, and *c* with apex *a* opposite side A and so on.

It is recommended that these rules are remembered and applied in this form to avoid confusion and to provide a logical basis for calculations. This rule is also summarized in Appendix 1.

In Figure 2.11A, the magnitude of C is unknown. This can be found by applying the cosine rule:

$$C^2 = A^2 + B^2 - 2AB \cos\gamma$$
$$C^2 = (780)^2 + (525)^2 - 2(780)(525)\cos(20)$$
$$C^2 = 608400 + 275625 - 769608.3 = 114416.7$$
$$C = 338.25 \text{ N}$$

In some textbooks, this is sometimes written as $|\underline{C}|$ the magnitude of the vector $\underline{C}$. In this book, the vector is shown in bold italics C and the magnitude of the vector is shown as just C or $|C|$.

To find the angle at which C acts at the hands, the cosine rule can be applied again, or a variety of other methods can be used. Applying the cosine rule:

$$\cos\beta = \frac{-B^2 + A^2 + C^2}{2AC} = \frac{-275625 + 608400 + 114416.7}{2(780)(338.25)} = \frac{447191.7}{528060}$$
$$= 0.8468$$

$$\beta = 32.1°$$

The reaction force at the hands acting on the sprinter's body is of magnitude 338 N and acts at an angle of 57.9° with respect to the horizontal.

▪ EXAMPLE 2.3

A sailboat moves 1200 m due east followed by 1500 m due northeast. What is the overall displacement?

Solution A: Graphical Method

Draw a vector diagram on graph paper showing the two displacements drawn to scale (e.g., 1 cm to every 100 m.) The initial position of the boat can be taken at the origin of coordinates (0,0) at the bottom lefthand corner of the graph paper.

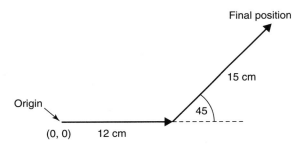

The angle of 45° for the second leg of 1500 m is drawn in accurately using a protractor. The resultant displacement is now represented by the line (not shown) joining the origin to the final position. By measuring with a ruler, this length is 25 cm (or 2500 m ± 10 m), and the angle of the resultant with the horizontal is 25 ± 1°.

Solution B: Cosine Rule

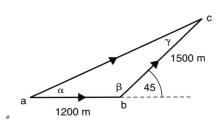

The angle β is $(180 - 45) = 135°$. α and γ are unknown. If the length ab = C, bc = A and ac = B, then:

$$B^2 = A^2 + C^2 - 2AC \cos \beta \text{ (cosine rule)}$$

so that:

$$B^2 = 1200^2 + 1500^2 - 2(1200)(1500) \cos (135)$$
$$B^2 = 1440000 + 2250000 - 3600000(-0.7071)$$
$$= 1440000 + 2250000 + 2545560$$
$$= 6235560$$
$$B = 2497.1 \text{ m}$$

For a complete solution, one of the angles α or γ (preferably α) would have to be specified in order to describe the direction of the resultant ac. It can be calculated from the cosine rule in this form:

$$A^2 = B^2 + C^2 - 2BC \cos \alpha$$

$$\cos \alpha = \frac{-A^2 + B^2 + C^2}{2BC} = \frac{-2250000 + 6235560 + 1440000}{2(2497.1)(1200)} = \frac{56425560}{5993040} = 0.9053$$

$$\alpha = \cos^{-1}(0.9053) = 25.1°$$

or, alternatively, it can be calculated using

$$\tan \alpha = \frac{(BC)\sin\phi}{(AB) + (BC)\cos\phi} = \frac{1500\sin(45)}{1200 + 1500\cos(45)} = \frac{1060.66}{2260.66} = 0.4692$$

$$\alpha = \tan^{-1}(0.4692) = 25.1°$$

2.2   Resolution of a Vector Into Components

2.2.1   RESOLUTION OF A VECTOR ALONG TWO PERPENDICULAR DIRECTIONS

We can **resolve** any given vector into two others in any two given directions by working the parallelogram rule backward, starting with the diagonal and drawing the adjacent sides in the chosen directions. The most important case is when the two directions are at right angles to each other; the two vectors then obtained are called the **components** of the original vector. When working in three dimensions, a vector can be resolved into three components along three perpendicular axes.

Thus, given a vector **R**, to find the components in two directions 1 and 2 at right angles to one another, OD is drawn to scale to represent **R**, the rectangle OADB is constructed where OA represents **P**, the component in direction 1, and OB represents **Q**, the component in the direction 2. This procedure is summarized in Fig. 2.12

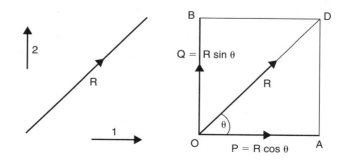

Figure 2.12   Resolution of **R** in directions 1 and 2 at right angles.

As $OA/OD = \cos \theta$
$P/R = \cos \theta$, or $P = R \cos \theta$
and as $OB/OD = AD/OD = \sin \theta$
$Q/R = \sin \theta$, or $Q = R \sin \theta$

See also Appendix 1 for a summary of mathematical techniques.

■ **EXAMPLE 2.4**

A javelin is thrown with an initial velocity of 20 m/s at an angle of 45° to the horizontal. Resolve this velocity into vertical and horizontal components.

Solution

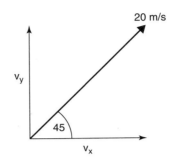

The horizontal and vertical components are shown on the diagram as v_x and v_y, respectively.

$$v_x = 20 \cos 45 = 20(0.7071) = 14.14 \text{ m/s}$$

and

$$v_y = 20 \sin 45 = 20(0.7071) = 14.14 \text{ m/s.}$$

In this example, v_x and v_y are equal. The original velocity of 20 m/s acting at 45° is entirely equivalent to the combined action of its components v_x and v_y and can be replaced by them in all calculations. It should be stressed, however, that you should only resolve once. Also, when components are taken, the original vector should then be forgotten about and ignored because it has been *replaced* by its components.

■ **EXAMPLE 2.5**

An athlete's foot produces a GRF of 410 N horizontally and 520 N vertically. What is the magnitude of the GRF and its angle with respect to the horizontal?

Solution

In this case, the angle θ that the force makes with the horizontal is unknown.

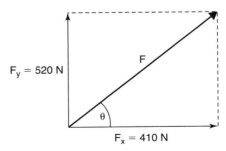

The magnitude of the force F is given by:

$$F = \sqrt{F_x^2 + F_y^2} = \sqrt{410^2 + 520^2} \text{ (by the Pythagorean theorem)}$$
$$F = 662.2 \text{ N}$$

The angle at which **F** acts is given by:

$$\tan \theta = \frac{520}{410} = 1.268$$

$$\theta = \tan^{-1}(1.268) = 51.7°$$

2.2.2 UNIT VECTORS IN THREE DIMENSIONS

Vectors can be conveniently expressed in terms of **unit vectors** (meaning vectors whose magnitude is one) pointing along the chosen coordinate axes. With rectangular righthanded x, y, and z axes (Fig. 2.13), the unit vectors are called **i**, **j**, and **k** and point along the positive x, y, and z axes, respectively. This means that any vector V can be written as:

$$V = V_x \mathbf{i} + V_y \mathbf{j} + V_z \mathbf{k}$$

where V_x, V_y and V_z are the components of V along the x, y, and z axes, respectively. This is sometimes abbreviated to just:

$$V = (V_x, V_y, V_z)$$

This means that any vector can be expressed as V_x units to the right, V_y units up, and V_z units perpendicular to the first two. It also follows that the magnitude of a vector V can be expressed as:

$$V^2 = V_x^2 + V_y^2 + V_z^2 \text{ or } V = (V_x^2 + V_y^2 + V_z^2)^{1/2}$$

To add two vectors A and B, the resultant can be written as:

$$R = A + B = (A_x + B_x)\mathbf{i} + (A_y + B_y)\mathbf{j} + (A_z + B_z)\mathbf{k}$$

2.3 Multiplication of Vectors

2.3.1 MULTIPLICATION OF A VECTOR BY A SCALAR

A vector can be multiplied by a scalar quantity to produce another vector. Thus, if we have a vector A and a scalar c, then the product of the two is another vector cA. The properties of cA are:

1. It has the same direction as the first vector A if c is positive and has the opposite direction to A if c is negative. If $c = 0$, clearly cA is 0 as well.

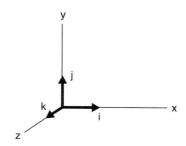

Figure 2.13 Unit vectors pointing along righthanded x, y, and z axes.

Figure 2.14 Illustration of the effect of multiplication by various positive and negative scalars on a vector **A**. The vectors in the lower half of this diagram represent vectors c**A** for $c = -2, -1, 0, 1$ and 2.

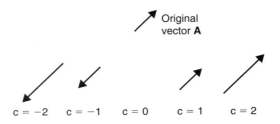

2. Its magnitude is increased or decreased by the magnitude of c. So, if $c = 0.5$, then the magnitude of the new vector will be one half the magnitude of **A**. If $c = -3$, then the magnitude of c**A** will be three times that of **A**.

Figure 2.14 shows an arbitrary vector and how it is altered for five different values of the scalar c.

CASE *Study 2.2*   **Higher Velocity with New Golf Club**

A new design of golf club enables professional players to achieve 15% more velocity off the tee on average than with the previous best golf clubs. An average velocity with the new club was 51.42 m/s compared with 44.72 m/s previously. The direction of hitting remains unchanged on average.

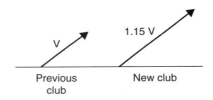

CASE *Study 2.3*   **Velocity of a Baseball at Different Times**

A pitcher pitches a ball in the game of baseball. The velocity components of the ball at three different subsequent times are given in Table 2.3. At $t = 0.675$ s, the ball is in the pitcher's hand and is being accelerated down. At $t = 0.800$ and 0.925 s, the ball is in the air and is moving down toward the ground. The velocity vectors at these times can be written as:

Table 2.3 The x, y, and z components of the ball velocity at three selected times

t (s)	V_x (m/s)	V_y (m/s)	V_z (m/s)
0.675	−2.733	−2.527	−1.863
0.800	−4.008	−4.062	−6.471
0.925	−3.911	−3.961	−7.405

$$v = -2.733\mathbf{i} - 2.527\mathbf{j} - 1.863\mathbf{k}$$
$$v = -4.008\mathbf{i} - 4.062\mathbf{j} - 6.471\mathbf{k}$$
$$v = -3.911\mathbf{i} - 3.961\mathbf{j} - 7.405\mathbf{k}$$

The magnitudes of the resultant velocity vectors are 4.162, 8.628, and 9.264 m/s, respectively.

■ **EXAMPLE 2.6**

A ball experiences two forces: its weight W = 5 N acting vertically down and a drag force directed in a direction opposite to the velocity of the ball. The velocity of the ball is given by $v = 15\mathbf{i} + 18\mathbf{j} - 20\mathbf{k}$. The drag force is given by:

$$F_d = 0.01 \times (\text{speed})^2$$

Figure out the weight of the ball and the drag force in terms of unit vectors **i**, **j**, and **k**. What is the resultant force on the ball in terms of unit vectors?

Solution

The weight of the ball can be written as:

$$\mathbf{W} = 0\mathbf{i} + 0\mathbf{j} - 5\mathbf{k}$$

The speed of the ball is given by the magnitude of its velocity:

$$v = \sqrt{(15)^2 + (18)^2 + (-20)^2} = \sqrt{225 + 324 + 400} = \sqrt{949} = 30.8 m/s$$

Therefore, the magnitude of the drag force is given by:

$$F_d = 0.01 \times (30.8)^2 = 9.49 N$$

In terms of unit vectors, it can be written as $F_d = (magnitude) \times \hat{v}$, where $\hat{v}$ is a unit vector along the direction of v.
A unit vector along the direction of the velocity would be

$$\hat{v} = \frac{15i + 18j - 20k}{30.8} = 0.487\mathbf{i} + 0.584\mathbf{j} - 0.649\mathbf{k}$$

We can write the drag force as:

$$\mathbf{F_d} = 9.49 \times (0.487\mathbf{i} + 0.584\mathbf{j} - 0.649\mathbf{k})$$
$$\mathbf{F_d} = 4.621\mathbf{i} + 5.542\mathbf{j} - 6.162\mathbf{k}$$

The overall force can be written as:

$$\mathbf{F} = \mathbf{W} + \mathbf{F_d}$$
$$\mathbf{F} = 4.621\mathbf{i} + 5.542\mathbf{j} - 11.162\mathbf{k}$$

2.3.2 SCALAR PRODUCT OF TWO VECTORS

If we have two vectors *A* and *B*, then their **scalar** (or **dot**) **product** is defined as:

$$\mathbf{A.B} = A\,B\cos\theta$$

where *A* and *B* are the magnitudes of the vectors and θ is the smallest angle (< 180°) between them when their tails touch, as in Figure 2.15. Because *A*, *B*, and cos θ are all

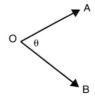

Figure 2.15 Two vectors, **A** and **B**, and the angle between them.

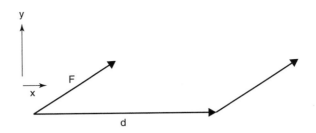

Figure 2.16 Work done by a force **F** acting at an angle θ to the ground is $W = \mathbf{Fd}$.

scalars, then so is the scalar product **A.B** (read as **A** "dot" **B**), hence the name scalar product. If the two vectors are expressed in terms of unit vectors, then:

$$\text{Scalar product} = \mathbf{A.B} = A_xB_x + A_yB_y + A_zB_z$$

This is useful in mechanics, particularly when it comes to defining the work done by a force, **F**, that is moved through a displacement, **d** (Fig. 2.16). We would then take the work done, W, as the scalar product of **F** and **d**:

$$W = \mathbf{F.d} = \mathbf{F}\,d\cos\theta.$$

If **F** and **d** are expressed using unit vectors, then the work done is:

$$W = \mathbf{F.d} = F_xd_x + F_yd_y + F_zd_z$$

The work done can then be viewed as the magnitude of the force (**F**) multiplied by the distance moved in the direction of the force (d cos θ). If **F** and **d** are collinear, (θ = 0), then cos θ = 1, and the work done is just force multiplied by distance moved.

■ **EXAMPLE 2.7**

A man pushing a bobsleigh exerts a force of 550 N acting at an angle of 20° to the horizontal. What is the work done on the bobsleigh over a 20-m distance along the bobsleigh run?

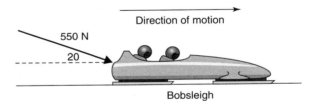

Direction of motion

550 N

20

Bobsleigh

Solution

The work done is **F.d** = F d cos θ where θ is the angle between **F** and **d**. **d** is a displacement vector parallel to the direction of motion of the bobsleigh. The work done, therefore, is:

$$W = 10336.7 \text{ Joules (or Newton meters)}$$

■ **EXAMPLE 2.8**

A man pushing a bobsleigh exerts a force of 516.8 N horizontally and a force of 188.1 N vertically downward. The bobsleigh moves horizontally a distance of 20 m down the track. What is the work done on the bobsleigh?

Solution

Using unit vectors **i**, **j**, and **k**, the force exerted on the bobsleigh can be written as:

$$\mathbf{F} = 516.8\mathbf{i} - 188.1\mathbf{j} + 0\mathbf{k}$$

assuming the bobsleigh is moving along the horizontal x axis and the upward vertical direction is the y axis.

The displacement of the bobsleigh can be written as:

$$\mathbf{d} = 20\mathbf{i} + 0\mathbf{j} + 0\mathbf{k}.$$

The work done can then be worked out as:

$$W = \mathbf{F}.\mathbf{d} = F_x d_x + F_y d_y + F_z d_z = 516.8(20) - 188.1(0) + 0(0)$$
$$W = 10336 \text{ J}$$

CASE *Study 2.4*   **Downward and Upward Movements in a Squat**

A weightlifter training for a competition squats 150 kg. On the downward movement, he allows the weight to fall at constant speed slowly to the lowest point by flexing his knees. He then pushes the weight upward at constant speed until his legs are straight. The total displacement is 0.9 m down and then 0.9 m back up. The weightlifter exerts a force **F** upward on the bar, which is roughly constant throughout the downward and upward movement, equal in magnitude roughly to the weight on the bar provided the upward and downward accelerations are small.

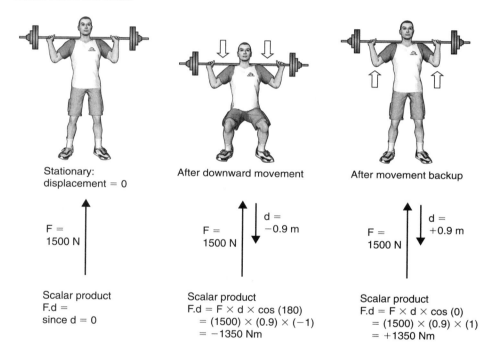

This illustrates that, after the downward movement, the force **F** on the bar and the displacement **d** of the bar are acting along the same straight line but in exactly opposite directions. In this case, the angle θ is 180°, the cosine of this angle is −1, and the work done by the weightlifter on the bar is −1350 Nm or Joules.

After the upward movement, the displacement of the bar is now upward, and **F** and **d** are pointing in the same direction. It follows that the angle θ is now 0, the cosine of the angle is 1, and the work done by the weightlifter on the bar is = 1350 Nm or Joules.

In the case of the downward movement, the work done by the weightlifter is negative, and it is natural to ask how this can happen and what it means. It is a difficult concept, but it can be made easier to understand by saying in this case that the bar is doing positive work on the weightlifter. During the upward movement, the reverse is true, and the weightlifter does positive work on the bar. Although the concept may appear a little artificial, it has important application in eccentric and concentric contraction of muscles. This idea of negative work being done actually occurs whenever the angle θ exceeds 90°. The functional dependence of cosθ on θ is shown in the following diagram for values of θ between 0 and 180°, where it can be seen clearly that cos θ is negative between 90° and 180°. Incidentally, angles are sometimes expressed in radians; if you need to convert between the two, the conversion factor is:

$$1 \text{ radian} = 57.29°$$

Radian measures are covered more fully in the chapters dealing with rotational motion.

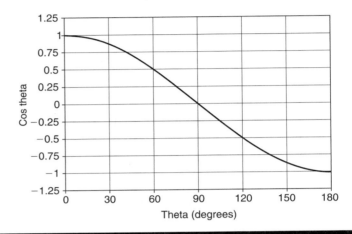

2.3.3 Vector Product of Two Vectors

The **vector** or **cross product** of two vectors *A* and *B* is defined as another vector:

$$C = A \times B$$

whose magnitude is:

$$|C| = |A||B|\sin\theta$$

where θ is the angle (< 180°) between *A* and *B*, and whose direction is perpendicular to both *A* and *B* in the sense of the righthand rule (Fig. 2.17).

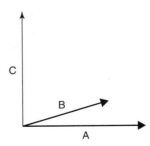

Figure 2.17   The vector **C** = **A** × **B** is perpendicular to the plane containing **A** and **B**; its direction is given by the righthand rule. The thumb of the right hand points along the direction of **C**; the fingers of the right hand curl around from **A** to **B**. Imagine **A** and **B** to be in the plane of the floor, perhaps. **C** would then be pointing vertically up in the air.

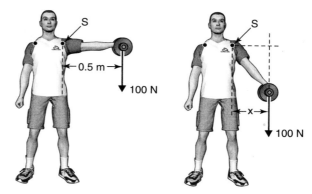

Figure 2.18 Someone holding a 100-N weight at arm's length. The length of the arm is 0.5 m. On the left, the arm is horizontal, and the line of action of the weight is 0.5 m from the shoulder joint. On the left, the arm has been lowered so that it is at 45° to the horizontal. The perpendicular distance between the line of action of the weight and the shoulder joint has now been reduced to x.

If the angle $\theta = 0$, then the crossproduct of two vectors is 0. Hence, $A \times A = 0$, for example. Also, if the angle between two vectors is a right angle, $\theta = 90°$, then $A \times B = AB$, the product of the magnitudes of the two vectors.

This concept is particularly useful when evaluating the moment caused by a given force. Consider someone holding a 10-kg mass at arm's length (Fig. 2.18). We can define a vector r to represent the displacement of the point of application of the weight W relative to the shoulder joint. The **moment** of the force is then given by:

$$M = r \times W$$

This is shown in Figure 2.19 for the two cases shown in Figure 2.18. The results for the vector cross product in the two cases are:

Arm horizontal: $M = r F \sin\theta = 0.5 \times 100 = 50$ Nm

Arm at 45° to horizontal: $M = r F \sin\theta = 0.5 \times 100 \times \sin(45) = 35.35$ Nm

The direction of the moments is clockwise in both Figures 2.18 and 2.19. This would be indicated formally in the vector crossproduct by saying that the vector M is in to the plane of the paper at right angles to both r and W. This is confirmed by using the righthand rule: the fingers curl around in the direction of r moving to the direction of W, meaning that the thumb is pointing in to the plane of the paper (Fig. 2.20).

Figure 2.19 The vector diagrams for the two cases shown in Figure 2.18.

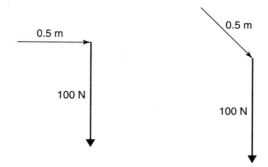

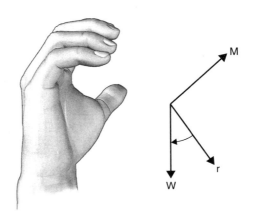

Figure 2.20 The right-hand rule for **r** × **W**, showing the thumb pointing in to the paper.

It is also possible to express the vector product of two vectors using unit vectors. Again suppose that:

$$\boldsymbol{A} = A_x\,\mathbf{i} + A_y\,\mathbf{j} + A_z\,\mathbf{k}$$

and

$$\boldsymbol{B} = B_x\,\mathbf{i} + B_y\,\mathbf{j} + B_z\,\mathbf{k}$$

then the cross- or vector product can be written as:

$$A \times B = \begin{vmatrix} i & j & k \\ A_x & A_y & A_z \\ B_x & B_y & B_z \end{vmatrix} = i(A_y\,B_z - A_z\,B_y) + j(A_z\,B_x - A_x\,B_z) + k(A_x\,B_y - A_y\,B_x)$$

The object:

$$\begin{vmatrix} i & j & k \\ A_x & A_y & A_z \\ B_x & B_y & B_z \end{vmatrix}$$

is known as a **determinant** and is useful in remembering the sequence of calculations required to evaluate the vector crossproduct. Think of it as a sequence of cross-multiplication and addition/subtraction operations (Fig. 2.21). For more information on determinants and the subject of vector analysis, see Spiegel (1959).

Figure 2.21 Calculation of components of vector crossproducts. To work out the **j** component, it helps to write the x components as an additional line to the right of the determinant.

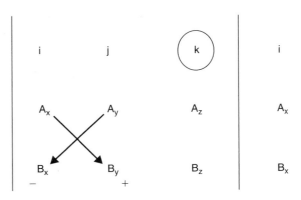

■ **EXAMPLE 2.9**   Torque can be expressed as a crossproduct. For example, take a thin wheel that is free to rotate about an axis through its center at point O. A force **F** acts at the edge of the wheel at a point whose position relative to the center of the wheel O is given by the position vector **r** as shown. The force **F** tends to rotate the wheel (assumed initially at rest) counterclockwise, so the angular velocity **ω** will point out of the page toward the reader.

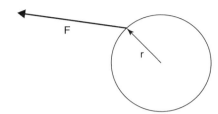

    The torque caused by **F** starts the wheel rotating counterclockwise so that **ω** points out of the page. The **torque** vector is defined as $\tau = r \times F$ and points out of the page. The magnitude of the torque is $\tau = r F \sin\theta$.

■ **EXAMPLE 2.10**   To work out the moment of a force about a point X, imagine a force **F** defined as:

$$F = 1i + 2.7j + 3.5k \text{ acting at a point } r = 10i + 0j - 3.7k$$

The moment of the force about the origin would be:

$$M = r \times F = (0 \times 3.5 - (-3.7) \times 2.7, -3.7 \times 1 - 10 \times 3.5, 10 \times 2.7 - 0 \times 1)$$
$$= (9.99, -38.7, 27)$$

This implies that the moment about the x axis is:

$$M_x = 9.99 \text{ Nm}$$

that about the y axis is:

$$M_y = -38.7 \text{ Nm}$$

and that about the z axis is:

$$M_z = 27 \text{ Nm}$$

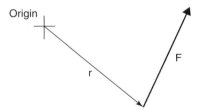

2.4 System of Units

This book is written using the SI (système internationale) system of units. This takes the fundamental units of mass, length, and time as the kilogram, meter, and second, respectively. In this section, the units commonly used in motion analysis and me-

Table 2.4 Commonly used units in the systéme internationale (SI) system

Physical Quantity	SI Unit	Alternative Unit Name	Conversion Factor to Other Units
Mass	kg	Kilogram	1 kg = 2.2 lb
Length	m	meter	1 m = 39 in
Displacement	m	Meter	1 m = 3.281 ft
Time	s	Second	1 s = 0.0002777h
Speed	m/s	ms^{-1}	1 m/s = 2.237 mph
Velocity	m/s	ms^{-1}	1 m/s = 3.281 ft/s
Acceleration	m/s^2	ms^{-2}	1 "gee" = 9.81 m/s^2
Force	N	Newton	1 N = 0.1 kg weight
Moment	Nm	Newton-meter	1 Nm = 0.72 lb/ft
Impulse	Ns	Newton second	
Pressure	N/m^2	Pascal	1 N/m^2 = 0.001422 psi
Linear momentum	kg m/s		
Angle or angular displacement	rad	Radians	1 rad = 57.3°
Angular speed	rad/s		1 rad/s = 57.3 °/s
Angular acceleration	rad/s^2	rad/s^{-2}	
Torque	Nm		1 Nm = 0.72 lb/ft
Angular momentum	$kg/m^2/s$		
Angular impulse	Nm		
Power	J/s	Watt	1 J/s = 0.001343 hp
			1 kW = 1.341 hp

chanics are summarized. Table 2.4 shows the physical quantity, its SI unit and any alternative names. The table also shows the conversion of some of the SI units to different systems in common use. Although very little use is made of alternative units in this book, it is useful to have a point of reference in case they are encountered in everyday situations. For example, a baseball pitcher releases the ball at 100 mph. In this case, miles per hour are used for two reasons:

1. The unit of miles per hour is well known by most people, so they can relate to it easily.
2. The unit of miles per hour is a convenient size so that the numbers obtained are neither too big nor too small.

Also, in this book, units such as m/s and ms^{-1} (meters per second) are used interchangeably. More information on SI units is given in Appendix 1.

SUMMARY

This chapter has introduced the fundamental concepts of scalar and vector quantities. Addition, subtraction, and multiplication of scalars and vectors are considered using graphical methods, trigonometric methods, and unit vectors. Three case studies are used to illustrate practical applications of the use of vectors to human movement situations. Scalar products are used for calculating the amount of work done when the force and displacement vectors are at some arbitrary angle to each other. Vector products are used for calculating the moment caused by a force acting at some position r using both formula and determinant methods.

REFERENCE

Spiegel MR: *Schaum's Outline of Vector Analysis.* New York. Schaum Publishing; 1959.

STUDY QUESTIONS

1. Classify the following as vectors or scalars:

    Force, torque, acceleration, velocity, mass, volume, displacement, area, length, and angular velocity

2. Add the following vectors *A* and *B* together by the tip-to-tail approach and draw in the resultant vector *C*.

    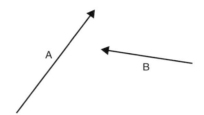

3. Use the polygon of vectors method to find the resultant of the following force vectors:

    20 N acting west

    35 N acting at 60° northeast

    25 N acting north

    15 N acting at 30° southwest

    Draw these on graph paper and do not forget to join them tip to tail. From the graph paper, measure the magnitude and direction of the resultant. Use a ruler and protractor for these measurements.

4. An ice hockey puck has a velocity of 15 m/s parallel to the edge of the rink. It also has a velocity of 5 m/s perpendicular to this edge. Use the Pythagorean theorem to calculate the magnitude of the resultant velocity of the puck to two decimal places.

5. Use the parallelogram rule to find the resultant of the following two vectors *A* and *B*.

    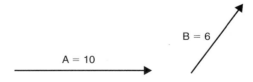

    The vector *B* makes an angle of 55° with *A*. Draw these on graph paper, form the completed parallelogram, and measure the size *and* direction of the resultant. Repeat the calculation of the resultant, this time using the cosine rule. Compare your answers to deduce something about the errors involved in the first method.

6. The following vectors represent the wind velocity at a point adjacent to the long jump area at an Olympic Games. In (a), the vector corresponds to a wind velocity of 10 km/h and is a tail wind. Comment on the wind velocities for (b), (c), and (d). The wind velocity has to be below 5 km/h

for the long jump competition to proceed. Under which condition (or conditions), (a) to (d), would you allow the competition to go ahead?

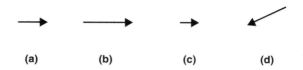

    (a)   **(b)**   **(c)**   **(d)**

7. A golf ball is projected with a velocity of 45 m/s at an angle of 10° with respect to the horizontal. What is the horizontal component of this velocity?

8. A javelin is projected with an initial velocity of 40 m/s. The vertical component of this velocity is measured as 29 m/s. What is its initial horizontal velocity?

9. The high bar of a piece of gymnastic equipment is subject to two forces as a gymnast swings around the bar. One is a vertical up force supplied by the vertical support members at the sides of the high bar. This force is 750 N upward on the bar itself. The other force is a force on the bar acting down and to the right at an angle of 30° to the horizontal applied by the gymnast's hands as he swings. This force amounts to 510 N. Draw these forces on a force diagram showing the two applied forces and the direction of the resultant. Use the cosine law to work out the magnitude and direction of the resultant. (It is assumed in this question that the two vertical supports have identical forces in them. In this case, 375 N each. These two forces are assumed to be combined into one 750-N force.)

10. An acceleration vector has a magnitude of 16 ms^{-2} and is directed upward at an angle of 35° to the horizontal. What are the vertical and horizontal components of the acceleration along the x and y axes? The *x* and *y* axes are directed horizontally and vertically such that the acceleration vector is in the *x*–I plane.

11. Unit vectors **i**, **j**, and **k** are set up along the *x*, *y*, and *z* axes.

    (a) A force is expressed as $F = 12\,\mathbf{i} + 25\mathbf{j} + 0\mathbf{k}$. What are the components of the force along the *x*, *y*, and *z* axes?

    (b) A displacement vector is given by $d = 2\,\mathbf{i} + 0\,\mathbf{j} + 3\,\mathbf{k}$. What is the total displacement in meters?

    (c) Two velocities given by $v_1 = 10\,\mathbf{i} + 5\,\mathbf{j} - 3\,\mathbf{k}$

    and $v_2 = -6\,\mathbf{i} + 3\,\mathbf{j} + 5\mathbf{k}$ are added vectorially to give a resultant.

    Write an expression for the resultant $v = v_1 + v_2$ using the unit vectors **i**, **j**, and **k**.

12. A rower exerts a force on his oars of $F = 200$ N acting horizontally while the displacement of the oars is 1.2 m at an angle of 15° above the horizontal.

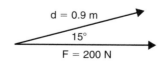

What is the work done as a result of this force and displacement?

13. A rower exerts a force on his oars given by $F = 150\,\mathbf{i} + 45\,\mathbf{j} + 0\,\mathbf{k}$. The displacement of the oar handles is given by $d = 0.8\,\mathbf{i} + 0.75\,\mathbf{j} + 0.15\,\mathbf{k}$. What is the work done?

14. A force of 50 N is applied tangentially to the outer rim of a discus (i.e., at right angles) to the line joining the center of the discus to the point on the rim. The diameter of the discus is 25 cm. What is the torque supplied by this force? Describe the effect of this torque on the discus.

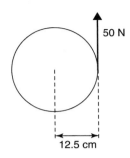

15. A force given by $F = 17i + 25j + 0k$ is applied to a point A on the surface of a ball. The position vector of the point A relative to the center of the ball is given by $r = 0.05i + 0.04j − 0.02k$. What is the torque supplied to the ball by this force?

16. Calculate the magnitude of the force in question 13. What is the diameter of the ball?

17. A soccer ball is moving with a velocity given by:

$$v = 10i − 2.5j + 3k$$

What is the speed of the ball? Write down an expression for a unit vector pointing along the direction of v. If the drag force on the ball is given by $F_d = 0.015 \times (\text{speed})^2$, write down an expression for the drag force in terms of unit vectors i, j, and k.

CHAPTER three

LINEAR KINEMATICS

CHAPTER *objectives*

The objectives of this chapter are to:

- Introduce the idea of the inertia of a body.
- Discuss the natural state of motion of objects.
- Introduce the study of kinematics.
- Describe motion in terms of displacement, velocity, and acceleration.
- Lay the foundations for the study of kinetics.

CHAPTER *outcomes*

After reading this chapter, the student will be able to:

- Understand the law of inertia.
- Apply several methods for finding an object's velocity.
- Use graphs to calculate velocity or acceleration.
- Use a trend line to estimate the velocity from experimental displacement–time data.
- Appreciate the affects of errors on calculated results.
- Understand and apply the following equations applicable to motion with uniform acceleration:

$$v = u + at$$
$$s = (u + v)t/2$$
$$s = ut + \tfrac{1}{2} at^2$$
$$v^2 = u^2 + 2as$$

- Differentiate between motion with uniform acceleration and other motions with non-uniform accelerations.
- Calculate instantaneous and average velocities or accelerations.
- Calculate the trajectories of projectiles with zero air resistance.

3.1   The Law of Inertia

Every body or object continues in its state of rest, or of uniform motion in a straight line, unless acted upon by an external force. This is equivalent to defining **force** as "that which causes acceleration" and implies that bodies have the property of inertia—that is, they do not accelerate unless acted upon by the agent called force. **Uniform motion** means constant velocity. This law is referred to again in Chapter 4, where it is referred to as **Newton's first law** and is discussed along with the other laws of motion initially formulated by Newton.

3.2   Measurement of an Object's Speed or Velocity

There are at least five ways of measuring an objects speed (usually with respect to the ground):

1. Observing the object going past a series of fixed marks at various distances along the path of the object and timing with a stopwatch or timer.
2. Attaching a long paper tape to the object and allowing it to pull the tape or string along as it moves. A fixed-frequency vibrator can make small ink marks on the tape as it passes through the vibrator. The distance between dots on the tape is then a measure of the object's velocity.
3. Allowing sound waves (or radar or microwaves) of a known frequency to strike the moving object and recording the sound waves reflected from the object. The frequency of the sound can be altered by reflection from a moving object in a known way (the Doppler effect) so the velocity of the object can be inferred.
4. Using a camera or cameras to follow the object's motion and inferring the velocity from a suitable calibration procedure.
5. Using infra-red light gates. The object's motion interferes with the passage of the light between transmitter and receiver, allowing the time to travel a given distance to be timed.

Whichever method is used to measure velocity, it is quite difficult to set up a demonstration of Newton's first law in action. This is because friction usually plays a dominant part in the proceedings and tends to slow down things or make things stick together. However, consider the experiment in Figure 3.1, where a moveable trolley can be supported on a track by means of a thin cushion of air.

With this arrangement, the friction force can be reduced to virtually zero. If the track is horizontal and level, the trolley will remain completely at rest provided it is not given any initial velocity to the left or right. If, on the other hand, the trolley is given a velocity, say to the right, then it will continue to move in this

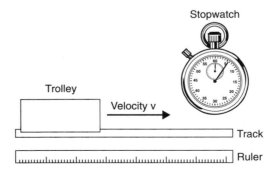

Figure 3.1   A trolley supported on a film of air on an air track.

Table 3.1	
Reading Taken From Ruler (cm)	**Time on Stopwatch (sec)**
0	0
10	5
20	10
30	15
40	20
50	25

direction at ostensibly constant speed. This can be checked by using a stopwatch and distance scale alongside the track or some other means of measuring speed. This would produce a set of readings similar to the ones shown in Table 3.1.

It can be seen that equal distances are being covered in equal intervals of time (e.g., 10 cm every 5 s). This is wholly consistent with Newton's first law and is an example of uniform motion or constant velocity. This motion would continue until the trolley reaches the end of the track, when the experiment must be deemed to have finished. The experiment would be unaffected by loading various small weights (masses) onto the trolley. The experiment would give similar results, but it would be noticeable that it is more difficult to get the trolley moving in the initial push to the left or right. Large weights would perhaps bring the surfaces of the trolley and track into contact so that friction would then come into play, slowing down the trolley.

3.2.1 GRAPHICAL MEANS OF DERIVING VELOCITY

Uniform motion, or motion with constant velocity, is conveniently displayed on a graph showing displacement against time. In this case, velocity can sometimes be calculated if displacement, initial velocity, and acceleration are known. Consider the graph in Figure 3.2, where the displacement of the trolley is plotted against time.

It is conventional to plot the **independent variable** (in this case, time) on the horizontal or x axis and to plot the **dependent variable** (in this case, displacement) on the vertical or y axis. The displacement of the trolley *depends* on the time elapsed, but the converse is not true; this latter time does not depend on the displacement.

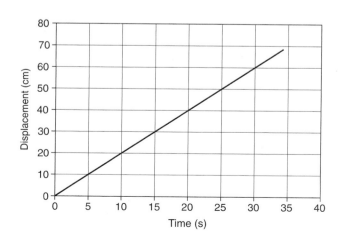

Figure 3.2 A graph of the data in Table 3.1: displacement versus time.

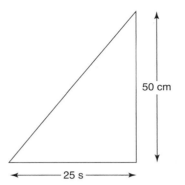

Figure 3.3 A triangle drawn from the graph of Figure 3.2 to calculate the velocity of the trolley.

It can be seen from Figure 3.2 that a straight line is obtained. In this case, the equation for a y versus x graph is shown as:

$$y = mx + c$$

where m is the **slope** or **gradient** of the line (a constant) and c is its **intercept** (also a constant) on the y axis. In this case, the line passes through the origin, so the value of $c = 0$. The equation of the straight line is thus of the simplified form:

$$y = mx$$

If we use the symbols s and t for the displacement and time, respectively, then the equation can be written as:

$$s = vt$$

where v is the slope of the s-t graph (a constant).

The slope of the graph is given by $\frac{\Delta s}{\Delta t}$, where Δs is the increment of s and Δt is the increment of t, so $v = \frac{\Delta s}{\Delta t}$. It can be seen that this quantity has the dimensions of length divided by time and represents, in fact, the velocity of the trolley (ms^{-1}).

Figure 3.3 is a graph of the displacement of the trolley as a function of time. In the particular case of the trolley on the air track and the data in Table 3.1, the slope of the straight line can be worked out by drawing a right-angled triangle with the straight-line graph as hypotenuse. Any size of triangle can be used, but in general, the bigger the triangle, the better for accuracy. The slope of this graph is 50 cm/25 s = 2 cm/ s or 0.02 m/s, so $v = 0.02$ m/s.

■ EXAMPLE 3.1

Draw the graph of s vs. t for the following data representing the motion of an ice hockey puck:

Distance (cm)	Time (s)
5	0
11	0.5
17	1.0
23	1.5
29	2.0
35	2.5
36	3.0

From the graph, calculate the velocity of the puck during the time interval between 0 and 2.5 seconds. (Use the slope of the graph to obtain the velocity.) Write down an equation for your straight-line graph in the general form $y = mx + c$. What are the values of m and c in your equation? Something happens to the puck between 2.5 and 3.0 s. Comment on what this is likely to be and the effect on the motion of the puck.

Solution

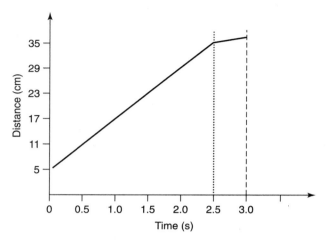

The graph is a straight line between 0 and 2.5 seconds; this is the **constant velocity**. The velocity of the puck is given by the slope of the straight line given by:

$$\frac{\Delta s}{\Delta t} = \frac{35 - 5}{2.5 - 0} = \frac{30}{2.5} = 12 cm/s$$

or 0.12 m/s if the distance is converted to meters. The equation of the straight line is:

$$s = 0.12\,t + 0.05$$

The intercept (at $t = 0$) is 5 cm (or 0.05 m), so the value of $c = 0.05$ and the value of m is 0.12. Between 2.5 and 3.0 s, the motion of the puck is interrupted, perhaps by the intervention of one of the players or hitting the side of the rink. The distance moved between 2.5 and 3.0 s is only 1 cm; previously it had been moving at the rate of 6 cm every half second.

CASE *Study 3.1*   **Velocity of a Toboggan Sliding Along a Track Measured by Students**

A class of 31 sports science students is asked to measure the speed of a toboggan as it slides slowly along a flat horizontal section of track near the start of its run. The toboggan is attached to a paper tape running through a vibrator that makes dots on a paper tape at a frequency of 50 Hz. Working in groups of three or four, each group is asked to take one paper tape measurement. Subsequently working from the paper tape, the velocity of the toboggan is worked out by taking a given number of dots on the tape and measuring with a ruler how far it has traveled in that time interval. The number of dots used could be between 11 and 100. For 11 dots, for example, the appearance of the paper tape might be as follows:

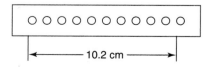

For 11 dots, there are 10 gaps in between dots, so the total time interval is 0.2 s. The distance moved in this example is 10.2 cm. Each group takes 10 pairs of distance–time measurements, and the data from all groups are amalgamated at the end of the day. The data are plotted as a graph with time on the horizontal axis and distance moved on the vertical axis.

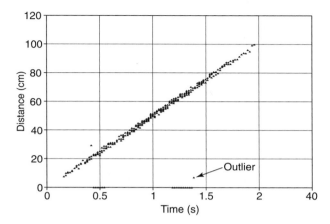

The graph shows a few important features involving errors or uncertainties in the measurement process:

1. The students make random errors when measuring the distances moved using a ruler or tape measure. The time measurement is assumed to be much more accurate because the vibrator is operated at mains frequency, which is tightly controlled to 50 Hz.

2. Two measurements are clearly suspicious: one at 1.38, 1.41 and another at 0.42, 5.9. These measurements are well separated from all the other measurements and could well be attributable to large-scale mistakes by the students when taking or recording their results. For example, a decimal point might be recorded in the wrong place so that a reading of 14.1 cm might be mistaken as 1.41 cm. A measurement such as this is called an outlier and can be rejected under certain circumstances. For more information on the statistical definition of an outlier, refer to Vincent (2005).

The velocity of the toboggan can be worked out using the first and last pairs of points, that is, 0.18 s, 1.5 cm and 1.96 s, 19.7 cm as:

$$\frac{\Delta s}{\Delta t} = \frac{19.7 - 1.5}{1.96 - 0.18} = \frac{18.2}{1.78} = 10.2 \ cm/s$$

Because each distance measurement is probably in error by as much as ± 0.1 cm, the value of $\Delta s = 18.2$ cm could be in error by as much as ± 0.2 cm, and the final velocity can be in error by as much as $\pm (0.2/1.78) = \pm 0.11$ cm/s. We assume here that the uncertainties in the times are very small, indeed. Expressing this in a different way, the percentage uncertainty in the velocity v ($\pm 1.1\%$) is equal to the sum of the percentage uncertainties in Δs ($\pm 1.1\%$) and Δt (0%). See Appendix 1 for a basic discussion of treatment of uncertainties.

However, the large number of measurements taken by the class means that the velocity can be estimated more accurately. The velocity of the toboggan is, in fact, equal to the slope of the s–t line. By taking a least-squares regression line on the data obtained by the 31 students, the velocity can be estimated as the slope of this line. See Appendix 1 for the definition of a least-squares regression line. This is easily done using a package such as Microsoft Excel; a trend line can be added to the data and the equation of the trend line can be displayed on the chart. The linear trend line generated using Excel is shown in the following graph with the two suspected outliers omitted:

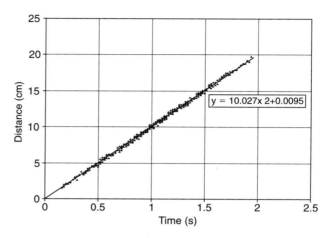

The slope of this trend line (i.e., the velocity of the toboggan) is 10.03 cm/s to two decimal places. This method has the advantage that the measurement is not based on just one pair of values, but is instead based on 310 pairs of values so that the effects of errors or uncertainties are minimized by a sort of "averaging" process. This approach is especially valuable if there are good grounds for believing that the points obtained lie on or close to a straight line and that there are at least 10 data points.

3.2.2 EQUATIONS FOR DISPLACEMENT AND VELOCITY FOR THE CASE OF UNIFORM ACCELERATION

Acceleration is the rate of change of velocity with time, and has units of ms^{-2}. A body moves with **uniform acceleration** (or constant acceleration) when it undergoes equal changes in velocity in equal successive intervals of time, however short these intervals may be. If a is the uniform acceleration, u the initial velocity, and v the final velocity after time t, then from the definition of acceleration:

$$v = u + at \qquad (1)$$

The velocity–time graph (Fig. 3.4) is thus a straight line, sloping upward, as shown if a is positive, and sloping downwards if a is a negative acceleration or

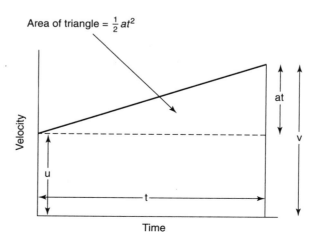

Figure 3.4 Velocity–time graph for an object moving with uniform acceleration a.

retardation. Remembering that the displacement is given by the area beneath the graph for the appropriate interval, we can see, regarding the area as a trapezium:

$$s = \tfrac{1}{2}(u + v)t \qquad (2)$$

Alternatively, regarding the area as a rectangle and a triangle:

$$s = ut + \tfrac{1}{2}at^2 \qquad (3)$$

These three equations contain all the information that the graph can give. However, sometimes it is convenient to calculate the velocity after the object has traveled a certain displacement s. This can be done by calculating t from equation (2) or (3) and then substituting into equation (1). This produces the result:

$$v^2 = u^2 + 2as \qquad (4)$$

It must be stressed that the equations (1) to (4) are only applicable in cases of uniform acceleration and when the motion is **rectilinear** (i.e., in straight lines) or if the motion can be resolved along two perpendicular axes and the accelerations along the two axes are constant and can be treated as independent.

■ **EXAMPLE 3.2**

A skier begins his descent of a downhill section. He gives himself a flying start by using his legs to propel himself from his starting position. As a result, his initial velocity is not 0 but is 2.5 m/s as he goes past the first marker on the downhill section. The clock is started when he goes past this first marker. Given that his acceleration is 3 m/s^2, calculate his velocity when he goes past the next distance marker, which is 10 m away from the first. How long (in seconds) will it take him to get up to a velocity of 25 m/s, assuming he maintains the acceleration of 3 m/s^2 as long as necessary?

Solution

$$\text{Initial velocity, } u = 2.5$$
$$\text{Acceleration, } a = 3$$

To do the first part, use $v^2 = u^2 + 2as$

$$v^2 = (2.5)^2 + 2\,(3)(10)$$
$$= 6.25 + 60$$
$$= 66.25$$
$$v = 8.14 \text{ m/s}$$

For the second part, use:

$$v = u + at$$
$$\text{Final velocity} = v = 25$$

It follows that:

$$25 = 2.5 + 3t$$

Therefore:

$$t = (25 - 2.5)/3$$
$$= 22.5/3$$
$$= 7.5 \text{ s}$$

■ **EXAMPLE 3.3**

In a direct measurement on the acceleration of a falling object, a spherical lead mass is released from O. It passes two light gates during its travel, one at a distance 0.5 m below O and the other at a distance 1.5 m below O. The first light gate starts a digital timer, and the second gate stops the timer.

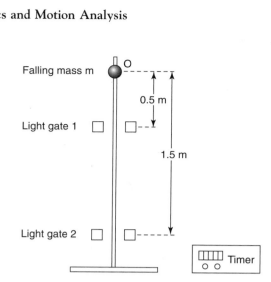

Falling mass m

0.5 m

Light gate 1

1.5 m

Light gate 2

Timer

  The distance fallen by the mass between light gates 1 and 2 is clearly 1 m. The result given by the digital timer is 0.2337 s. We have:

$$s_1 = \tfrac{1}{2} gt^2$$

and:

$$s_2 = \tfrac{1}{2} gt_2^2$$

so that:

$$t_2 - t_1 = \sqrt{\frac{2S_2}{g}} - \sqrt{\frac{2S_1}{g}}$$

Therefore:

$$0.2337 = \frac{1}{\sqrt{g}} \left(\sqrt{3} - \sqrt{1} \right)$$

$$\sqrt{g} = \frac{(0.732)}{0.2337} = 3.1322$$

$$g = 9.811 \, \text{m/s}^2$$

■ **EXAMPLE 3.4**

A downhill skier reaches the end of his run and is projected off the end of a ramp at high velocity. He is projected upward with a velocity of 20 m/s and falls freely under the influence of gravity.

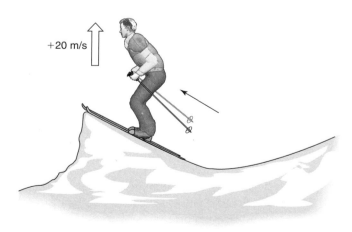

+20 m/s

Draw a graph of the vertical velocity of the skier as a function of time and a graph of her velocity as a function of displacement. Draw another graph of the displacement as a function of the time t and deduce the displacement after 5 s.

$$\text{Initial velocity} = u = +20\text{m/s}$$
$$\text{Acceleration attributable to gravity} = 9.81\text{m/s}^2$$

Because the question states that the skier falls freely, we can assume that there is no friction or air resistance. The following graphs are drawn using the equations:

$$v = u + at$$
$$v^2 = u^2 + 2as$$
$$s = ut + \tfrac{1}{2}at^2$$

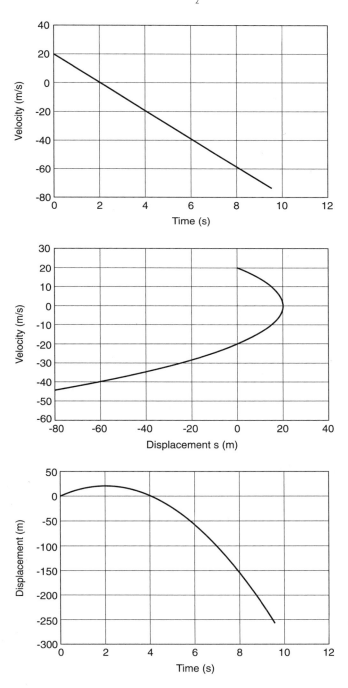

Table 3.2	Velocity of a falling object at 1 s intervals after release
Time (sec)	**Velocity (ms^{-1})**
0	0
1	9.8
2	19.6
3	29.4
4	39.2
5	49
6	58.8

The displacement after 5 seconds is $s = -22.6$ m, or 22.6 m below the skier's starting point. This example draws attention to the fact that the displacement s is a vector quantity. In this example, s becomes negative after a time of about 4 seconds, indicating that the skier is now beginning to fall below the level of her starting point.

3.3   Acceleration as the Slope of a Velocity–Time Graph

The most common example of uniform acceleration is that of free fall. An object in free fall accelerates with the **acceleration due to gravity**, that is, 9.81 ms^{-2} near sea level at the surface of the earth. This is true for all objects provided air resistance can be neglected. Such objects fall downward (towards the center of the earth) such that their velocities increase by 9.81 ms^{-1} every second. Table 3.2 shows the velocity of a falling object for the first 6 seconds of its motion after release from rest. Plotting the data of Table 3.2 on a velocity–time graph would result in a straight-line graph (Fig. 3.5).

The value of the acceleration in this case can be confirmed by measuring the slope or gradient of the v–t graph. By producing a right-angled triangle once again:

$$\text{Slope} = \text{Acceleration} = (58.8 - 0)/(6 - 0) = 9.8 \text{ ms}^{-2}$$

However, although constant accelerations produce nice linear graphs of v against t and lead to convenient calculations using equations (1) to (4), such constant

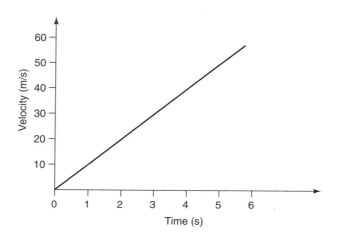

Figure 3.5   Plot of the v–t data in Table 3.2.

acceleration is a rarity in the real world unless special efforts are made to reduce or eliminate friction and air resistance. The case study presented here illustrates a case in which the acceleration is not constant.

| CASE *Study 3.2* | **Light Gates Used to Obtain Split Times in a 100-m Sprint** |

In a 100-m sprint, a series of light gates records the 10-m split times. The light gates operate by means of an infra-red beam traveling between a transmitter and a receiver; this signal can be interrupted by the passage of any object between the transmitter and receiver. The arrangement of the light gates is as follows:

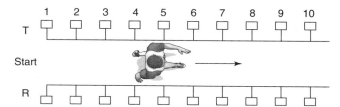

The light gates work in transmit–receive (T-R) pairs; number 1 starts a timer, and number 2 stops the timer and starts another timer. Thus, a split time for the first 10 m is obtained. When the sprinter reaches gate number 3, the timer that was started by gate 2 will be stopped and a split time for the second 10 m generated. The split times obtained for a training sprint were as follows:

Light Gate Number	Split Time (s)
1	1.50
2	1.20
3	1.05
4	0.94
5	0.92
6	0.9
7	0.89
8	0.9
9	0.93
10	0.94

This enables us to measure the average velocity over the 10-m split distances. To get the average velocity over the first 10 m:

$$v = \frac{\Delta s}{\Delta t} = \frac{(10 - 0)}{(1.50 - 0)} = 10/1.50 = 6.67 m/s$$

Over the second 10-m distance:

$$v = \frac{\Delta s}{\Delta t} = \frac{(20 - 10)}{(1.20)} = 10/1.20 = 8.33 m/s$$

Proceeding in this way for the other split times, we obtain average velocities of 6.67, 8.33, 9.52, 10.64, 10.87, 11.11, 11.24, 11.11, 10.75, and 10.64 m/s.

The next figures show three different ways of presenting this information. First, we can show how split times vary as a function of distance:

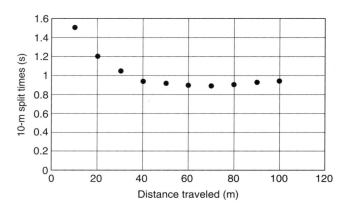

We can also show distance traveled as a function of cumulative time, obtained by adding the split times together, showing that the total time was 10.17 s:

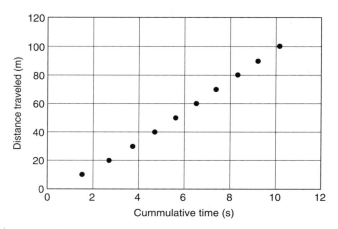

Finally, a plot of average velocity over a series of 10-m split distances versus distance traveled.

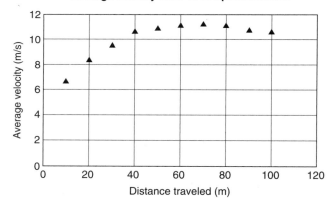

The average acceleration over the first 10 m is given by:

$$a = \frac{\Delta v}{\Delta t} = \frac{(6.67 - 0)}{(1.5 - 0)} = 4.45 \ ms^{-2}$$

The corresponding figure over the second 10 m is:

$$a = \frac{\Delta v}{\Delta t} = \frac{(8.33 - 6.67)}{(2.7 - 1.5)} = 1.38 \ ms^{-2}$$

Clearly, this illustrates a case in which the acceleration is not a constant but varies over the 100-m distance. The equations derived for uniformly accelerated motion (1) to (4) would *not* be applicable to this data except in modified form.

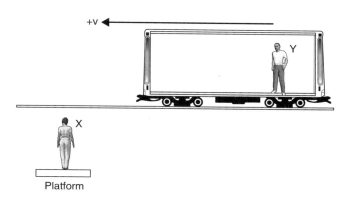

Figure 3.6 A train approaching a station with velocity +V relative to the observer standing on the platform.

3.4   Frames of Reference

Velocities are usually quoted without any mention of the frame of reference. In this case, the frame of reference is usually accepted as being fixed with respect to the surface of the earth. It is worth mentioning, however, that it is possible to use reference frames that are, themselves, moving with respect to the surface of the earth. Consider, for example, a train passing through a railway station. The platform is fixed, and the train is moving with a velocity +V relative to the platform (Fig. 3.6).

The observer X on the platform sees the velocity of the approaching train as +V, the plus sign being taken arbitrarily because this is a velocity directed from right to left as seen from X. The observer on the train, however, could quite legitimately claim that he is at rest (in his own frame of reference), and the woman on the platform X has a velocity +V.

What if the man on the train Y were to throw a ball in the direction toward the platform, as shown in Figure 3.7? Let us say the velocity of the ball is +v with respect to the man on the train Y. The velocity of the ball with respect to the woman on the platform X is (v + V), that is, the velocities of the train and the ball add together. To the man on the train, Y, the velocity of the woman on the platform X is +V, and the velocity of the ball is +v. This can be important in throwing

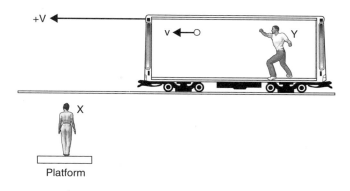

Figure 3.7 The man on the train throws a ball at velocity v with respect to the train in the direction of the platform.

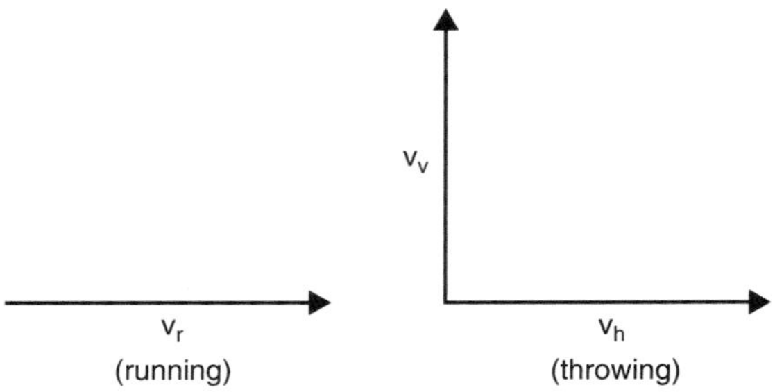

Figure 3.8 Addition of running and throwing velocities in the javelin throw.

events in which the athlete can be moving during the throwing action. In javelin, for example, Figure 3.8 shows that the velocity of the athlete running, v_r, must be added to the horizontal velocity, v_h, imparted to the javelin in the throw. The resultant velocity of the javelin (with respect to the ground) would then be $(v_h + v_r)$, and the vertical velocity is v_v.

3.5   Projectiles

Sport science is full of examples in which a body is projected into the air. In all cases, the body moves under the constant acceleration of gravity, about 9.81 m/s^2 vertically downward. Galileo was the first person to realize that all objects fall at the same rate, independent of their mass or weight. Thus, a sphere of lead falls at the same rate as a sphere of wood or a sphere of glass. Also, a small sphere of lead falls at the same rate as a large sphere of lead. This idea was at first difficult to accept, and many people still find it a tricky concept today. In practice, objects fall at different rates, caused mainly by the different frictional forces acting on them. A table tennis ball falls slower than a steel ball of the same diameter because the friction force has a greater effect on the table tennis ball. The mass of the table tennis ball is less and is affected more by the air resistance forces acting on the balls. If air resistance can be removed, all objects fall at the same rate. This was superbly confirmed by the Apollo astronauts, who dropped a feather and a metal tool on the Moon and found that they fell exactly together in the absence of air. In the sections that follow, we will ignore the effects of friction and treat projectiles as though they move with uniform acceleration. We can consider all of the following as examples for thinking of the moving body as a projectile:

- Shot putt
- High jumper
- Long jumper
- Soccer ball
- Tennis ball
- Golf ball
- Basketball
- Ski jumper

3.5.1 RESOLUTION OF VELOCITY INTO VERTICAL AND HORIZONTAL COMPONENTS

A projectile (e.g., ball, javelin, human body) launched (e.g., kicked, struck, thrown) with velocity v will generally have both vertical and horizontal components of that

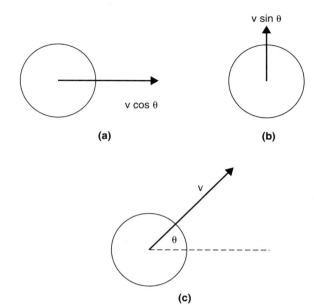

Figure 3.9 A ball projected with velocity (v) at some angle (θ). (A) The horizontal component of v. (B) The vertical component of v. (C) The overall vector (v) and its angle (υ) with the horizontal.

velocity. Let us consider the velocity v to be initially at some angle θ to the horizontal (Fig. 3.9).

Horizontal Motion

In the absence of friction, the horizontal component of velocity $v \cos \theta$ remains constant. This implies that to work out distance traveled horizontally, it is sufficient to use:

$$\text{Horizontal distance} = \text{Horizontal velocity} \times \text{Time}$$

This relationship can be used to find the range of the projectile (i.e., the distance moved horizontally), provided the flight time T is known. The flight time T can be found by considering the vertical motion of the projectile.

Vertical Motion

The vertical velocity of the projectile is $v \sin\upsilon$. In the absence of friction, the downward acceleration is the acceleration attributable to gravity, g. This implies that the downward velocity of the projectile increases at the rate of 9.81 m/s every second. Another way of looking at it is that the upward velocity decreases at the rate of 9.81 m/s every second. This indicates that the projectile moves upward initially, but its upward velocity gets smaller as time goes on. Eventually, at a time we will call t_{up}, the upward velocity becomes 0 (instantaneously), and the projectile has reached its maximum height, h. We can find t_{up} by using the equation $v = u + at$. It is important to note that this equation will now be applied purely to the upward components of the motion. For this reason and to avoid any confusion, we will define the upward direction as the $+y$ direction, so that the equation we will use to find t_{up} becomes:

$$v_y = u_y + a_y t$$

The initial velocity at time $t = 0$ is $v_{yi} = v \sin\upsilon$
The final velocity at time $t = t_{up}$ is $v_{yf} = 0$
The acceleration $a_y = -g$ (the acceleration attributable to gravity)
The time t_{up} is an unknown that we are trying to find.

Hence:

$$v_{yf} = v_{yi} + at$$
$$0 = v \sin \theta - gt_{up}$$
$$t_{up} = \frac{v \sin \theta}{g}$$

3.5.2 FINDING THE FLIGHT TIME T

To find the flight time, we also need to find t_{down}, the time the projectile takes to fall from maximum height down to the ground again. We will call the vertical displacement that the projectile undergoes during descent d. We will use the equation:

$$s = ut + \tfrac{1}{2} at^2$$

But again, to emphasize that we are dealing with vertical components only, we use a y suffix after s, u, and a. Thus:

$$s_y = u_y t + \tfrac{1}{2} a_y t^2$$

In this case:

Vertical displacement $= s_y = -d$

Vertical acceleration $= a_y = -g$

Initial velocity $= u_y = 0$

Time $= t = t_{down}$

We obtain:

$$-d = -\tfrac{1}{2} gt_{down}{}^2$$
$$t_{down} = \sqrt{\frac{2d}{g}}$$

The distance d depends on the level of the ground at which the projectile lands. This could be above the level at which it was released, at the same level as it was released, or below the level at which it was released. If the projectile lands at the same level as it was released, then $d = h$. Using $v_y{}^2 = u_y{}^2 + 2a_y s_y$ to find h, we get:

Displacement $s_y = h$?

Initial velocity $= u_y = v \sin\theta$

Final velocity $= v_y = 0$

Acceleration $= a_y = -g$

So that:

$$0 = (v \sin\theta)^2 - 2gh$$
$$h = \frac{(v \sin \theta)^2}{2g}$$

Because the vertical drop $d =$ height h, we can find t_{down} as:

$$t_{down} = \sqrt{\frac{2}{g} \times \frac{(v \sin \theta)^2}{2g}}$$
$$t_{down} = \frac{v \sin \theta}{g}$$

Thus, it is clear that, if the release and landing heights are the same, it follows that:

$$t_{up} = t_{down}$$

In this case, the flight time is T given by:

$$T = t_{up} + t_{down} = \frac{2v \sin \theta}{g}$$

Because g is fixed, varying T can only be achieved by altering the velocity v or the sine of the angle $\sin \theta$. The variation of $\sin \theta$ with θ is shown in the following table:

θ (°)	Sinθ
0	0.0000
15	0.2588
30	0.5000
45	0.7071
60	0.8660
90	1.0000

■ **EXAMPLE 3.5**

Calculate the time of flight of a rugby ball that has been kicked with a velocity of 15 m/s at an angle of 60° to the horizontal. (Assume that the projection and landing heights are the same.)

Solution

$$T = \frac{2v \sin \theta}{g} = \frac{2 \times 15 \times \sin(60°)}{9.81} = \frac{30 \times 0.8660}{9.81} = 2.65s$$

3.5.3 FINDING THE HORIZONTAL RANGE R

Using an x suffix to denote horizontal motion, to work out the horizontal range, we can use the equation:

$$s_x = v_x t$$

For landing height = release height, it follows that range:

$$R = v \cos \theta \times \frac{2v \sin \theta}{g} = \frac{2v^2 \sin \theta \cos \theta}{g}$$

Because of the nature of the trigonometric functions, this implies that the optimum angle for best range is 45°.

3.5.4 PROJECTILE RELEASED AT A HEIGHT ABOVE OR BELOW THE LEVEL AT WHICH IT LANDS

In this case, the descent distance is:

$$d = x + h$$
$$d = x + \frac{(v \sin \theta)^2}{2g}$$

where $x = x_2 - x_1$, x_2 and x_1 being the projection and landing heights respectively. Clearly, x is positive if x_2 is greater than x_1 (level of projection higher than the landing level), and x is negative if x_2 is less than x_1 (level of projection lower than the landing level). This altered descent distance will affect the time of descent t_{down}.

$$t_{down} = \sqrt{\frac{2x}{g} + \frac{(v \sin \theta)^2}{g^2}}$$
$$= \sqrt{\frac{2gx + (v \sin \theta)^2}{g^2}}$$

so that the total time of descent now becomes:

$$T = t_{up} + t_{down}$$

$$T = \frac{v \sin \theta}{g} + \frac{\sqrt{2gx + (v \sin \theta)^2}}{g}$$

$$= \frac{v \sin \theta + \sqrt{2gx + (v \sin \theta)^2}}{g}$$

The modified range of the projectile can now be calculated by:

$$R = v \cos \theta \times T$$

so that:

$$R = \frac{1}{g} \left(v^2 \sin \theta \cos \theta + v \cos \theta \sqrt{2gx + (v \sin \theta)^2} \right)$$

It can be seen that variations in v, θ, and x all affect the range R. It should be emphasized that this formula applies only if friction caused by air resistance can be ignored. This is usually the case for slowly moving objects in the air. A shot putt is a good example in which friction can be ignored. In this case, the optimum angle for getting the longest range depends on the speed of projection and on the height of projection. The optimum angle usually works out to be close to 45°.

■ **EXAMPLE 3.6**

A shot putt can be thrown with a velocity of 13.2 m/s from a height 2.15 m above the ground. What is the optimum angle of projection for maximum range, and what is the range in this case?

Solution

By setting up a spreadsheet, it can be shown that the optimum angle in this case is 41.9°, and the range is 19.795 m, assuming $g = 9.81$ m/s^2.

3.5.5 PARABOLIC PATH

The path traced out by a projectile in two dimensions is a **parabola**. Assuming that the motion of the projectile is restricted to the x–y plane and the object is projected from $x = 0$, $y = 0$, we have:

$$y = v_{yi}t - \tfrac{1}{2} gt^2$$

and

$$x = v_{xi}t$$

so that

$$y = \frac{v_{yi}}{v_{xi}} x - \tfrac{1}{2} \frac{g}{v_{xi}^2} x^2$$

This is the equation of a parabola in the x–y plane. Parabolic paths will always be obtained for projectiles provided air resistance is negligible. This may not always be the case, especially if the initial velocity of the projectile is high. Figure 3.10 shows a ball projected at an angle of 45° where the path of the ball has been illuminated stroboscopically at a frequency of 28 Hz. The projection velocity is roughly 4 m/s. This figure confirms some of the important features of projectile motion:

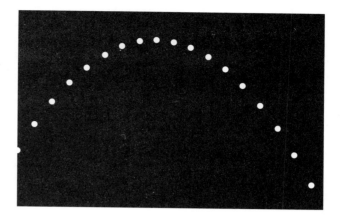

Figure 3.10 A ball is projected at an angle of 45° from the lefthand side. The strobe frequency is 28 Hz.

1. The horizontal velocity of the projectile is a constant once it is released. In Figure 3.10, the movement of the ball horizontally between strobe flashes is 0.1 m, and this does not vary across the figure.

2. The vertical velocity of the ball varies at a constant rate. In Figure 3.10, the vertical movement of the ball indicates that the vertical velocity starts off positive or upward, reduces to 0 after approximately the ninth flash, and finishes off negative or downward. It is also important to notice that the downward velocity is the same as the upward velocity on both sides of the apex of the trajectory.

CASE *Study 3.3*   **Motion of a Hockey Ball After Bouncing from Floor Using Motion Analysis**

A hockey ball is thrown downward toward a rigid floor, and the ball bounces back up from the floor at some angle. An optoelectronic motion analysis system is used to track the resulting trajectory of the hockey ball until it bounces again. The motion of the ball can be considered to be occurring in one plane (i.e., the ball can be considered to be moving in only two dimensions). The coordinate system is arranged so that the z axis is vertical, the x axis is horizontal, and the y axis is at right angles to both z and x (but the y axis will not be used in this case study). The origins of the coordinate system are arranged to be at the point of the initial bounce. The initial conditions ($t = 0$) are as follows:

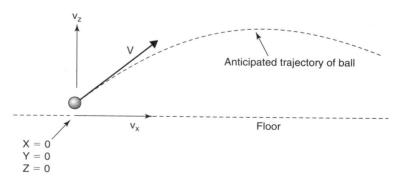

The x, y, and z coordinates of the center of the hockey ball are measured and recorded every $1/120^{th}$ sec by the measurement system. In principle, the horizontal velocity, v_x, of the ball should remain constant in the absence of air resistance. The vertical velocity will be subject to the acceleration attributable to gravity and, in principle, will increase downward at the rate of 9.8 m/s every second. Here is a graph showing the x and z velocities of the ball obtained by differentiation of the x and z displacement data:

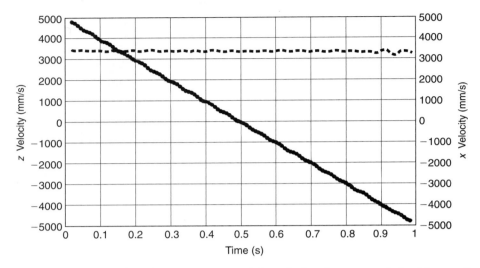

This graph shows that the x component of the velocity, shown as a dashed line on the graph, is indeed constant at a value close to 3400 mm/s throughout the duration of the experiment. The effects of air resistance are negligible over this time interval. At approximately $t = 1$ s, the ball bounces again, and the velocities will change as a result of the coefficient of restitution. The z component of the velocity, shown as a solid line, changes from a positive (upward) value of close to 5000 mm/s to a negative (downwards) value of -5000 mm/s.

To confirm the parabolic trajectory of the ball and to estimate the initial velocity components, consider the following figure and the graphs of the z coordinate (in millimeters) versus x shown by the discrete data points and z/x versus x (in millimeters) shown by the continuous line:

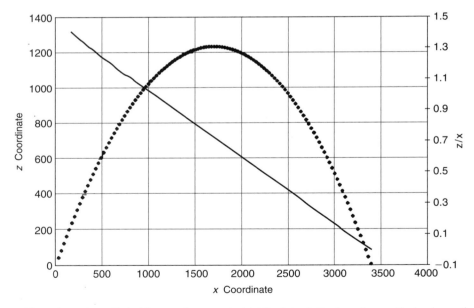

Here the value of z/x (the continuous straight line) is plotted on the vertical axis on the righthand side of the figure; the z coordinate (discrete points) is plotted on the lefthand axis. This confirms that the shape of the trajectory is parabolic. The intercept and slope obtained from the straight line are 1.4555 and -0.0004286 mm^{-1}, respectively. The slope yields a value for the initial $x -$ velocity, in meters per second, as:

$$-0.4286 = \frac{1}{2}\frac{g}{v_x^2}$$

$$v_x = \sqrt{\frac{g}{2(-0.4286)}} = 3.383 m/s$$

The intercept gives a value for the initial z velocity as:

$$1.4555 = \frac{v_z}{v_x} = \frac{v_z}{3.383}$$

$$v_z = 3.383 \times 1.4555 = 4.924 m/s$$

The range, estimated directly from the coordinate data, is 3394 mm, or 3.394 m. The range calculated using the equation $R = \dfrac{2v^2 \sin\theta \cos\theta}{g}$ is:

$$R = \frac{2(4.924) \times (3.383)}{9.81} = 3.396 m$$

SUMMARY

This chapter has summarized the important ideas of uniform motion and uniform acceleration in the study of kinematics. The "natural" motion of a body is constant velocity in a straight line, but in nature, we tend to see far more examples of objects that are stationary or moving with a constant acceleration. The equations applicable to uniform motion and uniform acceleration are explained and applied to the important case of a projectile moving with zero air resistance.

REFERENCE

Vincent, WJ: *Statistic in Kinesiology, Human Kinetics* 3rd Ed., Champaign, IL; 2005.

SUGGESTED READING

Hall S: *Basic Biomechanics.* McGraw-Hill Education—Europe; 2002.

STUDY QUESTIONS

1. The following table shows the progress of a Formula 1 racing car as it proceeds down a straight track. Distance markers are placed every 100 along the side of the track, and a timekeeper in the Team Observation Hut records the times at which the car is just passing the distance markers. The results are shown in the following table:

Distance Marker	Time (sec)
1	1.2
2	2.4
3	3.6
4	4.8
5	6.0
6	7.2
7	8.4
8	9.6

The distance markers are 100 m apart. Draw a graph using this data and measure the velocity of the car from the slope of the graph. Choose two of the following as an adequate descriptor for the motion of the car:

(a) The speed is not constant.

(b) The resultant force on the car is zero.

(c) The driving force exerted by the wheels on the ground must be zero.

(d) The velocity of the car is constant over the time interval from 0 to 9.6 s.

(e) The car is uniformly accelerated.

2. Write a short paragraph on the application of Newton's first law to the motion of the car. Explain the part played, if any, by the following: friction, gravity, driving force, air resistance, and torque.

3. Consider the following graph, which shows the distance covered by a runner along a straight track (x) as a function of time (t):

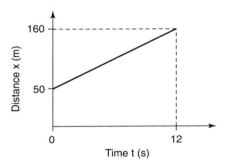

Write an equation for x as a function of t in the form:

$$x = mt + c$$

where m and c are constants. Evaluate m and c.

4. A man doing the luge event jumps on his luge trolley and begins to accelerate on a downhill section near the start of the course. His velocity at time, t, is 0. After 5 seconds, his velocity is 20 m/s. Using the equation $v = u + at$, work out his acceleration in ms^{-2}.

5. In a two-man toboggan run, the acceleration of the toboggan is 4 ms^{-2}. Given that its velocity passing the 100 m marker is 10 m/s, what will be its velocity as it passes the 200-m marker? Assume the acceleration is constant between 100 and 200 m.

6. A sprinter attempting a 60-m dash completes the distance in a time of 6.5 s starting from rest. What is the sprinter's average velocity over this distance?

7. A Manchester United center forward in soccer is tackled by a Liverpool defender, and the center forward loses the ball. Another Man Utd. player runs towards the ball at a speed of 6 m/s from 14 m away while a Liverpool player starts approaching at 5.5 m/s from a distance of 13 m. Which player gets to the ball first?

8. A canoeist accelerating uniformly from rest reaches a speed of 3.5 m/s in just 5 seconds. What is the canoeist's acceleration? What would the velocity be after 10 s?

9. A Formula 1 racing car traveling at a velocity of 20 m/s encounters a long straight section and accelerates uniformly from 20 m/s to 55 m/s in a time of 5.3 s. What is the acceleration? If this acceleration were to continue for a further 2 s, what would be the final velocity?

10. A toboggan run is displayed on the following plot of velocity, *v*, versus time, *t*:

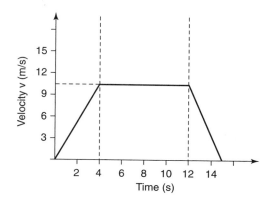

(a) Over what period of time is the acceleration uniform?

(b) Over what period of the time does the toboggan come to a stop?

(c) What is likely to be going on between 0 and 5 seconds?

(d) Over the period of uniform acceleration, what is the acceleration, *a*? (Measure this from the slope of a graph.)

11. The Cambridge rowing team is moving along at a steady speed of 4 m/s. The cox issues an order to increase the rate, and the boat accelerates uniformly to a velocity of 6 m/s over a distance of 5 m. What was the acceleration over that 5-m distance?

12. A 5000-m runner has a friend time her 400-m split lap times. The results are 1:27:0, 1:26.4, 1:25.8, 1:21, 1:18, 1:16.8, 1:16.8, 1: 17.4, 1:17.4, 1:18, 1:18, 1:19.2, and 40.2 s (last half lap). (The times are shown with a colon in between the minutes and seconds.) Work out the runner's average velocities for each lap. Sketch a graph of acceleration and deceleration during the course of the run. In between which laps did she accelerate the most? In between which laps did she decelerate the most?

13. A basketball is thrown vertically up in the air and travels up a distance of 6 m before stopping and coming back down. With what speed was the basketball thrown? Assume *g* is 9.81 ms^{-2}.

14. A long jumper projects himself with a velocity of 10 m/s and at an angle of 25° with respect to the horizontal. Assuming that his projection and landing heights are the same and ignoring friction, calculate the jumper's range and maximum height. Assume *g* is 9.8 m/s/s.

15. A shot putt is thrown with a velocity of 12.5 m/s from a height of 2 m above the ground. The angle measured with respect to the horizontal is 42°. Calculate the horizontal distance at which the shot putt hits the floor. Ignore friction *g* = 9.8 m/s/s.

16. A shot putt can be projected with an initial velocity of 14 m/s from a height 2.2 m above the floor. What is the optimum angle of projection for maximum range in this case? Ignore friction. *g* = 9.8m/s/s. (Set up a spreadsheet to answer this question.)

17. A baseball is thrown with a velocity of 15 m/s at an angle of 30° with respect to the horizontal.

(a) What are the horizontal and vertical components of the velocity just as the ball leaves the hand?

(b) What is the horizontal velocity of the ball when it reaches maximum height?

(c)   At what time after the throw does the ball reach maximum height?

(d)   How far has the ball traveled vertically and horizontally at this time?

If the ball is thrown from a height of 1.2 m above the floor and lands at a point 0.5 m below the level of the ground at which it was thrown, how far will the ball go?

18. The following three graphs show the velocity of a cyclist at three different stages of a 5-km time trial. Which of these corresponds to motion with uniform acceleration? To which of these would the equations (1) to (4) be applicable?

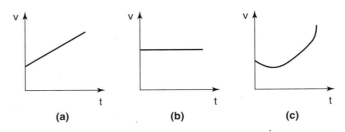

      (a)   (b)   (c)

CHAPTER four

EQUILIBRIUM

CHAPTER *objectives*

The objectives of this chapter are to:

- Introduce the concept of static equilibrium.
- Explain the force and moment conditions for static equilibrium.
- Elucidate the idea of the center of mass (CM) of a body of finite size.
- Explain the segmental method for estimating a person's CM.
- Introduce the concepts of hydrostatics and flotation.

CHAPTER *outcomes*

After reading this chapter, the student will be able to:

- Distinguish between a body that is in static equilibrium and one that is not.
- Apply the conditions for equilibrium to calculate unknown forces.
- Use the segmental method to estimate a person's CM from a two-dimensional image.
- Do simple calculations involving hydrostatic pressure and specific gravity.
- Draw and use free-body diagrams.

4.1 Conditions for Static Equilibrium

When all parts of a body are at rest or moving with the same constant velocity, the body is said to be in a state of **equilibrium**. One characteristic of a body in equilibrium is that the resultant of the components of force in any direction is zero. A second characteristic of such a body is that the resultant of the moments of force about any point in the same plane as that in which the forces act, is zero.

A precise definition of force is given in Chapter 5; however, for the purposes of this chapter on equilibrium, forces are vector quantities that tend to cause move-

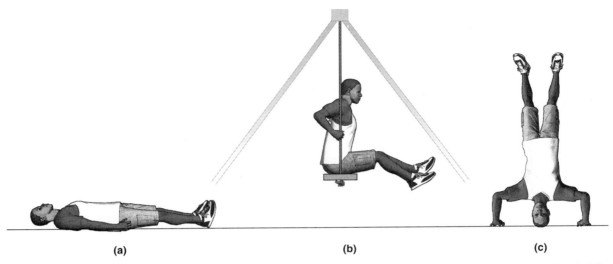

(a)   **(b)**   **(c)**

Figure 4.1   (A) Man lying on the floor (neutral equilibrium); (B) man sitting on a swing (stable equilibrium); (C) man in headstand position (unstable equilibrium).

ment in material objects. The **moment of a force** is defined in this chapter as a measure of the turning effect of a force.

In light of these ideas, we can summarize the requirements for a body to be in static equilibrium as:

$$\Sigma F = 0$$

and

$$\Sigma M = 0$$

That is, the sum of all forces acting on the body is zero, and the sum of all the moments of those forces are is zero. We can also distinguish between different classes of equilibrium for an object depending on its stability:

- **Stable equilibrium:** A slight disturbance of the object generates a restoring force to return it to its equilibrium position.
- **Unstable equilibrium:** A slight disturbance of the object leads to an increasing departure from equilibrium.
- **Neutral equilibrium:** A disturbance of the object simply moves it to a new position.

These three types of equilibrium are illustrated in Figure 4.1.

4.2   The Effect of Friction and Its Importance for Establishing Equilibrium

Many common everyday objects are in equilibrium because of the effects of the friction force. For example, a car parked on a slope relies on the friction in the brakes to prevent it from accelerating down the slope. If surfaces were frictionless, everyday objects would tend to slide in the direction of even the smallest downward slope and would tend to move around in response to even the smallest force or disturbance. Objects that are not moving with respect to the surfaces on which they are resting are affected by **static friction**.

Friction manifests itself as a braking force whenever real surfaces are moving relative to one another. We saw in Section 3.2 that a frictionless trolley on a horizontal air track would move with constant velocity forever unless some force interrupted

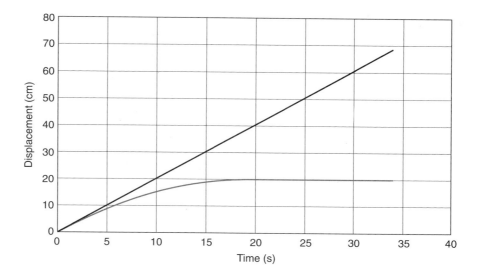

Figure 4.2 Displacement versus time for a trolley on a linear track in which friction is present shown by the *lower line*. The *top line* indicates what would happen if friction were absent (see Fig. 2.2).

that motion. If friction was present, however, the trolley would slow down as time progressed and would eventually stop. A graph of displacement against time might then appear as in Figure 4.2.

The trolley starts with a velocity of approximately 2 cm/s but soon loses this velocity. It is clear that the graph for the friction case looks quite different to that of the frictionless case of Figure 3.2. It can be seen that the curve of Figure 4.2 gradually reduces its slope as time progresses. The curve eventually becomes horizontal, indicating that the displacement has stopped changing with time; therefore, the velocity is zero. This is typical of a result produced by friction and, in this case, because surfaces are moving with respect to one another, this is described as **sliding friction**. Note that the trolley moving at constant velocity on a frictionless track is an example of a body in equilibrium. On the other hand, the trolley slowing down as a function of time represents a body not in equilibrium; however, as soon as it has come to a stop, then it will be in equilibrium.

Sliding friction is an example of **kinetic friction**. Examples of situations in which friction plays a part are:

The gradual slowing down of a golf ball as it rolls across a green

The brakes of a car getting hot as the car is brought to a stop

A stationary object on an inclined plane (if there were zero friction, it would slide to the bottom)

Somebody walking and not falling over

A bicycle and rider going round a corner

Friction is always present, sometimes in an obvious way, but at other times, friction is present in a way that is not that explicit. In special circumstances, friction can be reduced to very low values. Examples of very low friction situations are:

An ice skater going in a straight line

Curling (on an ice surface)

Skiing (on snow)

To summarize, friction is not essential for a body to be in equilibrium, but for most objects on the surface of the Earth, friction is the force that prevents objects from slipping and sliding and generally keeps them stationary.

CASE *Study 4.1*   **Hockey Ball Rolling Across a Flat, Level Synthetic Polymer Surface**

A rolling ball experiences friction because of its moving contact with the floor or surface it is moving on. A hockey ball was tracked using a motion analysis system during its rolling motion across a flat horizontal floor. The floor was a laboratory's concrete floor covered by a synthetic polymer surface. The following graph shows the velocity of the ball over a time interval of about 2.5 s. The velocity units are millimeter per second, and the velocity of the ball is directed along the negative y axis of the measuring system.

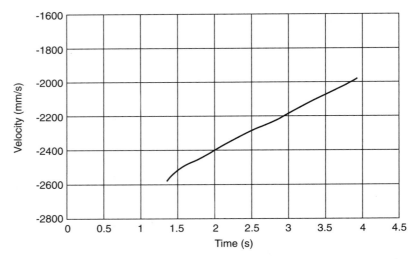

The initial velocity of the hockey ball was approximately -2575 mm/s at a time of 1.375 s, and the final velocity was -1977 mm/s at a time of 3.933 s. This is a reduction of about 23% in the velocity; this occurs over a total rolling distance of about 5.9 m. The relationship between velocity and time is approximately linear. The average deceleration of the ball over this time interval is:

$$a = (-1.977 - (-2.575))/(3.933 - 1.375) = 0.598 \text{ m}/2.558 \text{ s} = 0.233 \text{ m/s}^2$$

In this situation, the hockey ball is not in equilibrium because it is accelerating; however, as soon as it stops moving, at approximately $t = 12.41$ s, then it will be in equilibrium.

4.3 Moment of a Force

The **moment of a force** about a point (representing the intersection of a possible axis of rotation with the plane of the paper) is the tendency of the force to turn the body to which it is applied about that point. It is measured by the product:

Force × Perpendicular distance from the point to the line of action of the force.

The SI (international system of units) unit is the Newton meter (Nm). Moments are clockwise or counterclockwise. In Figure 4.3, if OZ represents a force F, the moment about the point X is $F \times d$, where d is the length of the perpendicular XY from X on OZ. For practical purposes, clockwise moments are taken as negative, and counterclockwise are taken as positive. The moment of the force in Figure 4.3 is negative.

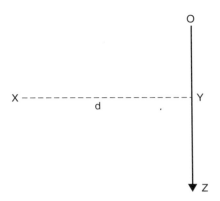

Figure 4.3 Moment of a force, F, shown as OZ, about a point, X.

■ **EXAMPLE 4.1**

A man supports a weight of 250 N (mass = 25 kg) with straight arms at right angles to his body. He holds the weight with both hands level with his shoulders. His arms are 75 cm long. What is the moment of the force?

Solution

$$Moment = F \times d$$
$$= (250 \text{ N}) \times (0.75 \text{ m})$$
$$= 187.5 \text{ Nm}$$

4.4   Adding and Subtracting Parallel Forces

The magnitude of the resultant of a set of parallel forces acting on a body is found by taking one sense as positive and the other as negative and finding the algebraic sum. The line of action of the resultant must be parallel to that of the individual forces and is determined by using the fact that it must be such that the moment of the resultant about any point is equal to the algebraic sum of the moments of the individual forces about that point. Thus, for **P** and **Q** acting at A and B in the same sense (Figure 4.4), the resultant is (**P** + **Q**) passing through a point C on AB such that (taking moments about A):

$$(P + Q) \times AC = Q \times AB$$

Similarly, if **P** and **Q** are in opposite senses, the resultant is (**P** − **Q**), and its line of action passes through C where:

$$(P - Q) \times AC = Q \times AB$$

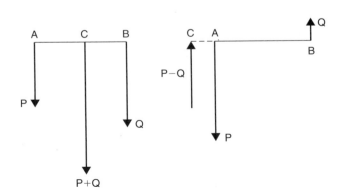

Figure 4.4 Resultant and line of action of parallel forces. P and Q acting at points A and B.

■ **EXAMPLE 4.2**   A canoe paddle is gripped with both hands with the left hand holding the end of the handle at A and the right hand gripping the paddle at a point 50 cm down the handle at B.

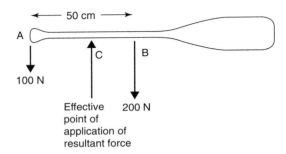

What is the resultant force on the paddle, and what is its effective point of application on the paddle?

Solution   The resultant force on the paddle is:

$$F = 100 + 200 = 300 \text{ N}$$

and its point of application of C is:

$$(100 + 200) \times AC = 200 \times (0.5)$$

so that:

$$AC = 100/300 = 0.33 \text{ m}$$

The point C is 0.33m from A.

CASE *Study 4.2*   **Weight Distribution Between the Left and Right Feet**

A male subject weighing 905 N is asked to step onto a device to measure ground reaction force (GRF). His left and right foot GRFs are measured by two load cells. The load cells have small zero errors amounting to − 10 N and − 8 N measured before his stepping onto the device.

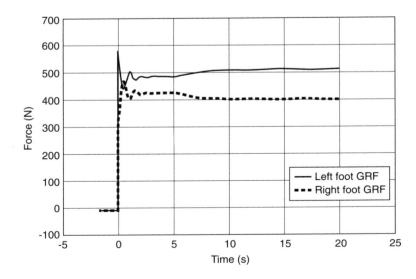

A number of features emerge from an examination of the results:

(a) The subject takes between 2 to 3 seconds to settle after the initial step on. During this time, a decrease in left foot GRF is accompanied by an increase in right foot GRF and vice versa.

(b) The subject appears to redistribute his weight after approximately 5 seconds transferring more weight to his left leg. However, this subject puts more weight on his left foot throughout the trial.

(c) The GRFs vary a little throughout the trial because of minor weight redistributions, swaying, and so on.

(d) The sum of the left and right leg GRFs is always the same, equal to the weight of the subject. This is illustrated below for five representative times.

Time (s)	Left Foot GRF (N)	Right Foot GRF (N)	Left + Right GRF (N)
0	577.5	327.5	905
1	501.9	403.1	905
3	483.6	421.4	905
6	489.9	415.1	905

4.5   Center of Gravity and Center of Mass

A body can be subdivided into very small portions. Each of these portions, taken alone, experiences a force toward the center of the earth, which is the weight of that small portion. The force that we call the weight of the whole body is really the resultant of a very large number of forces, namely, the weights of the individual particles comprising the body, which we can regard as parallel.

For each position of the body, this resultant has a definite line of action that can (in principle) always be found by applying the principle that the moment of the resultant weight about any point equals the sum of the moments of the individual weights about that point. All possible lines of action of the total weight pass through a point called the center of gravity of the body, which can be defined as follows:

The **center of gravity (CG)** of a body is that point, fixed with respect to the body, through which the line of action of the whole weight always passes, for all positions of the body. Consider a hypothetical, planar, elliptical body (Fig. 4.5).

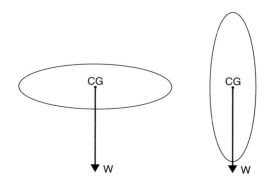

Figure 4.5   A hypothetical planar elliptical object has its center of gravity at the center of the ellipse. The weight of the body, W, can always be taken as acting vertically downward from this point irrespective of the orientation of the body.

Provided the body is materially homogeneous, the center of gravity will be at the center of the ellipse.

The term **center of mass (CM)** is also used, and perhaps more appropriately: if the line of action of the weight always passes through the point, it is as if the whole mass were concentrated at that point. Indeed, for most dynamical purposes, the body behaves as though the whole mass were concentrated at the CM.

■ **EXAMPLE 4.3**

For a particular individual, the CM is located at a position given by 0.52 H measured from the feet, where H is the person's height, provided the body is straight with the arms at the sides. The individual lies on a horizontal board with feet at one end, A. Given the data at the end of the question, calculate the moment of the person's weight about the point A.

Mass of individual = 80 kg
Height of individual = 1.9 m
Acceleration attributable to gravity = 9.8 m/s/s

Solution

The position of the CM is:

$$0.52 \times 1.9 \text{ m} = 0.988 \text{ m from A}$$

The weight is:

$$W = mg = 80 \times 9.8 = 784 \text{ N}$$

The moment is:

$$(784 \text{ N}) \times (0.988 \text{ m}) = 774.6 \text{ Nm}$$

CASE *Study* 4.3   Center of Mass of Human Body Found Using the Reaction Board Method

The reaction board method is often used to estimate the position of the CM of the human body in simple cases. Consider a man lying on a rigid, horizontal board (in equilibrium) with his feet at end A and her head at end B. The board is supported off the floor at A and is free to move at this point. The other end of the board, B, is supported by a load-measuring device, in its simplest form, a weighing scale.

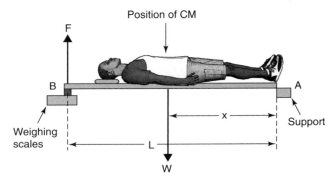

Let us take the length of the board to be *L*, measured from the support at A to the point at which the other end of the board B is supported on the weighing scales. With the subject lying on his back with his arms at his sides, we can assume that the CM will be somewhere along the axis of symmetry of the body at some distance *x* from end A. The weight, *W*, is shown acting vertically down from the CM. The weighing scales record a reading, *F*, with the subject lying in this position. The diagram shows the force *F* acting vertically upward on the underside of the board at end B. In this case, taking moments about point A, for equilibrium:

$$W \times x = F \times L$$

It follows that the CM is located at a distance x from end A is:

$$x = \frac{F \times L}{W}.$$

In this analysis, the weight of the board itself has been ignored. Although this would be clearly a source of error, in practice, the scales can usually be zeroed before the person lies on the board but with the board itself in place, so that the weight of the board is immaterial. Even if the scales cannot be zeroed, the initial reading can be subtracted from subsequent readings, thus giving the same result.

A series of trials on first-year undergraduate sport science students yielded the following results. In the table shown, the weight and height of the subjects are recorded in kilograms and centimeters, respectively; the x value is also shown in centimeters and as a percentage of the subject's height.

Subject	Mass (kg)	Height (cm)	Height of CM (cm)	Height of CM as a Percentage of Height
1	79	180	100.6	55.89
2	68	158	88	55.70
3	76	185	103	55.68
4	73	172.5	95	55.07
5	76	179	99.7	55.70
6	84	183	100	54.64
7	57	159	88	55.35
8	66	182	99	54.40
9	73.5	180	100	55.56
10	66	182	99	54.40
11	58	183	102	55.74
12	81	185	103	55.68
13	99	188	106	56.38
14	75	185	102	55.14

This shows that the center of gravity, expressed as a percentage of body height, is remarkably constant over a range of subjects with various heights and weights. The five-number summary of this data (minimum, first quartile, median, third quartile, maximum) is 54.40, 55.09, 55.62, 55.70, 56.38.

4.6 Couples: Two Equal and Opposite Forces Applied at Different Points

The resultant of two equal and opposite forces that are not acting in the same line is apparently zero. This does not mean that they have no mechanical effect but simply that no single force can be found to replace them.

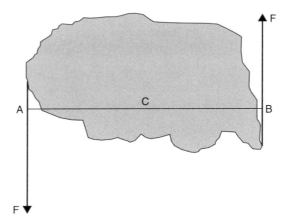

Figure 4.6 Two forces (F) forming a couple. AB is a line drawn perpendicular to the lines of action of the forces F.

In Figure 4.6, the forces tend to rotate the body in a counterclockwise direction. A pair of equal parallel forces, acting in opposite senses and not in the same line, is called a **couple**. Taking moments about C (any point along AB), the moment of *F* at A about C is:

$$F \times \text{AC}$$

The moment of *F* at B about C is $F \times \text{BC}$, both counterclockwise. The sum of these moments about C is:

$$F \times (\text{AC} + \text{BC}) = F \times \text{AB} \text{ counterclockwise (i.e., one force} \times \text{perpendicular}$$
$$\text{distance between the two forces)}$$

This is called the moment of the couple, and AB is called the arm of the couple.

■ **EXAMPLE 4.4**   Consider the rugby ball shown in the diagram. What is the moment of the couple?

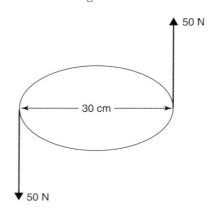

Solution   Moment of couple = 50N × 0.3 m = 15 Nm. The arm of the couple is 0.3 m. This rugby ball would, therefore, have a tendency to rotate and could not be said to be in equilibrium.

4.7   Bodies at Rest

A body at rest or in uniform rectilinear motion with respect to its surroundings, which we suppose to be fixed, is said to be in **equilibrium**. If we consider the body

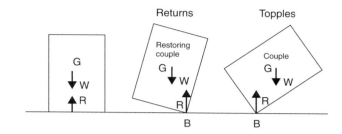

Figure 4.7 A body resting on a flat horizontal plane. G represents the center of gravity, W is the weight of the body and R is the reaction force exerted on the body by the floor.

as equivalent to a single massive particle located at the center of gravity, it follows that if it is at rest, there can be no acceleration of the center of gravity in any direction and, therefore, no resultant force in any direction. This means that the external forces acting must together combine to give a zero resultant. For equilibrium, another condition also has to be satisfied: the algebraic sum of the moments about any axis of all the external forces acing on a body in equilibrium must be zero.

4.8   Equilibrium Under the Action of Two Forces

Consider a body resting on a flat, horizontal surface (Fig. 4.7). The weight, **W**, of the body is matched by the reaction force, **R**. The object of Fig. 4.7 is in contact with the plane at a limited number of points determined by the flatness of the bottom surface of the object. The reaction forces at these contact points add together to form the resultant upthrust (resultant reaction force), **R**, whose line of action passes through G, the CM. The magnitudes of **W** and **R** is equal, so there are no resultant force on the body and no resultant turning moment.

If the object in Figure 4.7 is now displaced by lifting one of the bottom edges so that the only line of contact is now the opposite bottom edge (middle of Fig 4.7), the reaction force, **R**, is now immediately transferred to pass through point B, so that **R** and **W** constitute a couple. The magnitudes of **R** and **W** continue to be equal, but there is now a restoring couple that tends to return the body to its original position when released.

If the object is displaced in such a way that the center of gravity has been shifted up to or to the right of the vertical line through B, then the couple formed by **R** and **W** tends to make the object continue turning in the direction of the displacement, and the object will topple if released.

■ **EXAMPLE 4.5**   Any object resting on a rough, inclined plane experiences a vertical reaction force to ensure that equilibrium is maintained (assuming that the angle of inclination is not so great as to cause the object to slide).

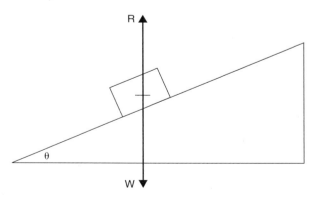

It can be seen that the reaction force, **R**, has a component up the slope and a component perpendicular to the slope. The component up the slope is just sufficient to counteract the component of the weight acting down the slope and thus stop it from sliding. This is the friction force, which is explained further in Chapter 5.

Calculate R, R_n and R_p if the weight, W, is 120 N and the angle $\theta = 40°$.

Solution

R is a force of 120 N magnitude acting vertically upward. R_n is:

$R_n = R \cos\theta = 120 (\cos 40) = 91.9$ N (acting up perpendicular to the surface)

R_p is:

$R_p = R \sin\theta = 120 (\sin 40) = 77.1$ N (acting down parallel to the surface)

4.9   Center of Mass of a Stationary Body

If we have a body in the form of an arbitrarily shaped thin sheet, several small suspension holes can be introduced in various positions round the edge of the sheet and the body suspended from a suitable smooth pivot through one of the holes A (Fig. 4.8). A plumb line of fine thread is also attached to the same pivot. Both are allowed to swing freely and come to rest. The direction of the plumb line is marked on the sheet. The CM hangs vertically below the point of suspension, so the CM must be somewhere on the line now marked on the sheet. The exercise is then repeated using another hole, B, about one quarter of the way round from the first. The two lines intersect at the CM, which must lie on both lines. This can be repeated at a number of other suspension points as a check.

Another method that can be applied to an object of the appropriate shape is the balancing method. An object will balance on a pivot provided the center of gravity is directly above the pivot. Hence, this method only works if the object is roughly straight and does not exhibit bends. For example, a baseball bat could be balanced, with difficulty, at a series of trial points before finding the balance point (Fig. 4.9).

The position of the center of gravity could be expressed as a percentage of the total length measured from the top of the bat, for example:

$$\frac{L_1}{L} \times 100\%$$

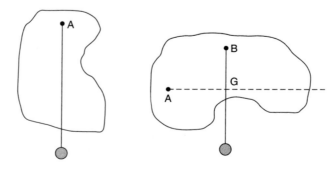

Figure 4.8   Locating the center of gravity (G) of a thin sheet. A and B are two arbitrary points of suspension.

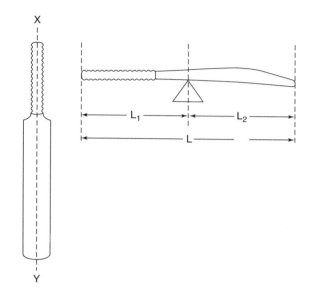

Figure 4.9 A baseball bat balanced on a pivot. By symmetry, the center of mass must lie on a plane XY at right angles to the face of the bat. Its distance from the top of the bat handle L_1 is found by the balance point.

4.10 Equilibrium Under the Action of Three Forces

If three external forces maintain a body in equilibrium, we can imagine that two of them, *P* and *Q*, are replaced by their resultant, *R*, so that only this resultant and the third force, *S*, need be considered. The resultant, *R*, of any two of the forces must thus be equal and opposite to the third force and must act along the same line as *S*. The lines of action of all three forces must all lie in the same plane; otherwise, *R* cannot act along the same line as *S*. The lines of action of all three forces must either all be parallel or pass through one point.

If *P* and *Q* are parallel, their resultant *R* is parallel to them; so *S*, acting along the same line as *R*, must be parallel to *P* and *Q*. If *P* and *Q* are not parallel, their lines of action must intersect at some point O; their resultant must also pass through O, but the third force is equal and opposite to *R*, so its line of action must also pass through O. Thus, all three lines of action are concurrent at O.

■ **EXAMPLE 4.6**

Consider a sprinter in the starting position. GRFs are acting at his hands and at his feet. We will assume, for simplicity, that the reaction forces at his right and left feet are amalgamated into one force at his feet and that the force at his right and left hands are amalgamated into one force at his hands.

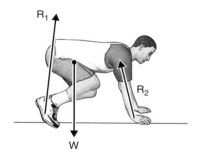

Note that, in this diagram, the forces shown are those acting on the sprinter, not those acting on the ground. In this case, for equilibrium, it is essential that the sum of R_1 and R_2 are equal and opposite to *W*.

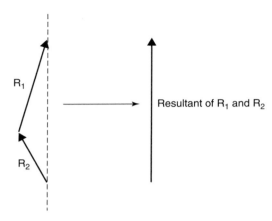

The resultant of R_1 and R_2 must be equal in magnitude to W but is oppositely directed.

4.10.1 Three Parallel Forces

The condition for the resultant force to be zero is that the algebraic sum of the forces must be zero (i.e., any one force is equal and opposite to the sum of the other two). The condition for the resultant moment about any point to be zero is that the algebraic sum of the moments of all the forces about any point in the plane shall be zero.

■ **Example 4.7**

A uniform beam, AB, which is 6 m long and weighs 400 N, is supported at the end, A, and at a point C, which is 2 m from point B. Find the reaction forces at the supports A and C.

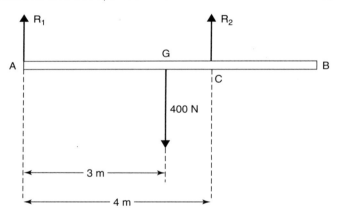

The diagram shows a uniform beam supported at points A and C. This free-body diagram shows the forces acting on the beam (not those acting on the supports). By the first condition:

$$R_1 + R_2 = 400 \text{ N}$$

Taking moments about A:
  Moment of 400 N wt at G = 400 × AG = 400 × 3 = 1200 Nm clockwise
  Moment of R_2 at C = R_2 × AC = R_2 × 4m counterclockwise
  Equating these (for equilibrium):

$$1200 = 4 R_2$$
$$R_2 = 1200/4 = 300 \text{ N}$$

It follows that R_1 is $R_1 = 400 - R_2 = 400 - 300 = 100$ N

■ **EXAMPLE 4.8**

A man weighing 700 N supports himself on his hands and toes in the press-up position with straight arms and legs. Because the man is in equilibrium, we can calculate the reaction forces

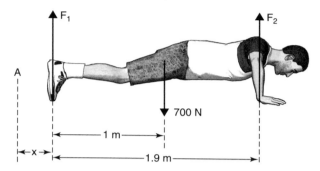

at the feet and hands, F_1 and F_2, respectively. Taking moments about the axis running through the toes, for equilibrium:

$$(700 \text{ N}) \times (1 \text{ m}) = F_2 \times 1.9$$

so that:

$$F_2 = 700/1.9 = 368.4 \text{ N}$$

Because the total resultant force must be zero for equilibrium, we also have:

$$F_1 + F_2 = W$$
$$F_1 + 368.4 = 700$$

so that:

$$F_1 = 331.6 \text{ N}$$

We can take moments about any convenient axis; the above results will still hold true. If we take the vertical axis through an arbitrary point, A, and take moments:

$$x \times 331.6 + (x + 1.9) \times 368.4 = (1 + x) \times 700$$

x will cancel from this equation, so that:

$$1.9 \times 368.4 = 700$$

That is, the equation balances, F_1 and F_2, are unchanged.

4.10.2 THREE NONPARALLEL FORCES

Consider the three forces D, E, and F in equilibrium (Fig. 4.10). F must be equal and opposite to the resultant G of D and E, represented by the diagonal OB of

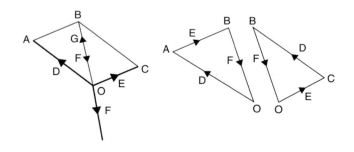

Figure 4.10 Triangle of forces. D, E, and F represent three forces in equilibrium. OABC represents a parallelogram of forces.

parallelogram of forces OABC. Because OB completely represents **G**, BO must completely represent **F**. We can use half this parallelogram to represent **D**, **E** and **F**; either of the triangles OAB or OBC will do this. Whichever triangle is taken, it can be seen that the arrows all follow the same way round. Thus, three nonparallel forces in equilibrium can be represented in size and direction by the three sides of a triangle taken in order. This is the **triangle of forces rule**. The condition for the resultant moment to be zero is automatically satisfied.

■ **EXAMPLE 4.9**

A child weighing 300 N is sitting on a swing suspended by ropes to a fixed point, P. A horizontal force, **F**, is applied to the seat of the swing, so that the ropes are inclined at an angle of 30° to the vertical. What is the value of F and what is the tension, T, in the string?

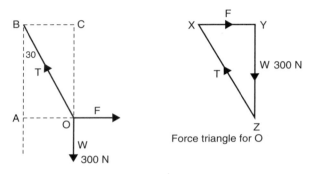

The child is in equilibrium under the action of the three nonparallel forces: her weight (i.e., 300 N) acting vertically downward; the horizontal force, **F**; and the tension, **T**, in the ropes directed along the string. These all meet at O. The force triangle for O is shown drawn to scale. The angle XZY is 30°.

Because tan 30° = XY/YZ = XY/300, it follows that XY = force **F** = 300 × (0.577) = 173 N

Also, because cos 30° = YZ/XZ = 300/XZ, it follows that XZ = tension T = 300/(0.866) = 346 N

■ **EXAMPLE 4.10**

An acrobat balances her weight on her hands using her partner as a support. The top acrobat

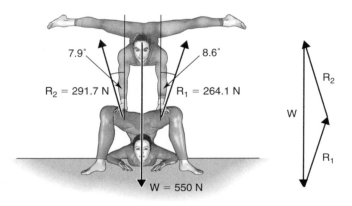

has a weight of 550 N. The reaction forces acting on the top acrobat are:

R_1 = 264.1 N acting upward at angle of 8.6° to the vertical
R_2 = 291.7N acting upward at angle of 7.9° to the vertical

It will be seen that these three forces form a closed triangle of forces when aligned correctly. The combined effect of R_1 and R_2 is a vertical upward force of 550 N to support the body weight. The vertical components of R_1 and R_2 (40 N and -40 N) cancel out each other.

4.11   Hydrostatics and Flotation

4.11.1 HYDROSTATIC PRESSURE AS A FUNCTION OF DEPTH

In any liquid, there is a variation in pressure as a function of depth of immersion in the liquid. Given that the liquid density is ρ kg/m^3, the pressure at depth h in N/m^2 is:

$$p = \rho g h$$

where g is the acceleration attributable to gravity and h is the depth below the surface.

■ **EXAMPLE 4.11**

Water has a density of approximately 1000 kg/m^3 and is the most commonly occurring liquid on Earth. Let us consider a diver in the sea at a depth of 20 m. What is the total pressure acting on him?

Applying the pressure formula, $p = \rho g h$, we find:

$$p = (1000 \text{ kg/m}^3).(9.81 \text{ m/s}^2)\,(20 \text{ m})$$
$$p = 196200 \text{ N/m}^2 \text{ or } 1.962 \times 10^5 \text{N/m}^2$$

Atmospheric pressure on Earth is approximately 1×10^5N/m^2 so that the total pressure on the diver is:

$$p_{total} = 1.962 \times 10^5 + 1.0 \times 10^5 = 2.962 \times 10^5 \text{N/m}^2$$

This total pressure amounts to almost 3 atm.

4.11.2 UPTHRUST ON AN IMMERSED BODY

Because there is a vertical pressure gradient in a fluid (a liquid or a gas) at rest, an immersed object is subject to forces at all points on its surface. Because the pressure increases with depth, the underside of the object experiences a greater force than the topside (Fig. 4.11). It follows that any solid body immersed in a fluid will experi-

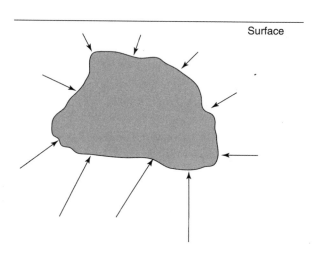

Figure 4.11 Forces acting at the boundary of an immersed object.

ence a force acting vertically upward (an upthrust), U, but there will be no horizontal force. The principle of Archimedes states:

> When a solid body is wholly or partially immersed in a fluid, it experiences an upthrust equal to the weight of the mass of the fluid, which is displaced. This upthrust acts vertically through the CM of the displaced fluid.

Note that for a body that floats in water (or fluid), the upthrust force is equal to the body's weight, $U = W$. For a body that sinks in water, the upthrust force is less than the body's weight, $U < W$. The ability of a body to float depends not only on its density but also on its shape. A body that is less dense than water will always float irrespective of its shape. Objects denser than water can still float provided they are shaped in such a way that they can displace at least their own weight of water.

4.11.3 SPECIFIC GRAVITY

The specific gravity (SG) of an object or substance is defined as:

SG = mass of a certain volume of that substance divided by mass of an equal volume of water

Or because masses are proportional to weights:

SG = weight of a certain volume of substance divided by weight of an equal volume of water.

The water is usually specified as being at a temperature of 4°C; which happens to be the temperature at which the density of water is a maximum, 999.97 kg/m^3.

■ **EXAMPLE 4.12**

Determination of Specific Gravity
A piece of flint has a weight of 131.5 g in the air and 81.5 g when immersed in water. What is the SG of the flint?

Weight of water displaced $= 131.5 - 81.5 = 50$ g wt

So the SG of the flint is:

SG = Weight of flint/Weight of equal volume of water $= 131.5/50 = 2.63$

Note that the SG calculated by this method is exactly the same as the density expressed in gm/cm^3, provided the density of water is taken as exactly 1000 kg/m^3 or 1 g/cm^3. As we have seen, the actual density of water at 4°C is 999.97 kg/m^3 or 0.99997 g/cm^3. The density of flint, therefore, is very close to 2630 kg/m^3 or 2.63 g/cm^3.

Note that the density of the human body is close to that of water, 1000 kg/m^3 (1 g/cm^3), so that its SG is close to 1.

4.12   The Segmental Method for Estimating a Person's Center of Mass

The **segmental method** may be used to determine the CM of an athlete from a knowledge of:

1. The position of the end points of all of the body's segments
2. The mass of each of the segments
3. The location of the CM within each segment

If working from a photographic image or a still frame from a video recording,

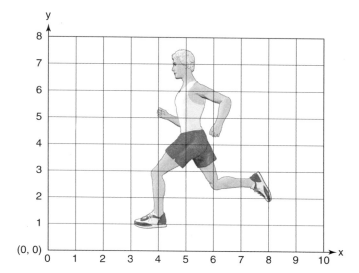

Figure 4.12 A still image of an athlete in a running position. An arbitrary origin is established (in this case, the *bottom left*), and an *x–y* coordinate system runs horizontally and vertically.

this yields a two-dimensional analysis and the CM location in a given plane. Figure 4.12 shows an example of a still image of an athlete running. This image could, for example, have been obtained from a still photograph and the outline traced using tracing paper and transferred onto graph paper. In the case of Figure 4.12, the numerical scales on the *x* and *y* axes correspond to centimeters on graph paper. The 14 body segments considered are:

Trunk

Head and neck

Right and left thighs

Right and left lower legs

Right and left feet

Right and left upper arms

Right and left lower arms

Right and left hands

Each body segment has its own CM and is usually expressed as a given fraction of the length of the segment from the proximal end.

The idea is, for each segment, to calculate the moment attributable to the weight of the segment about the *x* and *y* axes. These moments are then added together to find the total moment about the *x* and *y* axes. By dividing by the total body mass, the *x* (or *y*) coordinate of the CM is found. Figures 4.13 and 4.14 show the weights of the individual body segments and the total weight acting at the CM, respectively.

The masses of each of these segments (M_i) and the positions of the centers of mass of the segments (X_i and Y_i) are used to calculate the position of the whole-body CM.

$$X_{CM} = \frac{\Sigma M_i X_i}{M_{body}} = \Sigma \frac{\Sigma M_i}{M_{body}} X_i$$

and

$$Y_{CM} = \Sigma \frac{M_i Y_i}{M_{body}} = \Sigma \frac{M_i}{M_{body}} Y_i$$

In applying this method, it is common to use anthropometric information about

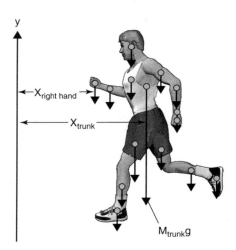

Figure 4.13 Taking moments of the weights of the 14 body segments about the y axis. Each small circle represents the center of mass of a segment. Only two distances (for the trunk and right hand) and only one segment weight (for the trunk) have been labeled for the sake of clarity.

human body segments to determine the location of each segment's CM and the mass. Body segment parameters (BSPs) are usually expressed as percentage values. The segmental CM is usually expressed as $FL\%$, the percentage of the segment length from the proximal end. Much of the information on $FL\%$ and M_i are based on the original work of Dempster (1955 and 1959).

The x coordinates of the distal and proximal ends of this right lower arm, shown as an example in Figure 4.15, are 4.1 and 4.9 U. It follows that the x coordinate of the CM is:

$$X_i = X_{proximal} + FL \times (X_{distal} - X_{proximal})$$

Because $FL = 0.43$ for the lower arm segment:

$$X_i = 4.9 + 0.43(4.1 - 4.9) = 4.56$$

A similar calculation would give $Y_i = 5.13$ for the lower arm. Table 4.1 gives the segment masses as a percentage of whole body mass ($FM\%$), and Table 4.2 gives the percentage distance of the CM from the proximal end of the body segment ($FL\%$). Table 4.3 shows a spreadsheet calculation for the CM of the male athlete shown in Figure 4.11.

Table 4.3 shows that the CM of the runner in Figure 4.12 is located at $x = 5.28$, $y = 4.86$. Sometimes it is desirable to convert this result into a different system of units. Although it is acceptable to quote a result in terms of centimeters on a graph paper, to convert this result into real distances requires a calibration of some

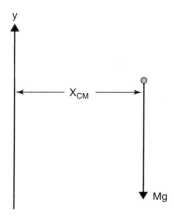

Figure 4.14 The 14 segments in Figure 4.13 are replaced by one mass at the center of mass. The center of mass is situated at a distance X_{CM} from the y axis. The force vector is equal to the body weight, Mg.

Figure 4.15 Calculating the center of mass (CM) of a single segment. For the lower arm, the CM is 43% of the way along the arm measured from the proximal end.

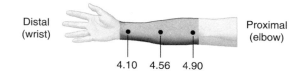

4.10   4.56   4.90

Table 4.1 Segment masses as a percentage of whole body mass *(FM%)*

Segment	Men	Women
Head and neck	8.96	8.20
Trunk	46.84	45.00
Upper arm	3.25	2.9
Forearm	1.87	1.57
Hand	0.65	0.50
Thigh	10.50	11.75
Lower leg	4.75	5.35
Foot	1.43	1.33

Table 4.2 Percentage distance of the center of mass from the proximal end of the body segment *(FL%)*

Segment	Men	Women
Head and neck	55	55
Trunk	50	50
Upper arm	43.6	45.8
Forearm	43	43.4
Hand	46.8	46.8
Thigh	43.3	42.8
Lower leg	43.4	41.9
Foot	50	50

Table 4.3 Center of mass calculated by a spreadsheet method[*][†]

Body Segment	F_{mi}	F_{li}	$X_{proximal}$	$Y_{proximal}$	X_{distal}	Y_{distal}	X_i	Y_i	$X_i \times F_{mi}$	$Y_i \times F_{mi}$
Trunk	0.468	0.500	5.5	4.2	4.9	6.5	5.2000	5.3500	2.433600	2.503800
Head and neck	0.090	0.550	4.9	6.5	4.8	7.6	4.8450	7.1050	0.436050	0.639450
Right tight	0.105	0.433	5.5	4.2	6.1	2.8	5.7598	3.5938	0.604779	0.377349
Right lower leg	0.048	0.434	6.1	2.8	7.6	2.5	6.7510	2.6698	0.324048	0.128150
Right foot	0.014	0.500	7.6	2.5	8.1	1.9	7.8500	2.2000	0.109900	0.030800
Left thigh	0.105	0.433	5.5	4.2	4.2	3.2	4.9371	3.7670	0.518396	0.395535
Left lower leg	0.048	0.434	4.2	3.2	4.1	1.5	4.1566	2.4622	0.199517	0.118186
Left foot	0.014	0.500	4.1	1.5	3.3	1.1	3.7000	1.3000	0.051800	0.018200
Right upper arm	0.033	0.436	4.6	6.2	4.1	5.4	4.3820	5.8512	0.144606	0.193090
Right lower arm	0.019	0.430	4.9	5.0	4.1	5.3	4.5560	5.1290	0.086564	0.097451
Right hand	0.007	0.468	4.1	5.3	3.7	5.4	3.9128	5.3468	0.027390	0.037428
Left upper arm	0.033	0.436	5.4	6.3	6.1	4.9	5.7052	5.6896	0.188272	0.187757
Left lower arm	0.019	0.430	6.2	5.9	6.1	4.9	6.1570	5.47000	0.116983	0.103930
Left hand	0.007	0.468	6.1	4.8	6.0	4.5	6.0532	4.6596	0.042372	0.032617

Sum of $X_i \times F_{mi}$ 5.284276
Sum of $Y_i \times F_{mi}$ 4.863742
$X_{CM} = 5.28$
$Y_{cm} = 4.86$

[*] The values of X_{distal}, Y_{distal}, $X_{proximal}$, and $Y_{proximal}$ are read off Figure 4.10. X_i and Y_i are calculated using the F_{li} values. The coordinates of the center of mass are obtained by summing the last two columns.

[†] All units are in centimeters.

CM = center of mass.

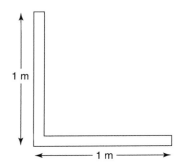

Figure 4.16 Calibration object for still two-dimensional image capture.

sort. It is possible, for instance, to take a still picture of a 1-m rule or, better still, two 1-m rules at right angles to one another, aligned with the x–y directions (Fig. 4.16) so that the picture can be calibrated. Provided these calibration objects are at the same distance from the camera as the runner, then the calibration will be accurate for the runner (see Chapter 1). In this way, for example, it might be established that the calibration for the image in Figure 4.12 is:

$$1 \text{ cm} \equiv 0.256 \text{ m}$$

It follows that the CM is $0.256 \times 4.8637 = 1.245$ m above the origin and displaced $0.256 \times 5.2843 = 1.353$ m to the left of the origin. However, the floor level is at a height of 0.95 cm above the origin, so the height of the CM above the floor would be $0.256 \times (4.8637 - 0.95) = 1.002$ m.

4.13   Free-Body Diagrams

By now, it should be clear that when considering whether a body is in equilibrium or not, it is usually necessary to draw a diagram, or diagrams, to show the forces acting on the body, taking into account the magnitude and direction of the forces acting.

4.13.1 CALCULATION OF UNKNOWN FORCES

Sometimes one or more forces acting may be unknown, so they must be put in as vectors with unknown magnitude and sometimes unknown angle. It is also necessary to be very clear as to what the "body" is. In biomechanics, the body is often defined as the whole of the human body, but in other situations, it could be defined as a baseball bat, a motor car, or a section of the human body (e.g., the foot segment). However the body is defined, for the purposes of a free-body diagram, it is important that only the forces acting on that body are considered and that other forces (e.g., forces that the body exerts on its surroundings) are excluded. As seen in Examples 4.6 to 4.10, unknown forces can sometimes be evaluated by invoking the conditions for equilibrium, $\Sigma F = 0$ and $\Sigma M = 0$. Figures 4.17 to 4.19 illustrate this idea with examples of free-body diagrams.

In the case of a man holding a bucket shown in Figure 4.17, the "force" condition for static equilibrium gives:

$$R_{1z} + R_{2z} = W + B \text{ and } R_{1x} + R_{2x} = 0$$

so that:

$$R_{1z} + R_{2z} = 950 \text{ N}$$

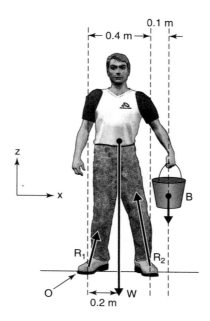

Figure 4.17 Free-body diagram for a man holding a bucket in a stationary position The man's weight is W, and that of the bucket is B. The reaction forces, R_1 and R_2, act at the man's feet and are not necessarily equal. The man's weight is 750 N, and the bucket's weight is 200 N. The x and z axes are horizontal and vertical respectively with origin at 0.

However, this condition on its own is not sufficient to find values for R_1 and R_2 separately. To do this, we would need to invoke the "moment" condition for equilibrium. Taking moments about the man's right foot at O:

$$-950 \times 0.2 + R_{2z} \times 0.4 - 200 \times 0.5 = 0$$

Note that R_{1z}, R_{1x} and R_{2x} do not make a contribution in this last equation because their lines of action pass through the point O. It follows that:

$$R_{2z} = (100 + 190)/0.4 = 725 \text{ N}$$

Therefore:

$$R_{1z} = 950 - 725 = 225 \text{ N}$$

In Figure 4.18, two people, R and S, are shown sitting on a see-saw. In this case, the body under consideration is most likely to be the see-saw itself. The construction of the see-saw itself clearly ensures that there is no bodily movement of the see-saw; only a rotation about the pivot is possible. The forces acting on this see-saw are the two weights, 600 N and 649 N, plus the reaction force, P, at the hinge. In Figure 4.18, this reaction force is shown acting vertically up, although this is not necessarily

Figure 4.18 Two people, R and S, sitting on a see-saw. The weight of R is 649 N and acts at a perpendicular distance of 2.20 m from the pivot. Likewise, the weight of S is 600 N and acts at a perpendicular distance of 2.38 m from the pivot.

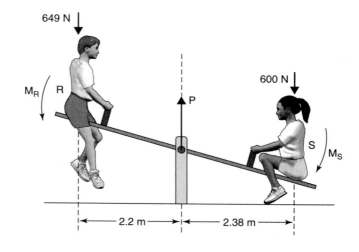

Figure 4.19 A free-body diagram for the lower leg showing the weight of the lower leg acting from the position of the center of mass together with unknown vertical reaction forces, A and C, and horizontal reaction forces, B and D, at the ankle and knee joints respectively. Also shown is the leg as a connected system of straight line segments: upper leg, lower leg, and foot. The lower leg (*circled*) is shown expanded.

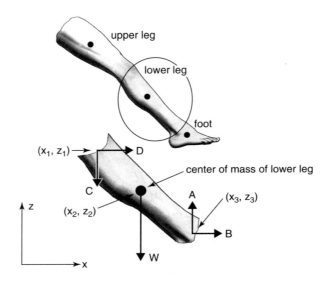

the case; it is probably fair to assume, however, that the bulk of the reaction force at the pivot will be vertical. Applying $\Sigma F = 0$:

$$P - 649 - 600 = 0$$

Therefore:

$$P = 1249 \text{ N}$$

Applying $\Sigma M = 0$ and taking moments about the pivot:

$$M_R + M_S = 0$$
$$-600 \times 2.38 + 649 \times 2.2 = 0$$

This last equality holds, at least to the nearest 0.2! Note that there will be little or no rotation of the see-saw, especially if there is any friction at the pivot. Also, the reaction force at the pivot, P, does not appear in the moments equation because its perpendicular distance from the pivot is zero.

The idea of equilibrium can also be applied to individual body segments in certain situations. To illustrate this, consider the lower leg segment shown in Figure 4.19, where it is supposed that the posture is one of equilibrium (i.e., the leg is at rest in this position or is moving at constant velocity with no segment rotation). If the lower leg shown in Figure 4.19 is in equilibrium, then:

$$\Sigma F = 0 \text{ yields}$$
$$A - C - W = 0$$
$$D + B = 0$$

To proceed further with this problem requires us to use the moments condition for equilibrium as well. Taking moments about the knee joint, $\Sigma M = 0$ yields:

$$-W \times (x_2 - x_1) + A \times (x_3 - x_1) + B \times (z_1 - z_3) = 0$$

Note that in this last equation, the weight is entered as $-W$ because it acts in the negative z direction. Similarly, B is entered as positive because the horizontal reaction force at the ankle is shown acting in the $+x$ direction. Writing the equation once more and identifying positive and negative moments:

$$[-W \times (x_2 - x_1)] + [A \times (x_3 - x_1)] + [B \times (z_1 - z_3)] = 0$$

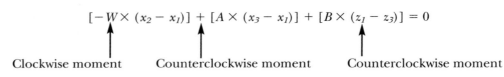

Clockwise moment   Counterclockwise moment   Counterclockwise moment

Suppose the x, z coordinates of the knee, CM, and ankle, measured in millimeters, are as follows:

$$(x_1, z_1) = (546.2, 1258.4)$$
$$(x_2, z_2) = (678.1, 1126.4)$$
$$(x_3, z_3) = (850.2, 954.3)$$

and that the value of C and W are 410 N and 39 N, respectively. This set of equations can now be used to find the other forces; A, B, and D. Hence:

$$A = C + W$$
$$A = 410 + 39 = 449 \text{ N}$$

Also:

$$[-W \times (x_2 - x_1)] + [A \times (x_3 - x_1)] + [B \times (z_1 - z_3)] = 0$$
$$[-39 \times (678.1 - 546.2)] + [449 \times (850.2 - 546.2)] + [B \times (1258.4 - 954.3)] = 0$$
$$-5144.1 + 136496 + 304.1 \times B = 0$$

Therefore:

$$B = (5144.1 - 136496)/304.1 = -431.9 \text{N}$$

So that:

$$D = -B$$
$$D = 431.9 \text{ N}$$

The fact that B turns out to be negative indicates that the **B** vector can be drawn in the opposite direction (i.e., acting from right to left).

4.13.2 CALCULATION OF JOINT MOMENTS

Free-body diagrams can also be used to estimate joint moments. Consider, for example, a gymnast standing on one leg. In Figure 4.20, we will consider the free-body diagram for the foot. The GRF is shown as R, and the weight of the foot segment is shown as mg. The turning effect of the force exerted by the calf muscles, F, and the associated turning moment about the ankle, M_a, are shown separately on the right for clarity.

The force acting down on the foot segment at the ankle joint has been omitted for clarity and because it does not have any moment about the ankle joint. Clearly, the calf muscles must produce a turning moment about the ankle joint in order to maintain equilibrium. If the distance from the ankle joint center to the CM of the foot is measured as 0.07 m and the distance from the ankle joint center to the reaction force is 0.3 m, then it is possible to calculate the moment about the ankle joint center:

$$M_a = (0.20 \times R) - (0.07 \times mg)$$

Figure 4.20 Calculation of ankle joint moment. mg represents the weight of the foot segment, R is the ground reaction force acting at the toe, F is the force exerted by the calf muscles and d is the moment arm of the force F.

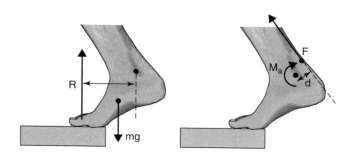

The force R must be equal to the weight of the subject. If the mass of the gymnast is 55 kg and the mass of his foot is 0.9 kg:

$$M_a = (0.20 \times 539) - (0.07 \times 8.82)$$
$$M_a = 107.2 \text{ Nm}$$

This ankle moment is generated by the force, F, of the calf muscles, shown as F in Figure 4.19. If the perpendicular distance from the ankle joint center to the force, F, is measured as $d = 0.04$ m, then F can be calculated as:

$$F = \frac{M_a}{d} = \frac{107.2}{0.04} = 2680N$$

| CASE *Study 4.4* | **Buoyancy and Stability in a Kayak** |

Consider a woman sitting in a kayak. The combined weight, **W**, acting at the CM, CM, pulls the boat down into the water until the upthrust force, **U**, generated by the submerged part of the boat, increases sufficiently to balance the weight. The upthrust force can be assumed to act at a point at the center of the submerged part called the **center of buoyancy** (CB) (see Section 4.11).

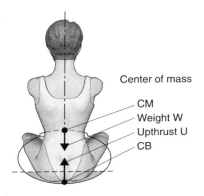

Center of mass
CM
Weight W
Upthrust U
CB

If the boat is tipped to one side, the shape of the submerged part of the hull changes, and the CB moves as shown. The effect of the two forces, now out of line, is to create a righting couple that tends to return the boat to the upright position; therefore, for small angles of tip, the boat is in stable equilibrium (see Section 4.1).

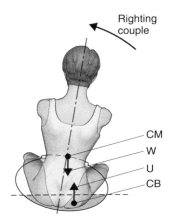

Righting couple
CM
W
U
CB

If the angle of tip is further increased, then the movement of the CB is insufficient to compensate for the movement of the center of gravity, and the boat will capsize. This is now a position of unstable equilibrium.

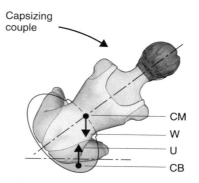

When fully capsized, the kayak again comes into stable equilibrium with the CB and the CM in line. An additional buoyancy force also acts on the torso from the moment it becomes immersed; this is shown as **UT**.

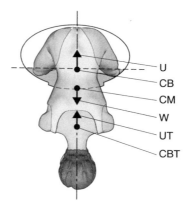

SUMMARY

This chapter on equilibrium focuses on the physical conditions necessary for static equilibrium to take place. This involves the conditions for force balance, $\Sigma F = 0$, and moment balance, $\Sigma M = 0$. The distinction between bodies in equilibrium and not in equilibrium is illustrated by a case study of the deceleration of a hockey ball rolling across a flat, level surface. The CM of the human body is estimated both by the reaction board method and the segmental analysis method. A second case study uses the reaction board method to find the CM among a number of individuals. Equilibrium is studied in a variety of common situations, including those involving two and three forces acting. This chapter also discusses hydrostatics and flotation and calculations involving the variation of hydrostatic pressure with depth. The chapter concludes by showing that the conditions necessary for equilibrium can be used to calculate unknown forces and moments on a human limb segment in certain circumstances. A case study of a kayak illustrates the varying nature of the stability of its equilibrium depending on the relative positions of the CB and CM.

REFERENCES

Dempster WT, Gabel WC, Felts WJL: The anthropometry of manual work space for the seated subjects. *Am J Phys Anthrop* 17:289–317, 1959.

Dempster WT: Space requirements of the seated operator" WADC-TR-55-159, Wright Patterson Air Force Base; 1955.

SUGGESTED READING

Hall S: *Basic Biomechanics.* McGraw-Hill Education—Europe; 2002.

STUDY QUESTIONS

1. An athlete holds a discus at arm's length in two different positions. In the first position, his arm is horizontal (**a**) and in the second position, his arm is 30° below the horizontal (**b**). The length of the athlete's arm

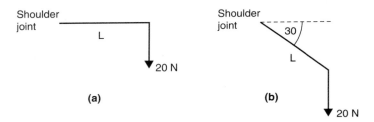

is 65 cm, and the weight of the discus is 20 N. Calculate the moment of this force about the shoulder joint in the two positions.

2. Two tobagganists are pushing a toboggan from behind in order to accelerate it before jumping in. Tobogganist 1 is pushing with a force of 650 N at a distance of 20 cm from the bottom edge of the toboggan, and tobogganist 2 is pushing with a force of 740 N at a distance of 30 cm

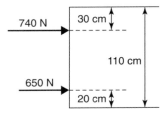

from the top edge. What is the resultant force on the toboggan, and what is its effective point of application?

3. To model someone's arm, the limb is considered as a circular cylinder. The density of the material making up the cylinder is taken as 1100 kg/m^3. Its length is 0.6 m, and its diameter is 0.1 m. Consider the position

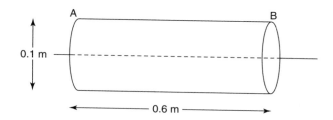

of the center of gravity (CG) of this body by using symmetry arguments. Mark the position of the CG on a diagram of the cylinder. If the arm is held out horizontal, what is the moment exerted about the shoulder joint? Assume that the acceleration due to gravity is 9.8 m/s² and the volume of a cylinder is $\pi r^2 h$.

4. A glider has control surfaces on its wings that enable the pilot to control the altitude of the glider. In a particular case, the lefthand wing is directing airflow downward, and the righthand wing is directing airflow upward, giving rise to an upward force on the lefthand side and a downward

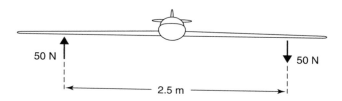

force on the righthand side. What is the couple acting on the glider, and what will the effect of this couple be?

5. A skier is stopped on a downward incline, as shown in the following diagram. The skier's weight is 800 N, and the angle of the incline is 35° with

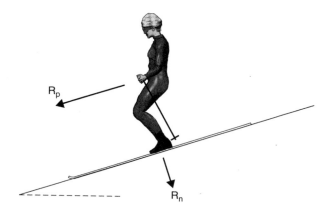

respect to the horizontal. Work out the components of the weight normal to the incline R_n and down the incline, R_p. If the skier is stationary at this point, explain how this can be. Why doesn't he accelerate down the slope?

6. A gymnast on the rings is hanging in the crucifix position. The gymnast's weight is 700 N, and the ropes are vertical. What is the tension in the suspension ropes?

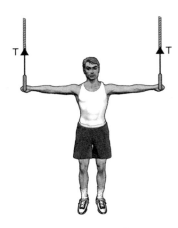

7. Consider the gymnast of question 6 but with the suspension ropes in-

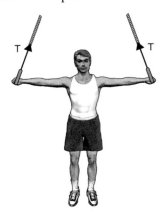

clined at an angle of 10° with respect to the vertical. What is the new tension in the ropes?

8. Calculate the moments of the following forces about the point O:

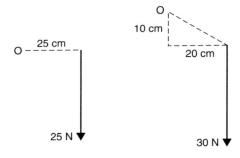

9. It is required to find out the CM of the following object: It is composed of three rectangular metal bars joined together to form a C shape. The

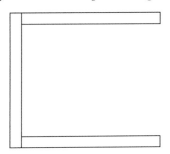

length of each bar is 20 cm, or 1 × 1 cm in cross-section. Each bar is of uniform material consistency and has its center of gravity exactly in the middle of the bar. Predict where the CM of this object is, and describe an experiment whereby the position of the CG can be measured.

10. Calculate the CM of the following person using the segmental method:

Segment	Center of Mass Coordinates	Mass (kg)
Head	(3.5, 7.0)	5.39
Trunk	(3.3, 5.8)	35.05
Left arm	(2.8, 5.7)	1.81
Right arm	(3.2, 5.8)	1.81
Left forearm	(3.1, 5.1)	1.06
Right forearm	(3.6, 5.2)	1.06
Left hand	(3.7, 5.0)	0.41
Right hand	(4.4, 5.3)	0.41
Left thigh	(3.6, 3.4)	6.58
Right thigh	(3.1, 3.4)	6.58
Left leg	(3.6, 3.5)	3.07
Right leg	(2.9, 2.0)	3.07
Left foot	(2.4, 2.4)	0.95
Right foot	(2.5, 0.5)	0.95

Refer to the following diagram for rough sketch of the person's position (distance units are arbitrary):

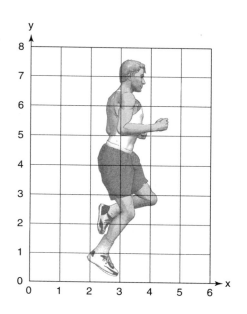

11. What is the moment of the couple on the following object?

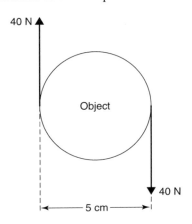

12. Consider someone's hand supporting a 10-kg mass in the position shown below:

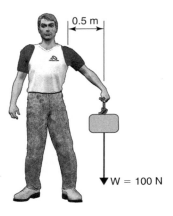

13. What is the moment exerted by a 100-N weight about the left shoulder joint?

CHAPTER five

DYNAMICS I

CHAPTER *objectives*

The objective of this chapter is to:

■ Give students a good introduction to Newton's laws and dynamics, including gravity, measurements of mass and force, friction forces and drag forces, fluid flow and Reynold's number, and motion of a projectile in the presence of drag.

CHAPTER *outcomes*

After reading this chapter, the student will be able to:

■ Understand and apply Newton's laws to motion in a straight line.
■ Do calculations on the gravitational force on objects.
■ Appreciate some of the methods used to measure forces.
■ Do calculations based on strain gauge and force plate outputs.
■ Link theoretical and experimental results for center of mass, force, and acceleration.
■ Do calculations based on friction coefficients.
■ Estimate trajectories for projectiles in air using a simple model for the drag force.

5.1 Inertia and Mass

Objects possess the property that if it they are at rest, they tend to resist being accelerated or made to move. Also, if an object is already moving, it has a tendency to continue moving and to resist changes in speed or direction. This property is described by the term **inertia**. It is clear from everyday experience that whereas large objects such as trains possess a great deal of inertia, small objects such as table tennis balls possess very small inertia. The quantity of matter that a body is composed of is called its mass and is a direct measure of its inertia. Using the SI (international system of units), mass is measured in kilograms. An adult human body has a mass in the range 45 to 100 kg corresponding to a weight of approximately 450 to 1000 Newtons. Weight is a force and is the result of the gravitational pull of the Earth on a body; converting mass to weight entails multiplying the mass (in kilograms) by the acceleration attributable to gravity, a value close to 9.8 ms^{-2} near sea level.

It is important to distinguish between an object's mass and its weight. This relationship between mass and weight is mentioned again in Section 5.7.

5.2 Force

Force is the agent that can change a body's state of motion. Force is a pushing or pulling action and can have the effect of altering a body's velocity in terms of its magnitude and possibly its direction. One of the simplest manifestations of a force is that of a weight being lifted against the force of gravity. All bodies have some weight that must be overcome in order to lift them off the floor. This means that any lifting force, whether it is exerted by a person, ropes, chains, and so on, must have a minimum value equal to the weight of the object in order to begin moving it upward. Force is a vector quantity because to specify it completely, its direction and magnitude must be given.

5.3 Newton's First Law

Every body continues in its state of rest or motion in a straight line unless compelled to change that state by external forces exerted upon it.

This law is also known as the law of inertia and was introduced in Section 3.1. For more information on Newton's laws and mechanics in general, the reader is directed to McCall (2000).

5.4 Gravitational Forces

In addition to forces that are the result of direct contact between bodies, other forces in nature occur in the absence of any contact. The most common example is that of gravity. Gravity is the force that keeps the moon orbiting around the Earth and the Earth orbiting around the sun. It is also the force that makes a shot putt heavy to lift and that brings a thrown javelin back down to the ground. The force is fairly weak as forces go and is usually negligible for interactions between everyday objects such as a bat and a ball. The only time gravitational forces are normally important is when one of the masses is the Earth. Newton stated his law of gravitation as follows:

The gravitational force between any two point masses is directly proportional to the product of the masses and inversely proportional to the inverse square of the distance between them.

The stipulation of point masses was important because Newton realized that the force of attraction between two extended masses can behave differently. Fortunately, Newton was able to show that for the Earth and for spherical masses generally, the force of attraction on an object could be calculated on the basis that the Earth behaved as though all of its mass were concentrated at the center of the Earth (the center of gravity). Objects such as the human body standing on the surface of the Earth are so small compared with the size of the Earth that they can be considered to be point masses. This law can be summarized in the form:

$$F = G\frac{m_1 m_2}{r^2}$$

where F is the force acting on each particle, m_1 and m_2 are the masses, r is the distance between the masses, and G is a universal constant with a value of $6.67 \times 10^{11} Nm^2 kg^{-2}$.

For the case of a body on Earth, let us assume that m_2 is the mass of the Earth and r is the radius of the Earth. It can be seen from this that at a given location on Earth, the force of gravity is proportional to the mass of the body concerned. It can also be deduced from this that the force of gravity on a given object will reduce as altitude increases. For example, in an aircraft flying at 10,000 m above sea level, the force of gravity is reduced from that at sea level. The altitude effect is fairly small, however, because the radius of the Earth is approximately 6,000,000 m.

The acceleration due to gravity measured at the surface of the Earth is approximately 9.81 ms^{-2}. However, this value varies slightly with exact location on Earth and varies with altitude, the presence of voids or mass concentrations underground, geographical latitude, and variations of the shape of the Earth from the spheroidal.

5.5   Newton's Second Law

Newton's second law establishes the relationship between force, mass, and acceleration. It states:

A force acting on a body gives it an acceleration which is in the direction of the force and has a magnitude directly proportional to the force and inversely proportional to the mass of the body,

$$a = \frac{F}{m}$$

or

$$F = ma$$

The SI unit of force is the **Newton** (1 N); this is the force that will give a standard mass of 1 kg an acceleration of 1 ms^{-2}. More information on the background to Newton's laws and dynamics is given in McCall (2000).

■ **EXAMPLE 5.1**   The jet-engined car Thrust SSC, which set a supersonic land speed record on the mud flats in the Black Rock Desert, Nevada, had a mass of 10,000 kg, and its engines could deliver a thrust of 200,650 N. What was the maximum acceleration the Thrust SSC could achieve?

Solution

$$\text{Acceleration} = a = \frac{F}{m} = \frac{200650N}{1000kg} = 20.065 \text{ ms}^{-2}$$

5.6   Measurements of Mass and Force

5.6.1 COMPARING UNKNOWN FORCES WITH KNOWN FORCES

In laboratories, the most common and precise mass measurements are carried out with beam balances that compare the weights of masses. Likewise, force measurements can be made by comparing an unknown force with a known weight. As an alternative, force can be measured with a spring balance by matching the unknown force with a known force supplied by a spring under tension. The spring balance can be calibrated by hanging known weights on it and checking how far it stretches.

5.6.2 STRAIN GAUGES

Electrical methods can also be used for measuring forces. A **strain gauge** is used to detect the linear deformation, or strain, of a material. When bonded to the surface of a structure such as a bone or a steel beam, a strain gauge can detect even the slightest bending in the structure. Because the degree of bending of the object is related to the force applied, the output from the strain gauge can be used to measure force. These gauges function on a principle first described by William Thomson (Lord Kelvin), who found that the resistance of a metal wire changes depending on the tensile strain in the wire. By attaching such a wire in the form of a strain gauge to the surface of an object, the wires will be stretched as the material is stretched. Many modern strain gauges are semiconductor varieties that have superior performance to the original metallic types. A typical strain gauge design is shown in Figure 5.1.

In some cases, such as with cantilever beams, a pair of strain gauges can be used above and below the cantilever beam so that as the beam is loaded (i.e., one gauge is stretched while the other one is shortened). This pair of strain gauges can be incorporated in a Wheatstone bridge circuit (Fig. 5.2) using a ''push–pull'' effect.

The strain gauge under tension SG1 has an increased resistance R + ΔR, and the one under compression SG2 has a decreased resistance R − ΔR. The resistance change ΔR is directly proportional to the strain. For more information on electrical instrumentation, the reader is directed to Regtien (2004). The gauge factor (GF) is defined as the fractional change in resistance to the fractional change in length strain along the axis of the strain gauge. Typical GFs are close to 2.0. Therefore:

$$\text{Strain} = \frac{\Delta l}{l} \text{ (i.e., the extension divided by the original length)}$$

Figure 5.1 Strain gauge. A and B represent pads that can be soldered to. The strain gauge is in the form of a thin film that can be bonded to most surfaces. The thick track is a metallic or semiconductor track whose resistance varies when the strain gauge is deformed.

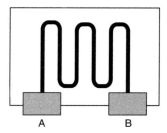

Figure 5.2 An example of one form of Wheatstone Bridge circuit. Assume for convenience that the unstrained resistance of SG1 and SG2 is R and that the other two fixed resistors in the circuit are also equal to R. The output voltage is:
$$V_0 = \epsilon \frac{\Delta R}{R}.$$

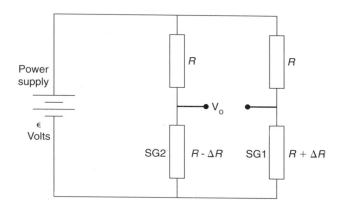

and:

$$GF = \frac{\Delta R/R}{\Delta l/l}$$

so that:

$$\Delta R = R \times GF \times \frac{\Delta l}{l}$$

The strain in an object is defined as the fractional change or deformation per unit length in a body resulting from applied force. Positive strain is defined as a tensile strain, and a negative strain is defined as a compressive strain. Microstrain is defined in parts per million, so that, for example:

$$\frac{0.001\,in}{in} = 0.1\%\,strain = 1000\,microstrain$$

In the Wheatstone bridge circuit, this gives double the output voltage compared with the output to be expected if just one strain gauge were used. Also, any other environmental factors affecting the first strain gauge would be expected to have an identical effect on the second strain gauge so that the effect on the output voltage would be minimized. For example, a temperature increase affecting SG1 would also affect SG2 equally so that any resistance change attributable to temperature variation would be the same for both strain gauges. This temperature effect would have a very small effect on the output voltage, V_0.

5.6.3 Load Cells and Force Platforms

Strain gauges are often incorporated into **load cells**, devices that enable a rapid and easy measurement of force to be made electronically. Load cells come in various shapes and sizes depending on the load to be measured. Many weighing scales are now of this type and often show a load in either kilograms or Newtons. Figure 5.3 shows two load cells being used simultaneously to both weigh an object being lifted and also locate its center of gravity, CGX.

Strain gauges are also used in **force platforms** for biomechanics, engineering, and medical research. For example, the AMTI OR6-7 platforms are the most commonly used force platforms for gait analysis. These platforms give F_x, F_y, and F_z force outputs and M_x, M_y, and M_z moment outputs (moments about the three axes)

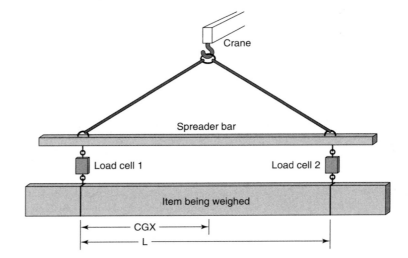

Figure 5.3 A typical load cell system used to locate the center of gravity of an object being weighed. The load cells are a distance L apart and the center of gravity of the object is at distance CGX from load cell 1.

and are ideal for measuring ground reaction forces (GRFs). The OR6 force platform (Fig. 5.4) has dimensions 463 × 508 mm. One version of this platform has a vertical F_z capacity of 4450 N, and an F_z sensitivity value of 0.17 μV/[VN].

5.6.3.1 Voltage Output Calculations

The equation required to calculate the output from each channel is:

$$V_0 = 0.000001 \times S \times \epsilon \times G \times (\textit{Force})$$

where:

$$
\begin{aligned}
V_0 &= \text{Output voltage from the amplifier used} \\
0.000001 &= \text{Volts/microvolt, units for sensitivity} \\
S &= \text{sensitivity} \\
\epsilon &= \text{the Wheatstone Bridge power supply voltage} \\
G &= \text{amplifier gain} \\
\text{Force} &= \text{Load applied in N (replace by ``moment'' in Nm if required)}
\end{aligned}
$$

■ **EXAMPLE 5.2**

Suppose a person who weighs 900 N stands on a force platform. What is the output expected from the F_z channel?

$$
\begin{aligned}
\text{Force} &= 900 \text{ N} \\
\epsilon &= 10 \text{ V (a normal value)}
\end{aligned}
$$

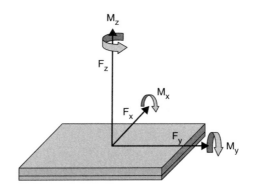

Figure 5.4 A biomechanics force platform with ground reaction force components F_x, F_y, and F_z together with moments M_x, M_y, and M_z about the x, y, and z axes.

$G = 4000$ (variable; other options are sometimes 2000 or 1000)
$S_{Fz} = 0.17$ μV/V/N
$V_0 = 0.000001 \times 0.17 \times 10 \times 4000 \times 900 = 6.12$ volts

Suppose that this system is connected to an **analogue to digital (A/D) converter** that converts the output voltage to a number of bits to be read by a computer. An A/D converter takes an analogue (smoothly varying) signal and converts in into a binary number consisting of N digits. Suppose the A/D converter has 12 bits with ± 10 V full scale input. This means that it has $2^{12} = 4096$ bits to represent an input range of 20 volts. This gives a conversion of 204.8 bits/volt. Therefore, a 900-N vertical force would give:

$$6.12 \text{ volts} \times 204.8 \text{ bits/volt} = 1253 \text{ bits output}$$

This also implies that the smallest change in load that could cause any change in the output (1 binary digit) would be:

$$900/1253 = 0.72 \text{ N}$$

For more information on A/D converters and binary numbers, refer to Regtien (2004).

5.6.3.2 COP Calculation

To calculate the **center of pressure** (COP) coordinates (x, y) for a single-force platform, the coordinates are as follows:

$$COP(x) = \left[\frac{(M_y + (z_{off} \times F_x))}{F_z} \right] \times (-1)$$

$$COP(y) = \left[\frac{(M_x - (z_{off} \times F_y))}{F_z} \right]$$

where

$COP(x) = x$ coordinate of the COP

$COP(y) = y$ coordinate of the COP

$z_{off} =$ vertical offset from the top plate to the origin of the force platform (negative number)

$F_x =$ force along the x axis

$F_y =$ force along the y axis

$F_z =$ force along the z axis

$M_x =$ moment along the x axis

$M_y =$ moment along the y axis

$M_z =$ moment along the z axis

The coordinates of the COP are quoted relative to a local origin at one of the corners of the force platform. The origin is located a vertical distance z_{off} below the top surface of the plate (Fig. 5.5). An example of the use of the COP is given in the following case study.

CASE *Study 5.1*   **Male Subject Wearing Sports Shoes Walking Across a Force Plate**

In normal walking gait, the COP moves from the heel in a smooth continuous fashion toward the toe during the stance phase. The diagram shows the COP plot as an $x-y$ diagram. The COP starts at the top of the diagram and moves toward the bottom of the diagram.

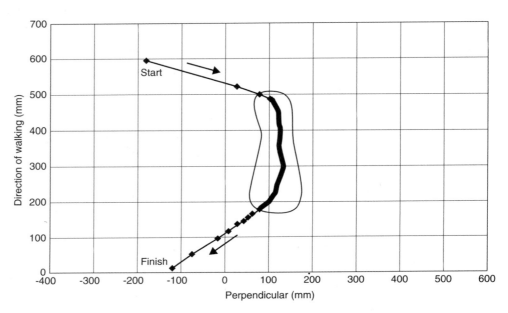

Figure 5.5 Location of origin for a typical biomechanics force platform.

It can also be seen that the COP moves perpendicularly to the direction of movement. However, in this real data set, the three points nearest "Start" and the eight points nearest "Finish" are spurious points caused by instrumental and calculational artefacts. The COP line is represented by the cluster of points between 75 and 125 mm on the "perpendicular" axis.

5.7   The Acceleration Attributable to Gravity and Weight

If we pretend that the Earth is a perfect sphere of mass, M, and radius, R, then we can calculate the force on a small object of mass m at the Earth's surface:

$$F = G\frac{Mm}{R^2}$$

If the object were raised through a small distance and released, it would accelerate at the normal rate of approximately 9.81 ms^{-2}. This value is known as g, and it is natural to ask what the relationship is between g and the formula above which Newton arrived at for the force between two point masses. Working from Newton's law of gravitation, the acceleration of an object released near the surface of the Earth is:

$$a = \frac{F}{m} = G\frac{M}{R^2}$$

This must be the same as g. As we have seen, the conditions in our example are such that the Earth and the small object can be thought of as point masses and that the distance through which the object is dropped is very small compared with the radius of the Earth. It also follows from these considerations that the weight of an object of mass, m, on the Earth is given simply by:

$$W = mg$$

where m is the mass in kilograms and g is the acceleration attributable to gravity. The units of g are ms^{-2} or N/kg.

■ **EXAMPLE 5.3**

Work out a value for g assuming $g = GM/R$ and using the following data:

Mass of the Earth $= 5.98 \times 10^{24}$kg
Radius of the Earth $= 6.38 \times 10^{6}$m
Gravitational constant $= 6.67 \times 10^{-11}$ Nm²/kg²

Solution

$$g = \frac{(6.67 \times 10^{-11}) \times (5.98 \times 10^{24})}{(6.38 \times 10^{6})^2}$$

$$= 9.81 \text{ ms}^{-2}$$

■ **EXAMPLE 5.4**

What is the weight of a person with a mass of 72 kg?

Solution

$$\text{Weight } (W) = mg = (72 \text{ kg}) \times (9.81 \text{ N/kg}) = 706.3 \text{ N}$$

CASE *Study 5.2*   **Vertical Jumping**

A man was selected for trials involving vertical jumps. He weighed 67 kg and was asked to perform vertical jumps from a force platform. A Vicon 512 system was used to perform simultaneous three-dimensional (3D) motion analysis at 120Hz. Thirty seven retro-reflective markers were applied to the subject's body in accordance with the anatomical locations defined by a marker set. The subject wore a wet suit during the trials with most of the markers being secured to the suit with Velcro attachments. The subject also wore a headband with four markers attached and two wrist bands, each with a double-marker wand attached. The force platform took 600 samples a second and recorded 3D force data of F_x, F_y, and F_z together with moment outputs of M_x, M_y, and M_z. The following figure shows a series of snapshot images of the subject at various stages of the vertical jump. In this trial, the subject was instructed to jump without using arm movement for assistance.

After running a suitable segmental model, the position of the subject's center of mass (CM) was calculated. The position of the CM can be seen in the above figure. In field 100, the CM position is labeled, and in subsequent fields, the CM is indicated by a *small circle*

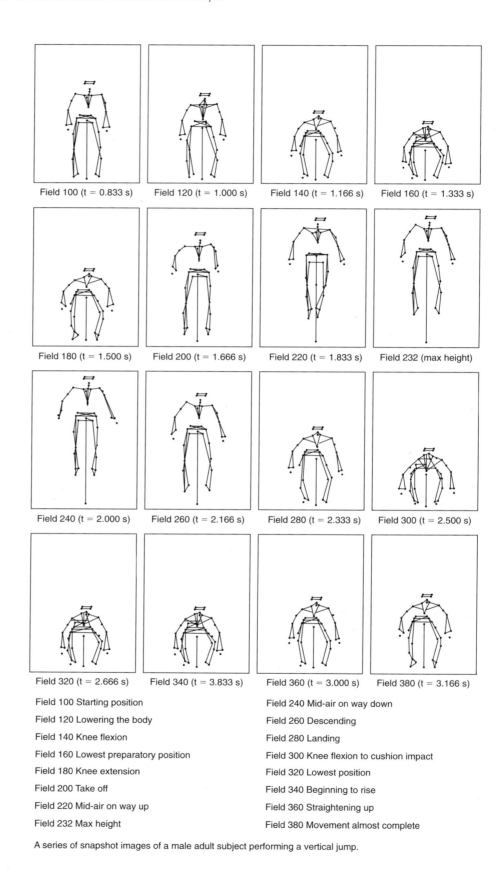

Field 100 (t = 0.833 s)   Field 120 (t = 1.000 s)   Field 140 (t = 1.166 s)   Field 160 (t = 1.333 s)

Field 180 (t = 1.500 s)   Field 200 (t = 1.666 s)   Field 220 (t = 1.833 s)   Field 232 (max height)

Field 240 (t = 2.000 s)   Field 260 (t = 2.166 s)   Field 280 (t = 2.333 s)   Field 300 (t = 2.500 s)

Field 320 (t = 2.666 s)   Field 340 (t = 3.833 s)   Field 360 (t = 3.000 s)   Field 380 (t = 3.166 s)

Field 100 Starting position

Field 120 Lowering the body

Field 140 Knee flexion

Field 160 Lowest preparatory position

Field 180 Knee extension

Field 200 Take off

Field 220 Mid-air on way up

Field 232 Max height

Field 240 Mid-air on way down

Field 260 Descending

Field 280 Landing

Field 300 Knee flexion to cushion impact

Field 320 Lowest position

Field 340 Beginning to rise

Field 360 Straightening up

Field 380 Movement almost complete

A series of snapshot images of a male adult subject performing a vertical jump.

at the top of the vertical line with the original position referenced by a *small cross*. This 3D coordinate data were exported to a text file for subsequent processing. This case study examines the vertical movement (*z* coordinate) of the CM only. The following chart shows the vertical position of the CM versus time:

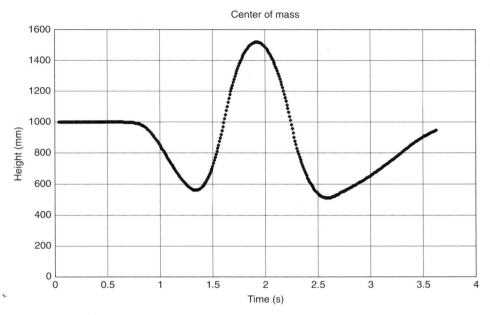

The following chart shows the vertical velocity (*black line*) and acceleration (dashed line) of the same point using a four-point smoothing method for both. Both the velocity and the acceleration have been calculated from the *z* coordinate and time data using the relationships

$$v_z = \frac{\Delta z}{\Delta t} \text{ and } a_z = \frac{\Delta v_z}{\Delta t}$$

but incorporating a certain degree of data smoothing, as stated. For comparison purposes,

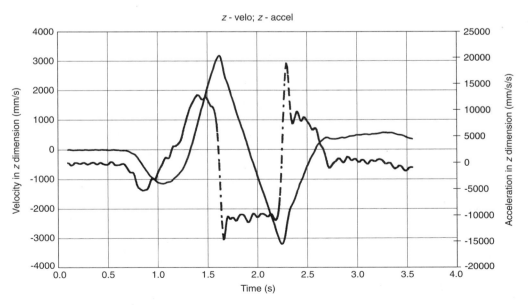

the *z* component of the force can be displayed over the same time interval. The following chart shows the resultant force acting on the CM in the *z* direction (in other words, with the bodyweight subtracted).

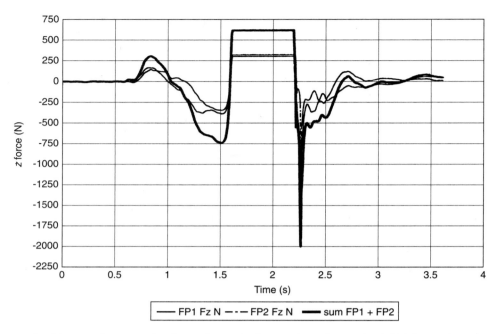

In this case, because the force shown is the resultant force, the initial force data are close to zero before the commencement of the jump (i.e., at times between 0.0 and 0.5 s). Two *curves* show the two force plates (left and right feet) separately, and the heavier *black curve* shows the sum of the two. The acceleration when the subject is in mid-air is close to 10,000 mm/s^2 (10 m/s^2 in SI units), as would be expected, between approximately 1.6 and 2.2 s. Also, the maximum excess upward force at time 1.5 s is about 750 N, so that the predicted acceleration would be $a = F/m = 750$ N/67 kg $= 11.2$ m/s^2. As can be seen from the acceleration curve, this is approximately the same as the measured upward acceleration at the same time, about 12 m/s^2. Therefore, this verifies that force equals mass times acceleration.

5.8 Newton's Third Law

When someone paddles a canoe, the paddles push backward against the water, propelling the canoe forward (Fig. 5.6). These action and reaction forces occur whenever the paddle is moved through the water and are reciprocal—that is, they are equal and opposite to each other. Another example is a tennis ball being struck

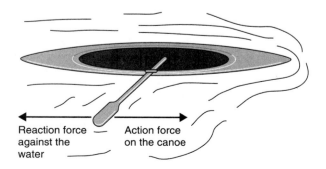

Figure 5.6 Forces acting on a canoe.

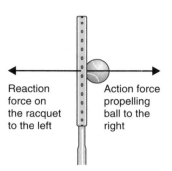

Figure 5.7 Tennis ball being struck by a tennis racquet.

by a tennis racquet (Fig. 5.7). Again, in this tennis example, the action and reaction forces always occur together in pairs and are equal and opposite to each other. Newton's third law is usually stated in the form:

Whenever a body exerts a force on another body, the latter exerts a force of equal magnitude and opposite direction on the former.

It is normal to describe these forces as the "action" and "reaction," although it.is by no means clear sometimes which force is which. Sometimes the effect produced by the action force is more noticeable than that produced by the reaction force. In the case of the canoe, the action force is clearly pushing the canoe forward, but the reaction force is merely propelling a certain mass of water backward, which is not so noticeable. In the tennis example, the ball is propelled to the right at high velocity as a result of the action force that was present briefly during the ball–racquet collision. However, the racquet is merely slowed down slightly by the reaction force, and the change in the velocity of the racquet head would not normally be noticed because the mass of the racquet is greater than that of the ball.

Newton's third law also applies to objects resting on the ground or on inclined surfaces. A person of mass 80 kg standing on level ground, for example, has a weight of 800 N approximately acting vertically down from the CM. Fig. 5.8 shows that the reaction forces at the feet act vertically upward and together are sufficient to exactly balance the weight, **W**. If an object is resting on an inclined surface, then the weight, **W**, has to be resolved into components normal to the surface and tangential to the slope.

Fig. 5.9 shows a weight, **W**, on an inclined plane with an inclination of θ with the horizontal. If the interface between the object and plane is frictionless, then the object will slide down the plane with an acceleration that can be worked out from Newton's second law:

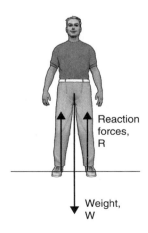

Figure 5.8 Weight and normal reaction forces at the feet. The two reaction forces together add up to be equal (and opposite) to *W*.

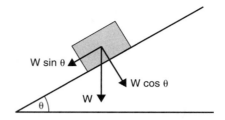

Figure 5.9 A weight, *W*, on an inclined plane.

$$a = F/m = (W\sin\theta)/m$$

but:

$$m = W/g$$

so that:

$$a = g\sin\theta$$

The normal reaction force would be $W\cos\theta$ throughout the slide. If the interface is not frictionless, then two possibilities exist:

(a) The coefficient of friction is large enough to provide a friction force acting on the object up the incline equal and opposite to $W\sin\theta$. The object will remain at rest.

(b) The coefficient of friction is too small to prevent sliding, and the object will slide down the incline.

Friction, the effects of which were mentioned in Section 4.1, is an important topic in biomechanics and is discussed further in Section 5.9.

5.9 Friction

Consider the object now resting on a rough plane in Figure 5.9.

CASE (A)

The coefficient of friction is large enough so that the object remains at rest. The maximum friction force available can be worked out from:

$$F = \mu R$$

where R is the **normal reaction force** and μ is the **coefficient of static friction**. In other words, the force of friction is usually proportional to the force that presses the surfaces together as well as the roughness of the surfaces. The amount of force required to move an object starting from rest is usually greater than the force required to keep it moving at constant velocity after the motion has been started.

$$R = W\cos\theta$$

In this case, for the object to remain at rest, we must have:

$$W\sin\theta < \mu W\cos\theta$$

or

$$\sin\theta < \mu\cos\theta$$

or

$$\tan\theta < \mu$$

■ **EXAMPLE 5.5**

An object that weighs 50 N rests on a rough plane with angle of inclination 50°. The coefficient of friction between the object and plane is 0.5. Will the object slide down the plane?

Solution

The weight of the object is irrelevant to the solution. For the object to remain stationary:

$$\tan\theta < \mu$$
$$\tan 50° = 1.1917, \text{ which is greater than } \mu$$

So the object will slide down the plane.

Case (a) illustrates that the friction force increases as the angle θ is increased. However, at a certain critical angle, sliding is about to commence and the friction force, F, has then reached its limiting value (**limiting friction**) and then

$$\mu = \tan\theta.$$

These considerations lead to some fairly straightforward conclusions about the limiting value of the static friction force:

(a) It can be increased by increasing the normal reaction force, R. This can be achieved by pressing the two surfaces together by whatever means is available.

(b) The maximum friction force available cannot be varied by altering the (macroscopic) area of contact between the objects.

(c) The static friction force is useful in preventing objects from slipping or sliding when this is not desirable. Once sliding has started, the friction force is then called sliding friction and is illustrated by Case (B). The frictional force is independent of the velocity of motion.

CASE (B)

The friction force is not large enough to prevent the block from sliding down the inclined plane.

In Figure 5.9, if the angle θ is too great, the component of the weight, $W\cos\theta$, acting tangentially down the plane becomes greater than the limiting value of the static friction force. The object will then start sliding down the plane and is subject to **sliding friction** (or kinetic friction). Sliding friction is governed by the equation:

$$F_s = \mu_s R$$

where R is the normal reaction force and μ_s is the **coefficient of sliding friction**. The sliding friction force is less than the static friction force so that μ_s is less than μ. As soon as the block has started sliding, its acceleration can be worked out using Newton's second law:

$$\begin{aligned}
\text{Force} = ma &= W\sin\theta - \mu_s R \\
&= W\sin\theta - \mu_s W\cos\theta \\
&= W(\sin\theta - \mu_s \cos\theta)
\end{aligned}$$

So:

$$Acceleration = a = \frac{W}{m}(\sin\theta - \mu_s \cos\theta)$$

This equation indicates that the block would accelerate down the plane with a constant acceleration. In practice, this might or might not be true depending on variations in the value of μ_s attributable to changes in the roughness of the contacting surfaces.

5.9.1 FRICTION AND AREA OF CONTACT

One of the assumptions of the standard model of surface friction is that the frictional resistance between two surfaces is independent of the area of contact. However, friction is a complex phenomenon, and most assumptions can be shown to be faulty under certain circumstances. In the case of a crate that is being shifted across a floor by pushing, it is true that the orientation of the crate is of no consequence because the friction force is the same (Fig. 5.10(a) and (b)).

In the case of the triangular-shaped load of Figure 5.10(c) and (d), there is an obvious contradiction to this assumption. In Figure 5.10(d), the load digs into the surface and causes the force required to slide the object to increase. However, the independent of area assumption has a lot of merit in it and implies correctly, for example, that wide tires are no better than narrow tires in providing better traction, and will not provide a shorter stopping distance for a car. Better traction can still be provided by wider tires or by tires with reduced pressure, if the coefficient of friction is increased, as might happen on snow. The wider tires will not pack the snow as much, so the coefficient of friction will be higher.

5.9.2 FRICTION AND VELOCITY

The assumption that the kinetic friction force is independent of velocity is usually a good one. However, as the speed increases and air friction is encountered, the friction increases as the square of the speed, or even higher powers of speed. In some circumstances, fluids can show a friction force proportional to speed, known as viscous resistance. There are some situations in sports when friction forces (generally, sliding friction) need to be increased. The following are some examples in which attempts are made to increase friction:

- Use of chalk on hands in some gymnastics events and in weightlifting
- Drying the hands to improve grip on the ball in cricket
- Use of resin in some ball games to provide better grip
- Design of sports shoes to provide good grip on various types of flooring
- Design of tires in car racing to enable corners to be taken at high speed

Alternatively, some situations demand a low friction force to facilitate sliding when this is required. Some examples of reducing friction are:

Figure 5.10   (A) Crate on narrow end requires force, *F*, to move it along the floor. (B) Crate on wide end requires same force, *F*, to move it. (C) A different object resting on its large area end requires a force, *G*, to move it. (D) The object resting on its sharp end requires a force much larger than *G* to move it.

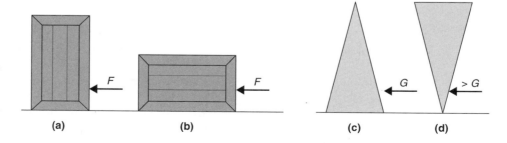

Table 5.1	Static and sliding friction coefficients	
Materials	μ	μ_s
Waxed ski on snow		
At 2108C		0.20
At 08C		0.05
Steel on steel	0.70	0.60
Croquet ball on lawn		
Fast lawn	—	0.48
Heavy lawn	—	0.53
Copper on glass	0.70	0.50
Rubber on concrete	~1.00	~1.00

- Use of wax on skis to reduce friction on snow
- Curling and the use of brushes to alter the path
- The use of shark skin suits for swimmers
- Ice skating

Table 5.1 lists some static and sliding friction coefficients. The values given in Table 5.1 are only approximate, and it should be kept in mind that friction depends on temperature and on the condition of the surfaces. The low friction of ice and snow is caused by the formation of a lubricating film of water between the ice surface and the other surface. It is also worth noting that, although the friction force is independent of the area of (macroscopic) contact for metals and many other substances, the coefficient of friction depends on the shape of the sliding surfaces for other materials such as plastics and rubber.

5.9.3 SUMMARY OF STATIC FRICTION AND KINETIC FRICTION

Friction is normally characterized by a coefficient of friction equal to the ratio of the frictional resistance force to the normal force pressing the surfaces together. Typically, there is a considerable difference between the coefficients of static and dynamic friction. Two cases of static and dynamic friction are summarized in Figure 5.11.

Figure 5.11 In the static friction case, the friction force resists motion and opposes any applied force up to a threshold value, and the object begins to slip. In the kinetic case, with an object moving with constant velocity, the force of kinetic friction resists the motion, but this resistance is taken to be independent of velocity.

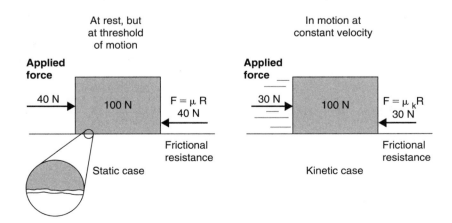

■ **EXAMPLE 5.6**   A man pushes a toboggan on a level ice field. The mass of the toboggan is 60 kg, and the coefficient of sliding friction is $\mu_s = 0.15$. The man pushes down on the toboggan at an angle of 30° to the horizontal. What force must the man exert to keep the toboggan moving at constant velocity?

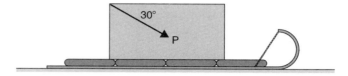

Solution

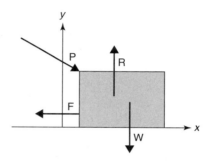

The above diagram is a free-body diagram for the toboggan. The forces acting on it are the push (**P**) of the man, the weight of the toboggan (W), the normal reaction force (R), and the friction force (F) attributable to sliding friction. Because the man is pushing the toboggan down against the snow, the magnitude of the reaction force, R, is increased above and beyond the value mg (the weight of the toboggan).

The horizontal and vertical components of the forces are

$$P_x = P \cos 30°$$
$$P_y = - P \sin 30°$$
$$W_x = 0 \qquad W_y = -mg$$
$$R_x = 0 \qquad R_y = R$$
$$F_x = - \mu_s R \qquad F_y = 0$$

The acceleration of the toboggan is zero in both the x and y directions, so the net force in each of these directions is zero.

$$P \cos 30° + 0 + 0 - \mu_s R = 0$$
$$-P \sin 30° - mg + R + 0 = 0$$

These are two equations for the two unknowns, P and R. Multiplying the second of these equations by μ_s and adding to the first equation:

$$P (\cos 30° - \mu_s \sin 30°) - \mu_s mg = 0$$

so that:

$$P = \frac{\mu_s \, mg}{\cos 30° - \mu_s \sin 30°}$$

$$= \frac{0.15 \times 60kg \times 9.8m/s^2}{\cos 30° - 0.15 \times \sin 30°} = 111.5N$$

| CASE *Study* 5.3 | Maximum Speed on Banked Race Track |

As the racing car takes a corner, the centripetal force required to take it around a circular arc of radius (r) has to be provided by the friction force at the wheels. There will be a maximum speed at which the car will be on the threshold of sliding up the incline. At this maximum speed, v:

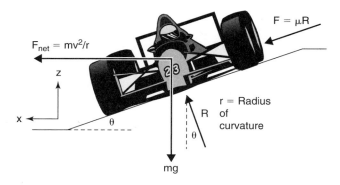

$$\Sigma F_x = m\frac{v^2}{r} = R\sin\theta + \mu R\cos\theta$$

$$\Sigma F_z = R\cos\theta - \mu R\sin\theta - mg = 0$$

Solving this pair of equations for the maximum speed, v:

$$v_{max} = \sqrt{\frac{rg\,(\sin\theta + \mu\cos\theta)}{\cos\theta - \mu\sin\theta}}$$

In a particular case, $\mu = 0.5$, the angle θ of the bank is 15°, and the radius of the curve is 10 m. Therefore, the maximum speed that can be used around this corner is:

$$v_{max} = \sqrt{\frac{10 \times 9.81 \times (0.2588 + (0.5 \times 0.9659))}{(0.9659 - (0.5 \times 0.2588))}} = \sqrt{87.03} = 9.32 m/s$$

We can compare this case with two other limiting cases:

$$\text{Frictionless case: } v_{max} = \sqrt{rg\tan\theta} = 5.12 m/s$$

and

$$\text{Flat, level road: } v_{max} = \sqrt{rg\,\mu} = 7 m/s$$

Rolling friction occurs whenever an object on wheels or castors rolls across a surface. Balls such as golf balls and pool balls also suffer rolling friction when they roll across the green or the pool table. With rolling balls, this type of friction occurs because both the ball and the surface on which it is rolling are deformed to some extent in the rolling process. Golf is a good example in which the player must gauge the amount of rolling friction present before playing a shot. The golfer assesses the length of the grass, whether it is wet or dry, how soft or hard the ground is, and the way the grass is lying (the grain). All of these factors influence the ball as it rolls across the green. Rolling friction is normally a lot smaller than sliding or static friction. For this reason, shifting heavy loads is usually accomplished by using a vehicle fitted with wheels or rollers to reduce friction. Coefficients of rolling friction are of the order 0.001; in other words, rolling friction is about 100 to 1000 times smaller than sliding and static friction. Rolling friction, similar to sliding friction, depends on the normal reaction force, but it can also depend on the diameter of the ball, the nature of the ball, and the nature of the surface.

CASE *Study 5.4* | **Rolling Friction on Hockey Ball**

In Chapter 3, the case study of the rolling hockey ball showed a deceleration of 0.233 m/s² attributable to rolling friction. The mass of the hockey ball is 0.14 kg. The magnitude of the decelerating force is mass multiplied by deceleration, given in Chapter 3 as −0.233 m/s/s. Hence, the friction force is:

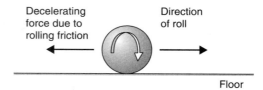

$$F = 0.14\,kg \times -0.233\ m/s/s = 0.0326\ N$$

The coefficient of rolling friction is:

Ratio of friction force/Normal reaction force

so that:

$$\mu = 0.0326N/(0.14kg \times 9.81\,m/s^2) = \frac{0.0326}{1.3734} = 0.0237$$

5.10 The Momentum of a Body

Newton's laws can be expressed very conveniently in terms of momentum. **Momentum** is defined as mass multiplied by velocity. Bearing in mind that velocity is a vector quantity and mass is a scalar quantity, it can be seen that momentum p is a vector quantity

$$p = m\,v$$

Momentum p is a vector that has the same direction as the velocity, but its magnitude is m times as large as that of v. The units are kg.m/s in the SI system of units. Newton's first law simply states that in the absence of external forces, the momentum of an object remains constant:

$$p = \text{constant}$$

In science, if a quantity has a value that does not change, we say that the quantity is conserved. Thus, the momentum of a body that is not subject to any external forces is conserved. This situation does not happen very often in sports. An astronaut in outer space would not have any gravitational forces acting on him or her, so the momentum would be constant. On Earth, someone standing still on firm ground does not experience any net external force because the person's weight is exactly balanced by the normal GRF. A train moving along at constant speed on a level frictionless track would have a constant momentum.

Newton's second law can be expressed in terms of momentum as well. Provided the mass of an object is constant, which is normally the case, we can transform mass times acceleration as follows:

$$m\boldsymbol{a} = m\frac{d\boldsymbol{v}}{dt} = \frac{d}{dt}(m\boldsymbol{v}) = \frac{d\boldsymbol{p}}{dt}$$

The second law can be written:

$$\boldsymbol{F} = \frac{d\boldsymbol{p}}{dt}$$

This states that the rate of change of the momentum of a body equals the net external force acting on it.

■ **EXAMPLE 5.7**

A runner exerts a constant horizontal backward thrust of 60 N to propel himself forward along a level track. Ignore all other forces acting on his body. What is the rate of change of his momentum? Given that his mass is 60kg, what will his velocity be after 5 seconds?

Solution

The rate of change of his momentum $= dp/dt =$ force $F = 60$ kg.m/s^2
His momentum changes at the rate of 60 kg.m/s^1 every second, so after 5 seconds, his momentum will have changed by 300 kg.m/s^1.

His velocity will then be $v = \dfrac{1}{60kg}\left(300\ kg.m/s\right) = 5m/s$

The momentum concept can also be used to express Newton's third law. Because the action force is exactly equal and opposite to the reaction force, the rate of change of momentum generated by the action of the force on one body is exactly opposite to the rate of change of momentum generated by the reaction force on the other body. Also, the time for which the force acts is the same for both bodies. Therefore, whenever two bodies exert forces on one another, the resulting changes of momentum are equal and opposite.

■ **EXAMPLE 5.8**

A tennis player plays a forehand drive shot at a ball that is approaching her at 40 m/s. The tennis ball, which has a mass of 0.06 kg, travels at 45 m/s away from her after the shot. What was the change in momentum of the tennis racquet? If the ball was in contact with the racquet for 0.01 s, what was the average force on ball (and racquet) during that time?

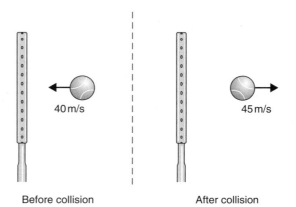

Before collision   After collision

Solution

Initial momentum of ball $= p_x = mv_x = 0.06kg \times (-40m/s) = -2.4$ kg.m/s
Final momentum of ball $= p_x = mv_x = 0.06kg \times (+45\ m/s) = +2.7$ kg.m/s

We can use $\frac{dp}{dt} = F$ to calculate the average force in the collision. We will have to assume that the force was constant during the time ball and racquet were in contact. This is obviously not entirely true but will, in any case, give us the average force that we seek. We will rewrite the differential form of the equation using:

$$\Delta p = \text{change in momentum} = p_{final} - p_{initial}$$
$$\Delta t = \text{time interval} = t_{final} - t_{initial}$$

so that:

$$\frac{\Delta p}{\Delta t} = \bar{F}$$

where $\bar{F}$ is the mean or average force. Therefore:

$$\bar{F} = \frac{p_{final} - p_{initial}}{t_{final} - t_{initial}} = \frac{2.7 - (-2.4)}{0.01} = \frac{5.1}{0.01} = 510 N$$

It is clear that this force is exerted to the left on the racquet and to the right on the ball. The change in momentum of the ball is 5.1 units to the right; for the racquet, it is 5.1 units to the left. The velocity of the racquet will change during the impact with the ball to reflect this momentum change.

5.11   Projectile Motion, Taking Into Account the Drag Force

5.11.1 INTRODUCTION

The equations given so far ignore the frictional force represented by air drag. Any object moving through the air has a friction force proportional to the square of the velocity or proportional to the velocity if the velocity is very low. For most projectiles we are concerned with in sports science, the velocities are such that the **drag force** is proportional to the square of the velocity. This has the effect of modifying the range of the projectile and altering the shape of the trajectory in the horizontal–vertical plane.

5.11.2 REYNOLDS' NUMBER

The flow of air around a sphere changes its detailed pattern with the velocity, but this also depends to some extent on the size of the sphere. It is possible to characterize the air flow around the ball by using Reynolds' number. In the case of a spherical ball, Reynolds' number is determined by the velocity of the ball, the diameter of the ball, and the physical properties of the air. For spherical balls moving through the air, it can be shown that **Reynolds' number (R)** is:

$$R = 64000 \; dv$$

where d is the diameter of the ball in meters and v its velocity in meters per second. Thus, for a cricket ball of diameter 0.072 m traveling through air at 30 m/s, the value of Reynolds' number is:

$$R = 64000 \times (30) \times (0.072) = 138240$$

Experiments on balls in wind tunnels have shown that over a wide range of Reynolds' numbers from 1000 to about 150,000, the air resistance increases as the square of the velocity of the flow. However, if the velocity is increased further to raise R to about 200,000, the smooth ball experiences a sudden dramatic reduction in the drag force to about one quarter of the value previously found. The reason for this sudden decrease in air resistance as the velocity is increased beyond this critical

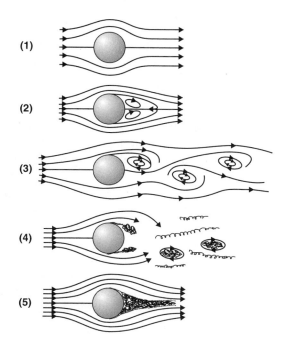

Figure 5.12 Flow of air around a ball as the air speed and, therefore, Reynolds' number increases. (1) $R = 10^{-2}$, (2) $R = 20$, (3) $R = 100$, (4) $R = 10^4$, and (5) $R = 10^6$.

value is the behavior of the boundary layer of air around the ball. The variations of air flow around the ball are illustrated in Figure 5.12 for various flow velocities.

Figures 5.12(1) to (3) show Reynolds' numbers below 2000. In Figure 5.12(4), the Reynolds' number is 10,000. In Figure 5.12(5), it is 1,000,000. Figures 5.12(1) and 5.12(2) show laminar flow at low speed. The air in front and behind the ball comes to a stop so that the pressure is at its highest at these points, but the net force on the ball attributable to pressure differences is approximately zero. There is no pressure drag. Figure 5.12(4) shows a turbulent wake with the air behind the cylinder no longer slowing down and the pressure no longer increases behind the ball. Because of the high pressure in front of the ball, it now experiences a large pressure drag. This happens for values of R between 2000 and 100,000. As the speed increases still further, Figure 5.12(5) shows that the turbulent region works itself around toward the front of the ball. This is now a turbulent boundary layer. The flow lines separate from the ball and follow the turbulent boundary layer. The pressure behind the object increases again, and the pressure drag is much smaller.

In many cases, we are concerned with the motion of balls through the air, which can include golf balls, baseballs, shot putts, and soccer balls. In most games, the maximum ball velocity encountered is about 30 m/s. Taking this figure for the ball velocity, the corresponding Reynolds' numbers for a selection of balls can be calculated:

Soccer ball: 425,000

Tennis ball: 122,000

Golf ball: 79,000

Squash ball: 78,000

Table tennis ball: 73,000

It can be seen from this that the air flows for all sports balls are turbulent. For the soccer ball, the Reynolds' number is above the critical value and will benefit from a reduced drag force. The velocity of the golf ball may well be higher than 30 m/s when the ball is driven off the tee.

5.11.3 Drag Force and Its Effect on Motion

It has been shown experimentally that, for $R > 1$, the drag force increases as the square of the velocity. In each of these cases, therefore, the drag force can be written as:

$$F_d = \tfrac{1}{2} C_D \, \rho \, A v^2$$

where ρ is the density of air, A is the cross-sectional area of the ball, v is its velocity, and C_D is a dimensionless empirical quantity called the *drag coefficient*. For spherical objects, the drag coefficient has a value of about 0.5. This implies that, for any object in free fall, including projectiles, the net downward force is:

$$F_y = mg - F_d = mg - \tfrac{1}{2} C_D \, \rho \, A v_y^2$$

So that the mass (ball) has a net downward acceleration of:

$$a_y = g - \left(\frac{C_D \, \rho \, A}{2m}\right) v_y^2$$

When the object begins to accelerate downward, its velocity, v_y, will eventually reach a limiting value determined by the net downward force on the object becoming zero. The velocity at which this happens is known as the terminal velocity and is:

$$v_t = \sqrt{\frac{2mg}{C_D \, \rho \, A}}$$

This is useful to know and leads to the interesting conclusion that the terminal speed of a sphere increases with the square root of the radius of the sphere. This is also true for some types of balls provided the ball is of uniform solid construction throughout. In sports, we are invariably faced with the question of what the range is for a ball struck or thrown with a velocity v. How is this range modified by the presence of friction or drag? Although the presence of the drag force is universally recognized, it is ignored in many cases because the mathematics do not allow for a simple analytical solution. In the next section, a numerical solution is given to this problem, which is of great significance in ball games.

5.11.4 Numerically Modeling a Ball's Motion

For a ball moving through the air, the acceleration vertically upward (in the y direction) is:

$$a_y = -g - \frac{C_D \, \rho \, A}{2m} v_y^2$$

where v_y is the y component of the velocity of the ball at any instant. Likewise, its acceleration horizontally (in the x direction) is:

$$a_x = -\frac{C_D \, \rho \, A}{2m} v_x^2$$

where v_x is the x component of the velocity at any instant. A numerical solution to these equations can be found by the Euler method using small time steps, Δt, and calculating velocities as:

$$\Delta v_x = a_x \times \Delta t \text{ and } \Delta v_y = a_y \times \Delta t$$

and calculating displacements as:

$$\Delta x = v_x \times \Delta t \text{ and } \Delta_y = v_y \times \Delta t$$

This can be achieved simply using a spreadsheet such as Excel or by writing a short program in BASIC, FORTRAN, or another programming language. For a short introduction to calculus, please refer to Appendix 1. The data required for the calculation on a baseball are as follows:

Radius, $r = 3.66$ cm

Mass, $m = 0.145$ kg

Cross-sectional area, $A = 0.0042$ m^2

Density of air $= \rho = 1.29$ kg/m^3

Dimensionless constant $C_D = 0.5$ roughly for a sphere

Note that the value of C_D may be modified in the case of a ball with a seam or with dimples. The success of the calculation rests on obtaining the correct sign for the drag force in the spreadsheet or program. The acceleration in the y direction, for example, can be calculated as:

$$AY = -G - K \times VY \times ABS(VY)$$

where K is $\dfrac{C_D \, \rho \, A}{2m}$ and $ABS(VY)$ is the absolute value of VY. This gives the positive magnitude of VY regardless of whether VY is negative or positive. The value of K for a baseball turns out to be very close to 0.01, so this value has been taken for the following calculations. Table 5.2 assumes an initial x velocity of 20 m/s and an initial y velocity of 20 m/s and gives the values of t, x, and y obtained for a baseball projected from $x = 0, y = 0$ using time steps of $\Delta t = 0.01$ s.

The last row in Table 5.2 gives the first result obtained for which y is negative. That is, the range obtained is 55.67 m, assuming that the landing and projection heights are equal. In the absence of drag, the range would have been 81.63 m, so

Table 5.2	x and y coordinates versus time for a projected baseball with $v_x = 20$ m/s, $v_y = 20$ m/s*	
Time (s)	**x Coordinate (m)**	**y Coordinate (m)**
0.2	3.92	3.72
0.4	7.69	6.92
0.6	11.32	9.64
0.8	14.83	11.91
1.0	18.21	13.75
1.2	21.49	15.16
1.4	24.66	16.17
1.6	27.73	16.78
1.8	30.71	16.99
2.00	33.61	16.81
2.20	36.42	16.25
2.400	39.16	15.29
2.60	41.82	13.96
2.80	44.42	12.26
3.00	46.95	10.19
3.20	49.41	7.79
3.40	51.82	5.07
3.60	54.17	2.03
3.73	55.67	− 0.09

* It is assumed that the baseball starts from $x = 0$, $y = 0$ and that the projection and landing heights are the same.

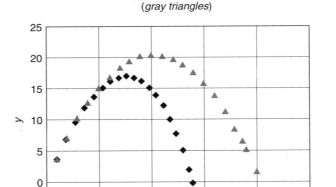

Baseball with drag (*black diamonds*) and without drag (*gray triangles*)

Figure 5.13 Using data from Table 5.2, a comparison of the trajectories for a projected baseball with and without drag. Initial velocities are the same for both trajectories.

that the range obtained with drag is just 68.2% of what it would have been with no drag. The x–y trajectory can also be calculated for the baseball in the absence of drag, giving a parabolic shape (see Section 3.5). This can be compared with the trajectory for the baseball subject to the drag force. Figure 5.13 shows the comparison between the two cases. Notice that the ''with drag'' trajectory is asymmetrical about a vertical axis passing through the point of maximum height. The curve is ''snub nosed'' in the sense that it approaches the baseline more steeply on the righthand side of the maximum because the drag term is reducing the horizontal velocity but the ball continues to accelerate downward.

We can see the effect of velocity on the drag term in Table 5.3, which shows the range computed for a baseball projected at a number of different velocities, all at an angle of 45°. It can be seen that the effect of the drag is almost negligible when the vertical and horizontal velocities are 5 m/s. However, the effect of the drag increases dramatically with velocity so that at 25 m/s, the range has decreased to 58.8% of the range to be expected with no drag.

The variation of range with projection angle is also different when drag is acting on the ball. Table 5.4 shows the variation of range with angle θ for angles close to 45°. This shows that for $v_x = 20$ m/s, $v_y = 20$ m/s, the angle for maximum range is about 43.5°. The same data are shown in the graph of Figure 5.14.

Table 5.3	The computed range for a baseball projected at various speeds and at an angle of 45°*			
V_x (m/s)	V_y (m/s)	Range (with Drag) (m)	Range (Without Drag) (m)	Range (with Drag; %)
5	5	4.92	5.10	96.50
10	10	18.14	20.41	88.00
15	15	36.08	45.92	78.60
20	20	55.67	81.63	68.20
25	25	75.03	127.50	58.8

* $K = 0.01$, $g = 9.8$ ms^{-2}. It is assumed that projection and landing heights are the same.

Table 5.4	Variation of range with projection angle*
Angle $\upsilon°$	**Range (m)**
42	56.79
43	56.82
44	56.82
45	56.77
46	56.58

* The baseball is projected with velocity of 28.28 m/s and angle υ measured with respect to the horizontal. The value of k is taken as 0.00934 m^{-1}.

For a golf ball, the ball parameters are:

Mass, m = 0.046 kg

Area, A = 0.0042 m^2

Radius, r = 3.66 cm

So that the value of k is:

$$\frac{0.5 \times 1.29 \times 0.0042}{2 \times 0.046} = 0.00982 \text{ m}^{-1}$$

By coincidence, the values of k for the baseball and the golf ball are very similar; this is because the ratio A/m is almost the same for both balls. This implies that the results we have obtained for a baseball are equally valid for a golf ball. However, this ignores the effect of dimples on a golf ball and the effect of spin, which is introduced in Chapter 11.

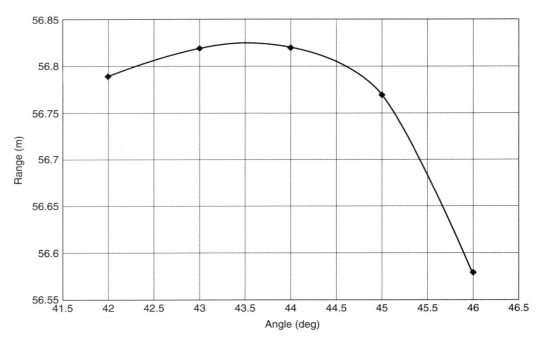

Figure 5.14 Using data from Table 5.4, variation of range with projection angle for a projected baseball.

SUMMARY

Chapter 5 begins by considering the inertial properties of material objects and their natural motion. The chapter also introduces Newton's first and second laws and thus formally establishes the relationship between mass, force, and acceleration. The means by which mass and force can be measured are explored, particularly by reference to modern measurement devices such as strain gauges, load cells, and force platforms. Some typical biomechanics applications are discussed, including COP measurements and GRF measurements during vertical jumps. The relationship between action forces and reaction forces is summarized through a discussion of Newton's third law. This is particularly useful when considering the frictional forces at work in everyday situations such as objects standing on inclined surfaces and cars driving around curves. Newton's laws are also explored from the alternative viewpoint of linear momentum. Finally, the motion of a projectile in the presence of a drag force is considered as an illustration of a case in which motion cannot be considered as uniform.

REFERENCES

McCall MW: *Classical Mechanics. A Modern Introduction.* New York: John Wiley & Sons; 2000.

Regtien PPL: *Electronic Instrumentation.* Delft, The Netherlands: Delft University Press; 2004.

STUDY QUESTIONS

1. A ball is rolled across a flat level floor with a speed of 2 m/s. If there is zero friction between the floor and the ball, what is the speed of the ball?

    (a) after 1 s

    (b) after 2 s

    (c) after it has rolled for 10 m?

    This is an idealized case that would probably never happen in practice. Discuss a few ways in which a real ball might be slowed down after a certain length of time or after rolling a certain distance.

2. Work out the gravitational force on the body of an athlete of mass 80 kg at sea level. Assume the Earth is a perfectly spherical body with a radius of 6.38×10^6 m corresponding to sea level. Newton's law of gravitation is $F = G\frac{m_1 m_2}{r^2}$. If the athlete were at an athletics stadium 5000 m above sea level, calculate the difference this would make in your answer.

3. A sprinter taking part in a 100-m race accelerates from rest to a final speed of 10 m/s in a time of 1.5 s. If his body mass is 65 kg, what is the net force acting on his body averaged over this 1.5-s time interval?

4. A soccer ball is kicked from the penalty spot toward the goal. Draw a diagram showing the instantaneous forces acting on the sneaker and on the ball while the two are in contact. Estimate the magnitude of the forces involved given that the mass of the ball is 0.2 kg and it is accelerated from 0 to 20 m/s in a time of 0.01 s. State any assumptions that you have to make.

5. What is the weight of a 25-kg mass?

6. The coefficient of static friction between a sled and the snow is 0.18, with a coefficient of dynamic friction of 0.15. A boy weighing 250 N sits on the 250-N sled. How much force parallel to the horizontal surface is required to start the sled in motion? How much force is required to keep the sled in motion?

7. A 70-kg box is to be slid across the floor. The coefficient of static friction between the box and the floor is 0.65, and the coefficient of dynamic friction is 0.62.

   (a) How much force is required to start the box in motion?

   (b) How much force is required to keep it in motion?

   The acceleration attributable to gravity = 9.81 m/s^2

8. A 150-kg sled is pulled across a horizontal surface. If the coefficient of dynamic friction is 0.3, what is the force required to accelerate the sled by 3 m/s^2?

9. A 20-kg box resting on a horizontal surface is pulled by a horizontal force of 100 N. If the resulting acceleration is 4 m/s^2, what is the coefficient of dynamic friction?

10. A 1000-kg car negotiates a curve in a track with a radius of curvature of 7.5 m. The angle of banking on this section of track is 20°. The coefficient of friction between the tires and the road surface is 0.65. What is the maximum speed at which the car can take the corner? What is the centripetal force acting on the car at this speed?

11. A golf ball rolling across an artificial surface encounters a coefficient of rolling friction of 0.002. How far will the ball roll across the surface given that the starting speeds are (a) 2.5m/s and (b) 5 m/s? The mass of the golf ball is 0.046 kg.

12. What is the momentum of a sprinter running at 9 m/s? The mass of the sprinter is 70 kg.

13. A tennis player returns a 120 mph serve with a return speed of 85 mph. What is the change in momentum of the tennis ball? Assume the mass of the tennis ball is 0.1 kg and that 1 mile is 1.6 km. (Convert the speed to meters per second first.)

   If the time of racquet contact was 5 ms (5 milliseconds = 0.005 s), calculate the average force acting on the ball (or racquet) during this time. Sketch a vector diagram showing the forces on the ball and on the racquet.

14. Use a spreadsheet method to calculate the trajectory of a football kicked at an angle of 45° with initial speeds of (a) 5, (b) 10, (c) 15, (d) 20, and (e) 25 m/s. Assume the mass of the ball is 0.3 kg, its radius is 12.5 cm, and its C$_D$ value is 0.5. Work out the range achieved by each kick assuming that projection and landing heights are the same.

CHAPTER six

DYNAMICS II

CHAPTER *objectives*

The objectives of this chapter are to:

■ Continue the discussion of dynamics to include energy, work, power, momentum, conservation laws, and application to oscillations.

CHAPTER *outcomes*

After reading this chapter, the student will be able to:

■ Calculate the work done by constant and varying forces.
■ Perform calculations of kinetic energy, potential energy, and strain energy.
■ Apply the law of conservation of mechanical energy.
■ Work out the power in simple movements.
■ Understand conservation of momentum and impulses.
■ Distinguish between elastic and inelastic collisions.
■ Understand and do simple calculations on damped and undamped oscillations.

6.1   Work Done by a Constant Force

Let us consider a force, F, being applied to a load that can be moved. Under some circumstances, the load will move in the same direction as the force applied. This implies that a displacement vector d exists that is parallel with the vector F. It can be shown that such a displacement requires the expenditure of energy, a quantity that is of fundamental importance in human movement. We say that *mechanical work is done* by the force F. Energy can be used in general for a wide variety of tasks; some examples where energy is put to use are:

Lifting a weight up to a given height
Charging a battery
Heating an object to a given temperature

Figure 6.1 Force (F) and displacement (d) acting along the same straight line. The work done is simply $W = F \times d$.

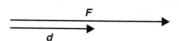

Boiling water

Accelerating an object to a given speed

In these examples, it may appear that the energy involved is different in some cases; for example, whereas heating an object and boiling water are both said to involve a form of energy called *heat*, lifting a weight and accelerating an object involve application of a force to a moveable point on the object and use a form of energy that we might describe as *mechanical energy*. In the case of a battery being charged, it would appear that the energy is in yet a different form, *electrical energy*. All these different forms of energy can be shown to be equivalent to each other and, in fact, in certain circumstances, energy can be converted from one form into another. Examples of this energy conversion are apparent in the examples we have already considered. In the case of a mass being lifted, mechanical work is being done to increase the potential energy (PE) of the mass. With a battery being charged, electrical energy from a generator is being stored as chemical energy in the battery. Heating or boiling water with an electrical heater involves conversion of electrical energy into heat energy. Accelerating an object involves performance of work to increase the kinetic energy (KE) of the object.

Considering a force, **F**, moving through a displacement, **d**, (Fig. 6.1), when the applied force and the displacement are in the same straight line, the **work done** can be calculated as:

$$\text{Work done} = \text{Force} \times \text{Distance moved}$$

In other cases, the force **F** and displacement **d** are acting along different directions (Fig. 6.2). Consider a man pushing against a toboggan at some angle θ to the direction of motion of the toboggan. In the case of the force **F** and displacement **d** shown in Figure 6.2, the work done is given by the force multiplied by the distance moved in the direction of the force, that is, $W = F\,d\cos\theta$.

In terms of the scalar product of the vectors, as explained in Section 1.7, this can be expressed simply as:

$$W = \boldsymbol{F} \cdot \boldsymbol{d}$$

In the SI (international system) of units, forces are measured in Newtons (N) and distances in meters (m) so that work, W, can be expressed in units of Nm. These units can also be referred to as Joules (J). One Joule would, therefore, be the work done when a force of 1 N moves through a distance of 1 m in the same direction as the force.

Figure 6.2 Man pushing toboggan with a force (F) at some angle (θ) to the direction of motion. The work done is $W = F\,d\cos\theta$.

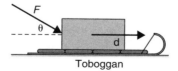

Toboggan

■ **EXAMPLE 6.1**

During a throw, a discus is subject to a force of 60 N for a distance of 50 cm. What is the work done on the discus? Assume the force acts along the same direction as the displacement.

Solution

The work done is:

$$W = F \times d$$
$$= (60 \text{ N}) \times (0.5 \text{ m})$$
$$= 30 \text{ Joules}$$

■ **EXAMPLE 6.2**

A rugby player in the scrum applies a force of 1000 N, but the scrum moves 1.5 m in a direction at 30° to the force (Fig. 6.3). What is the work done by the rugby player in this move?

Solution

The work done is:

$$W = Fd \cos\theta = (1000 \text{ N}) \times (1.5\text{m}) \times (0.866) = 1299 \text{ J}$$

6.2   Work Done by a Force That Varies

In most cases of practical interest, the force **F** is not fixed but is varying to a greater or lesser degree. In this case, the work done cannot be calculated by the method outlined in Section 6.1 because there is no single value that can be attributed to the force **F**. Let us consider the case where the varying force **F** and the displacement **d** are both acting along the same straight line, the x axis. Such a case might occur if someone is trying to compress a spring, for example, when the force required increases as the spring is compressed.

Another example is throwing a javelin when the throwing force is not constant but instead increases from zero, reaches a maximum, and then decreases back to zero as the javelin is released. Let us assume that F varies with x in some arbitrary fashion (Fig. 6.4). In Figure 6.4(**a**), the force is shown varying in a smooth and continuous manner over the range of x that is of interest (i.e., between the initial and final values x_i and x_f). We can imagine dividing up this range of x values in Figure 6.4(**a**) into a number of equal intervals of width Δx. Within each x interval, we can further imagine that the force F can be approximated by a constant value, equal to the average value of the force F over this interval. This has been done in Figure 6.4(**b**) for an arbitrary number of 10 such intervals. Thus, in interval 1, the value of the force is F_1. In interval 2, the value of the force is F_2, and so on, finally ending with the tenth interval and force F_{10}. The work done in each of these intervals

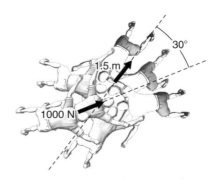

Figure 6.3   Rugby player applying force of 1000 N at 30° to direction of movement of scrum.

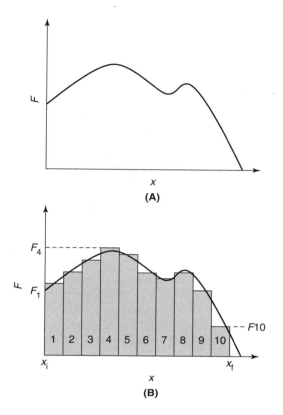

Figure 6.4 (A) A graph of force (F) that varies in an arbitrary manner with distance (x). (B) The same graph envisaged as being approximated by a force that varies in a stepwise manner (see text).

can then be calculated because the force is constant within each interval. Thus, the work done in interval 1 is (F_1) $\times$ (Δx), the work done in interval 2 is (F_2) $\times$ (Δx), and so on, finally finishing with the work done in the tenth interval, which is (F_{10}) $\times$ (Δx). It follows that the total work done can be approximated as:

$$W = (F_1) \times (\Delta x) + (F_2) \times (\Delta x) + \ldots\ldots\ldots + (F_{10}) \times (\Delta x)$$

or

$$W = (F_1 + F_2 + \ldots\ldots\ldots + F_{10}) \times (\Delta x)$$

where $\Delta x = (x_f - x_i)/10$ is the width of each interval on the x axis.

There might well be a small error in our answer for the work done because of the approximation we have been using to calculate it. However, the error will be quite small and can be reduced even further if we take a greater number of intervals (e.g., 100). In this case, the widths of the intervals are clearly far narrower, the answer obtained is even closer to the true value, and we would write this sum of 100 terms as:

$$W = \sum_{i=1}^{100} F_i \, \Delta x$$

where $\Delta x = (x_f - x_i)/100$

Mathematically, it is clear that the number of intervals must be allowed to extend to infinity (∞) and then the summation becomes identical with the mathematical operation of **integration** (see Appendix 1). The work done is then written as:

$$W = \int_{x_i}^{x_f} F \times dx$$

The integral may be worked out analytically if there is an exact solution or numerically using an approximation technique if there is no exact solution.

6.3   Kinetic Energy

A moving object carries **energy** with it. This can be demonstrated by measuring the amount of energy necessary to stop a moving object. Moving objects thus possess the ability to increase the temperatures of other bodies and themselves, raise masses to a higher level, compress or stretch springs, or make other objects move. It is natural to ask, therefore, if a body is moving with velocity v, how much energy does it possess? Let us consider a cricket ball of mass m being thrown starting from a stationary position. Let us assume that the force, F, accelerating the ball, exerted by the hand, is constant in magnitude until the ball leaves the hand and is the total resultant force on the ball. This implies that the acceleration of the ball will be uniform. Let us also assume that the time of acceleration is t. We may assume that the ball leaves the hand with velocity v at the end of time t. The work done by F is given by $F \times$ Distance moved in direction of force.

The distance moved can be estimated from the time, the final velocity, and the force. The acceleration of the ball is:

$$a = F/m$$

The final velocity of the ball is:

$$v = at$$

The distance moved is:

$$s = \tfrac{1}{2}at^2 = \tfrac{1}{2}a\left(\frac{v}{a}\right)^2 = \tfrac{1}{2}v^2\,\frac{m}{F}$$

Thus, it can be seen that the work done on the ball is:

$$F \times \tfrac{1}{2}v^2\,\frac{m}{F} = \tfrac{1}{2}mv^2$$

This quantity can be taken as a useful expression for the **kinetic energy** (KE) of the ball. A similar type of analysis could also be undertaken for the work that would be required to stop a moving ball, with identical results. A final expression for KE is:

$$KE = \tfrac{1}{2}mv^2$$

■ **EXAMPLE 6.3**   Calculate the KE of a sprinter of mass 70 kg moving at 10 m/s.

Solution

$$KE = 0.5 \times (70\ \text{kg}) \times (10\ \text{m/s})^2 = 3500\ \text{Joules}$$

■ **EXAMPLE 6.4**   How much work would have to be done to stop a ball of mass 0.5 kg traveling at 20 m/s? If the stopping force is applied over a distance of 0.4 m, what is the magnitude of the stopping force, assuming that it is constant?

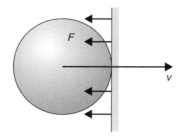

Figure 6.5 Ball being stopped by a braking force.

Solution

Work required = 0.5 × (0.5 kg) × (20 m/s)^2 = 100 Joules

Let us call the stopping force F (Fig. 6.5). The work done is calculated as F × d, so that:

$$100 \text{ J} = (F) \times (0.4 \text{ m})$$
$$F = 100/0.4 = 250 \text{ N}$$

Before leaving the subject of KE, it is worth mentioning that the formula KE = $\frac{1}{2}mv^2$ is widely applicable in general and is not restricted to cases in which the accelerating force is constant. Rotating objects (e.g., spinning balls, turntables) also have rotational KE; this is discussed further in Chapter 8.

6.4   Gravitational Potential Energy

Gravitational potential energy, often abbreviated as PE, is the energy attributable to an object by virtue of its position in a gravitational field. We saw in Section 5.7 the relationship between the acceleration attributable to gravity and the weight of an object. It is quite simple to calculate the work done on an object as it is moved up or down near the surface of the Earth. Consider an object of mass m lifted from the floor (height = 0) up to a new height, h, above the floor (Fig. 6.6).

The weight of the object, given by mg, is assumed to be constant over the range of movement of the object, and this holds true provided h is much less than the radius of the Earth. Because the radius of the Earth is about 6000 km, this is not a serious restriction on the height. Lifting this object to height h will require work to be done on the object:

Work done = Force × Distance moved in direction of force
= (mg) × h

This amount of work is then assumed to reside permanently as PE in the object, so that:

$$PE = mgh$$

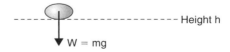

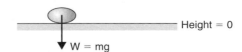

Figure 6.6   A mass (m) being raised from the floor up to a height (h).

Figure 6.7 A mass (*m*) being moved from the floor to a height (*h*) along a complex trajectory. The potential energy of the object is still *mgh* even though it has taken a complicated route to acquire its height.

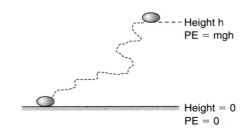

Height h
PE = mgh

Height = 0
PE = 0

It also follows from this that the PE does not depend on the path taken connecting the points at height 0 and height *h*. In the above instance, the weight was moved vertically upward a distance *h*, but the movement could have included side-to-side displacements without altering the PE. Figure 6.7 shows a mass being moved along a complicated trajectory but still ending up at a height *h* above the ground.

■ **EXAMPLE 6.5**

A pole vaulter of body mass 70 kg succeeds in clearing a bar that is 6 m above the ground. Calculate his PE at the top of the vault. (Assume $h = 6$ m and $g = 9.81$ m/s^2.)

Solution

$$PE = mgh = (70 \text{ kg}) \times (9.81 \text{ m/s}^2) \times (6 \text{ m})$$
$$= 4120.2 \text{ Joules}$$

6.5   Conservation of Mechanical Energy

It has been found in experiments that energy is a conserved quantity in nature. In mechanical systems, the energy of the system or constituent parts of the system can usually be identified as follows:

KE (as in objects that are moving)
Gravitational PE (as in the lifting or lowering of masses)
Strain potential energy (SE, as in the compression or extension of a spring)

In such a mechanical system, if the system is isolated, meaning no work is being done on or by the system involving external sources, then the sum total of all the mechanical energies in the system is a constant quantity. Putting this another way, if 1 represents a time, t_1, and 2 represents a later time, t_2, then:

$$KE_1 + PE_1 + SE_1 = KE_2 + PE_2 + SE_2$$

This equation is merely saying that if KE is reduced for whatever reason, then the sum of gravitational PE plus strain PE must be increased by the same amount. Such a mechanical system could be any system involving masses being increased or decreased, masses moving with varying speeds, pulleys with strings, or with springs being compressed or stretched. However, such a system is somewhat idealized, and it would not be very easy to find a system anything like this in practice. A real system would inevitably involve friction, as discussed in Section 5.9. The presence of friction implies that some of the mechanical energy in the system would be converted into different forms of energy not accounted for so far, mainly heat and sound. An example of this is a pulley wheel whose bearing is not perfect (not frictionless); if a string under tension causes such a pulley to rotate, the friction will cause a slight temperature rise in the pulley wheel, causing an increase in the thermal energy (heat) of the wheel and eventually the whole system. This thermal energy can be accounted for simply by including a **thermal energy** (ThE) term in the energy balance sheet. It may also be of interest that the temperature increase ΔT of an object of mass m can be worked out simply in terms of the amount of heat energy deposited in it and the specific heat capacity, c, of the material.

$$\Delta T = \frac{ThE}{c \times m}$$

where ΔT = temperature rise in degrees Celsius; c = specific heat capacity in Joules per kilogram; m = mass in kilograms; and ThE = thermal energy deposited in the object.

■ EXAMPLE 6.6

A skier begins a downhill section starting at 3 m/s. A short time later, as he is passing the judges' vantage point, his drop (height reduction) has been 15 m. Assuming his descent on the downhill section was frictionless, what was his final speed as he is passing the judges?

Solution

Assuming conservation of mechanical energy, because there is no mechanical strain energy in this case:

$$PE_1 + KE_1 = PE_2 + KE_2$$

We can assume for convenience that the PE at the start of the run is 0. The PE after the 15-m drop will be negative. Therefore, if the velocity after descent is v
Dividing throughout by m and rearranging:

$$v^2 = (9) + (2 \times 15 \times 9.81) = 303.3$$

so that:

$$v = 17.4 \text{ m/s}$$

■ EXAMPLE 6.7

A trapeze artist (mass, 75 kg) falls from a high-wire position a distance of 22 m to make a soft landing on a safety mattress. On landing, he rebounds to a distance of 1 m above the mattress.

(a) Calculate the trapeze artist's KE just before he hits the mattress for the first time, assuming no air resistance is present.
(b) Discuss what happens to this energy as the trapeze artist lands on the mattress, causing the mattress to deform. Would you expect the temperature of the mattress to increase? Explain your reasoning.
(c) When the trapeze artist is at a height of 1 m above the mattress with zero velocity (first bounce), what has happened to the energy in the system?

Solution

The trapeze artist's initial gravitational PE is:

$$mgh = (75 \text{ kg}) \times (9.81 \text{ m/s}^2) \times (22 \text{ m}) = 16186.5 \text{ J}$$

If no air resistance is present, this will be the same as his KE just before hitting the mattress for the first time.

(a) KE = 16186.5 J

(b) As he lands on the mattress, some of the energy may be converted into mechanical strain energy, especially if there are springs or springy materials making up the structure of the mattress. Also, it would be expected that a lot of the energy would go into thermal energy, thus increasing the temperature of the mattress. There may also be some sound energy created so that there would be an audible noise when he hit the mattress.

(c) If he rebounds to a height of 1 m, some mechanical strain energy was, indeed, stored in the mattress, albeit a fairly small amount. It would be reasonable to assume that the new gravitational PE:

$$(= 75kg) \times (9.81 \text{ m/s}^2) \times (1 \text{ m}) = 735.75 \text{ J})$$

is equal to the strain energy that was stored in the mattress. It is clear that a large fraction of the initial PE has been apparently "lost," but most of it is probably still present as thermal energy or heat in the mattress. The thermal energy is difficult to convert back efficiently into KE and PE, so it is natural to regard this energy as being "lost" and irrecoverable, although some of it might be recovered if special steps were taken.

6.6 Power

Power is the rate of doing work or the rate of energy transfer. The units of power are Joules per second (J/s), also known as Watts (W).

$$Power(W) = \frac{Energy(J)}{Time(s)}$$

In a previous system of units, energy was measured in units called calories defined as the amount of heat required to increase the temperature of 1 g of water by 1°C under specified ambient conditions. You will recall from Section 6.1 that 1 Joule is the work done when the point of application of a force of 1 N moves through a distance of 1 m. Experiments have shown that a calorie is equivalent to 4.186 J. It is still advantageous to remember this conversion because many foods are still quoted as "calories or kilocalories per 100-g portion".

■ **EXAMPLE 6.8**

A person doing a squat exercise raises a 180-kg mass by a distance of 1.2 m in a time of 2.1 s. What is the power?

Solution

The question is asking for the rate of doing work on the bar. We can assume that this can be worked out from the increase in the PE of the mass divided by the time taken, so:

$$power = \frac{(180kg) \times (9.81m/s^2) \times (1.2m)}{2.1s} = 100.9W$$

6.7 Impulsive Forces and Collisions

6.7.1 THE IMPULSE–MOMENTUM RELATIONSHIP

Forces that occur over very short time intervals are called **impulsive forces**. They occur, for example, when a football is kicked or a golf ball is struck by a club. The force only occurs when the two bodies are in contact; this usually occurs on a

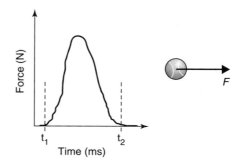

Figure 6.8 A ball under the influence of a short-duration force (F) such as might be encountered in kicking or striking.

timescale of milliseconds with both bodies deforming to a greater or smaller extent during the collision. Let us consider an object, for example, a ball of mass m being subjected to a short-duration force such as being hit with a bat (Fig. 6.8). The initial velocity of the ball is 0, and the force is applied along a direction from left to right. We will call this direction the x axis.

Clearly, the effect of this impulsive force will be to make the ball move to the right. The question is by how much? The force is clearly not constant because it increases from 0 to some maximum value and then decreases back to 0 again in a time of a few milliseconds. If we could divide up the interval between t_1 and t_2 into a lot of very small time intervals, then we could approximate and say that the force was constant over each of the intervals. If we say that the force is F exerted between t and $t + \Delta t$, then from Newton's second law, we can calculate the change in the velocity of the ball during this time interval. If the velocity of the ball at time t is v, then the acceleration of the ball is given by force divided by mass:

$$\frac{\Delta v}{\Delta t} = \frac{F}{m}$$

You will recall from Section 2.5 that acceleration is velocity divided by time. That the change in velocity is:

$$\Delta v = \frac{F}{m} \Delta t$$

It makes of sense to let the number of time intervals tend toward infinity so that Δt becomes an infinitesimally small interval or differential, dt. The differential velocity change is then:

$$dv = \frac{F}{m} dt$$

To get the total effect of the force, we would evaluate the total velocity change by the mathematical process of integration (Appendix 1) between limits t_1 and t_2

$$v_2 - v_1 = \frac{1}{m} \int_{t_1}^{t_2} F dt$$

The result of this integration depends on the magnitude of F and its variation with t. Rearranging this equation slightly gives:

$$m v_2 - m v_1 = \int_{t}^{t_2} F dt$$

The force function integrated over time between t_2 and t_1 is defined as the **impulse**. Therefore:

Change in momentum of the ball $=$ Impulse

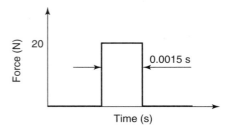

Figure 6.9 A graph of a force of 20 N applied to an object for 0.0015 s.

6.7.2 SPECIAL CASE OF A CONSTANT IMPULSIVE FORCE

Consider a ball struck with an implement such that the force applied is constant over the time interval between t_2 and t_1. Let us consider a ball of mass 0.2 kg and an impulsive force of 20 N applied for a time of 0.0015 s. This force as a function of time is shown in Figure 6.9. Such a constant impulsive force is highly unlikely to occur in practice, but it may be useful to think of this case as a useful approximation when dealing with forces that can be considered to be almost constant. In this case:

$$mv_2 - mv_1 = \int_t^{t_2} F dt$$

so that

$$0.2 \times (v_2 - v_1) = \int_0^{0.0015} 20\, dt = \left[20t\right]_0^{0.0015} = 20 \times 0.0015 - 20 \times 0$$

$$= 0.03 kg.m.s^{-1}$$

This number is equal to the area enclosed between the F–t curve and the t axis. (See Appendix 1 for an explanation of integration.) It follows that the velocity change is 0.15 m/s, so that if the ball started from rest, its final velocity would be 0.15 m/s.

6.7.3 COLLISIONS IN ONE DIMENSION

Many events in sports rely on collisions between objects as an integral part of the action. Consider the following collisions:

Ice hockey puck with hockey stick
Golf ball and golf club
Hand and ball in volleyball
Ball and bat in baseball
Foot and ball in soccer
Ball and ball in billiards

In each of these cases, the force between the colliding partners only exists for a short time and, by Newton's third law, is equal and opposite on the two objects. Consider, for example, Figure 6.10 and the forces acting on a bat and a ball during

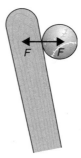

Figure 6.10 Two objects in collision (e.g., a bat and a ball) and subject to equal and opposite forces (*F*) as determined by Newton's third law.

a collision. The impulse on the two objects will thus also be the same but clearly of opposite sign because the force on the ball is in the opposite direction to the force on the bat. The change in the momentum of the ball will then clearly be same numerically as the change in the momentum of the bat but will be, of course, in the opposite direction. If we assign symbols m_{bat} and m_{ball} for the masses of the bat and ball, respectively, then we can say that:

$$m_{bat}\,(v_{bat}(2) - v_{bat}(1)) \; = \; -\,m_{ball}\,(v_{ball}(2) - v_{ball}(1)) \; = \; \int_{t_1}^{t_2} F dt$$

where $v_{bat}(1)$ and $v_{bat}(2)$ are the initial and final velocities of the bat and $v_{ball}(1)$ and $v_{ball}(2)$ are the initial and final velocities of the ball, respectively.

6.7.4 CONSERVATION OF LINEAR MOMENTUM

It follows from the discussion in Section 6.7.3 that linear momentum is conserved. In the example on the collision between the bat and the ball, the decrease in the momentum of the bat is the same magnitude as the increase in the momentum of the ball. Therefore, the total momentum (i.e., that of the bat and ball together) is unchanged. This can be viewed as a general law that is just as valid as Newton's second law from which it is derived. It must be applied with caution, however, because we have to be quite clear what "system" is being referred to. In the case of the example in Section 6.7.3, the bat and ball are considered as isolated from everything else so that there were no other forces to be considered. In a real case, perhaps the hand holding the bat would exert additional forces not accounted for by this analysis.

To reinforce the point about momentum being conserved, let us take the simple case of two billiards balls colliding head on a pool table (Fig. 6.11). If we assume that the cue ball is projected at a speed of 2 m/s from left to right toward a stationary object ball, the outcome may be two billiards balls that are both moving after the collision. In this case, we would expect conservation of momentum to apply, so that:

Total momentum before collision = Total momentum after collision

Taking momentum to the right to be positive:

total momentum before collision = $2m + 0 = 2m$

where m is the mass of a billiards ball.

Total momentum after collision = $v_2\,m + v_1\,m$

$$2m = v_2\,m + v\,m$$
$$2 = v_2 + v_1$$

Any combination of v_2 and v_1 giving this result is acceptable in the sense that conservation of momentum applies. For example, $v_1 = 0.5$, $v_2 = 1.5$, or $v_1 = 0$,

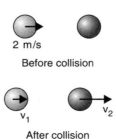

2 m/s

Before collision

v_1 v_2

After collision

Figure 6.11 A collision between two billiards balls.

$v_2 = 2$, or even $v_1 = -1$, $v_2 = 3$. The real outcome will be determined by energy conservation or otherwise (see Section 6.5) in the collision plus other factors such as whether spin is applied to the cue ball.

6.7.5 ELASTIC AND INELASTIC COLLISIONS

It is noted in Section 6.5 that mechanical energy can often be said to be conserved within certain systems. In some systems, this means interchange of energy between the various kinetic, potential, and strain energy forms. During collisions between two or more objects, it is possible to distinguish between collisions in which KE is conserved and those in which it is not conserved. Collisions in which KE is conserved are known as **elastic** collisions. In these kinds of collisions, the total KE of the system after the collision is the same as the total KE before the collision. The simplest example of this is probably a rubber ball bouncing on a solid surface such as concrete. If the ball is dropped from a height h_0 and returns to the same height after bouncing, the collision with the floor is clearly elastic. The velocity of the ball just before the bounce is:

$$v_1 = \sqrt{2gh_0}$$

and its corresponding KE is:

$$\tfrac{1}{2}mv_1^2 = mgh_0.$$

For an "elastic" bounce, the velocity just after the bounce is clearly the same as the velocity just before the bounce, except that the direction is reversed. We can define a **coefficient of restitution** e such that it is equal to the ratio of the speeds of the ball just after (v_2) and just before (v_1) the collision:

$$e = \frac{v_2}{v_1}.$$

For an elastic collision:

$$v_2 = v_1 \text{ and } e = 1$$

Moreover, different balls and surfaces exhibit different bounces and hence different values of the coefficient e. For most real cases, the value of e will be less than 1, and the collisions (or bounce) will be **inelastic**. An example of an inelastic bounce is a ball bearing dropped on a soft and compliant floor, something like putty, for example. In this case, the bounce may be very small, and the coefficient of restitution would be close to 0. The value of e will be in the range $0 \leq e \leq 1$ with $e = 0$ corresponding to a completely inelastic (or plastic) collision and $e = 1$ corresponding to a perfectly elastic collision.

■ **EXAMPLE 6.9**

A good example to begin with is probably the example of two billiards balls colliding on a pool table. Let us assume initially that, in the collision, both linear momentum and KE are conserved. Initially, the cue ball is moving with velocity v_1, and the object ball is at rest. After the collision, let us assume that the velocities of the cue and object balls are v_2 and v_3, respectively. The situations before and after the collision are shown in Figure 6.12. What are the velocities of the two balls after the collision?

Analysis

Conservation of linear momentum is:

$$mv_1 = mv_2 + mv_3 \tag{1}$$

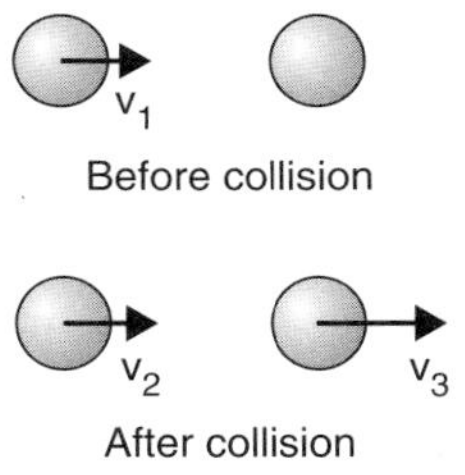

Before collision

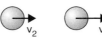

After collision

Figure 6.12 A collision between two billiards balls assuming that both linear momentum and energy are conserved.

Conservation of KE (perfectly elastic) is:

$$\tfrac{1}{2}mv_1^2 = \tfrac{1}{2}mv_2^2 + \tfrac{1}{2}mv_3^2 \tag{2}$$

Dividing (1) by m gives:

$$v_1 = v_2 + v_3 \tag{1*}$$

Dividing (2) by $\tfrac{1}{2}m$ gives:

$$v_1^2 = v_2^2 + v_3^2 \tag{2*}$$

Substituting for v_1 from (1*) into (2*) gives:

$$(v_2 + v_3)^2 = v_2^2 + v_3^2$$

so that:

$$v_2^2 + v_3^2 + 2v_2v_3 = v_2^2 + v_3^2$$

implying that:

$$2v_2v_3 = 0.$$

The only way this can be true is if $v_2 = 0$ or if $v_3 = 0$. Clearly, this only makes sense if $v_2 = 0$ and $v_3 = v_1$. In other words, the cue ball has been stopped dead, and the velocity v_1 has been transferred to the object ball.

■ **EXAMPLE 6.10**

Let us now consider the two billiards balls colliding in a similar fashion: head on and with the object ball initially stationary. This time, let us consider an inelastic collision between the balls (Fig. 6.13).

Relative velocity before collision $= v_1$

Relative velocity after collision $= (v_3 - v_2)$
Assuming that we now have a coefficient of restitution e (< 1), we have:

$$ev_1 = v_3 - v_2 \tag{3}$$

while conservation of linear momentum still gives

$$mv_1 = mv_2 + mv_3 \tag{4}$$

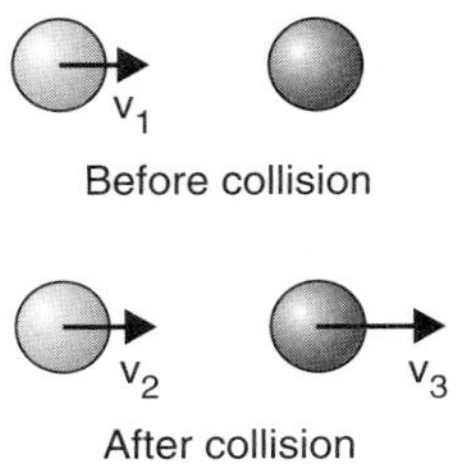

Before collision

After collision

Figure 6.13 An inelastic collision between two billiards balls.

Dividing (4) by m gives:

$$v_1 = v_2 + v_3 \tag{4*}$$

Rearranging (3) for v_1 gives:

$$v_1 = \frac{1}{e}(v_3 - v_2) \tag{3*}$$

Substituting for v_1 in terms of v_2 and v_3 yields:

$$\frac{1}{e}(v_3 - v_2) = v_2 + v_3$$

So that:

$$\frac{v_2}{v_3} = \frac{1 - e}{1 + e}$$

Also, it can be shown that:

$$v_2 = \frac{(1 - e)}{2} v_1$$

and:

$$v_3 = \frac{(1 + e)}{2} v_1$$

Clearly, if $e = 1$, $v_2 = 0$, and $v_3 = v_1$, we are dealing with the perfectly elastic case. If the collision is inelastic, there is a loss of KE determined by the coefficient of restitution. In this case, the total KE after the collision is:

$$\tfrac{1}{2}mv_2^2 + \tfrac{1}{2}mv_3^2 = \tfrac{1}{2}m\left(\frac{1-e}{2}\right)^2 v_1^2 + \tfrac{1}{2}m\left(\frac{1+e}{2}\right)^2 v_1^2 = \frac{mv_1^2}{2}\left(\frac{1+e^2}{2}\right)$$

CASE *Study 6.1*

Coefficient of Restitution of a Ball Measured by Incident and Rebound Velocities from a Steel Surface

A solid ball of rigid polymer construction and mass 0.25 kg is bounced off a flat, horizontal steel plate that is rigidly fixed to the ground. The initial and final velocities of the ball are measured by analysis of coordinate–time data obtained by optoelectronic motion measurement methods. For convenience, the ball can be considered to be moving in the x–z plane, with the z axis being the upward vertical and the x axis being in the plane of the steel plate aligned such that x points in the direction of horizontal motion of the ball. The initial and final velocity components are shown in Table 6.1. The coefficient of restitution can be calculated from the ratio of the incident and rebound velocities in the vertical direction:

$$e = \frac{4.7986}{9.3614} = 0.5126$$

The ratio of the horizontal velocities gives almost exactly the same value.

Table 6.1 Vertical and horizontal velocities of a ball before and after bouncing

	Time, t (s)	Vertical Velocity v_z (m/s)	Horizontal Velocity v_x (m/s)
Before bouncing	0.510	−9.3614	−6.7218
After bouncing	0.535	4.7986	−3.4117

Table 6.2	Height of bounce and coefficient of restitution for various types of balls with a drop height of 1.83 m	

Type of Ball	**Height of Bounce (m)**	**Coefficient of Restitution**
"Superball"	1.44	0.89
Basketball, football, or volleyball	1.06	0.76
Tennis ball: Old	0.91	0.71
Tennis ball: New	0.81	0.67
Hockey ball	0.46	0.50
Cricket ball	0.18	0.31

The KE before bouncing is

$$T = \tfrac{1}{2}mv^2 = \tfrac{1}{2} \times (0.25) \times (11.525)^2 = 16.6J$$

and after bouncing it is reduced to

$$T = \tfrac{1}{2}mv^2 = \tfrac{1}{2} \times (0.25) \times (5.888)^2 = 4.333J$$

The final value of T is e^2 times the initial value

For the case of a ball bouncing on a solid floor, the coefficient of restitution is conveniently calculated from the drop and rebound heights. If the height from which the ball is dropped is h_d and the height to which it bounces is h_b, then"

$$e = \sqrt{\frac{h_b}{h_d}}$$

The coefficient will depend on the ball and the surface. Table 6.2 shows some coefficients of restitution for balls dropped from 6 ft (1.83 m) onto a hardwood floor. Table 6.3 gives some coefficients of restitution for a volleyball dropped from 6 ft (1.83 m) onto various surfaces.

There is also a temperature effect on coefficients of restitution, as illustrated in Table 6.4.

Table 6.3	Height of bounce and coefficients of restitution for a volleyball dropped onto various surfaces with a height of drop of 1.83 m	

Surface	**Height of Bounce (m)**	**Coefficient of Restitution**
"Proturf"	1.05	0.76
Wood	1.03	0.75
Steel	1.02	0.75
Concrete	1.00	0.74
Tumbling mat (2.5 cm thick)	0.83	0.67
Gravel	0.67	0.61
Grass	0.34	0.43
Gymnastics landing mat	0.33	0.42

Table 6.4	Coefficients of restitution for a solid rubber ball and a golf ball under different temperature conditions		
Ball	**Cold (1 hour in freezer)**	**Normal**	**Hot (15 min at 225°)**
Solid rubber	0.57	0.73	0.80
Golf ball	0.67	0.80	0.84

6.7.6 Oblique Impacts

As well as direct or right-angle impacts, oblique impacts play a major part in many ball games. It is possible to resolve the velocity into two components, one parallel to the surface and one perpendicular to the surface. In the case of a ball bouncing on the floor, we can resolve into horizontal and vertical components (Fig. 6.14).

u = Velocity before impact

v = Velocity after impact

u_h = Horizontal component of velocity before impact

u_v = Vertical component of velocity before impact

v_h = Horizontal component of velocity after impact

v_v = Vertical component of velocity after impact

It follows that the coefficient of restitution is:

$$e = -\frac{v_v}{u_v}$$

If the ball and floor are perfectly smooth:

$$u_h = v_h$$

but friction will reduce v_h. For rough surfaces, therefore, u_h is greater than v_h. Figure 6.15 shows that, for a rough surface, the angle of incidence is not equal to the angle of reflection. In general, the angle of incidence is not equal to the angle of reflection. In fact, the two angles are equal only when the effect of friction on the horizontal velocity exactly balances the effect of elasticity on the vertical velocity.

6.7.7 Bat-and-Ball Games and the Effect of Spring

In bat-and-ball games, the speed of a ball after impact can be increased by:

1. Increasing the mass of the bat
2. Decreasing the mass of the ball
3. Increasing the initial velocity of the bat
4. Increasing the initial velocity of the ball
5. Increasing the angle of incidence (e.g., by hitting a glancing blow)
6. Increasing the value of the coefficient of restitution

The effect of spin on the bounce of balls is to vary the horizontal component of the initial velocity. This has the effect of changing the frictional effects. For example, if a ball has backspin, the frictional effects are increased (Fig. 6.16). But if the ball has topspin, the frictional effects are decreased (Fig. 6.17).

Consider a tennis ball projected with (a) no spin, (b) topspin, and (c) backspin (Fig. 6.18). The trajectories after bouncing with a surface would resemble those shown in Figure 6.19. Whereas the ball with topspin has considerably greater range than the ball with no spin, the range for a backspinning ball is reduced.

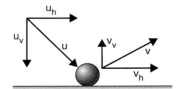

Figure 6.14 An oblique impact.

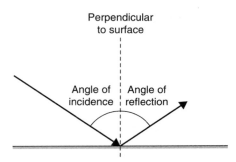

Figure 6.15 Angles of incidence and reflection.

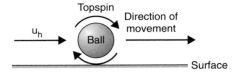

Figure 6.16 A ball with backspin bouncing off a surface.

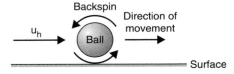

Figure 6.17 A ball with topspin bouncing off a surface.

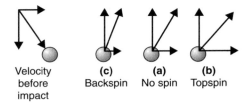

Figure 6.18 Velocity components before and after impact for a ball with (A) no spin, (B) topspin, and (C) backspin.

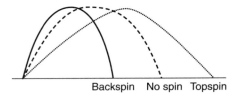

Figure 6.19 Possible trajectories for a tennis ball with no spin, backspin, and topspin.

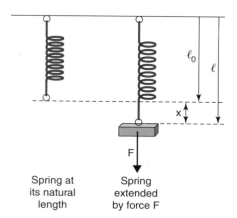

Figure 6.20 A spring being subjected to a stretching force (F) and extending by an amount (x).

Spring at
its natural
length

Spring
extended
by force F

6.8   Oscillations

6.8.1 SPRINGS AND HOOKE'S LAW

Springs and springy materials are useful for storage of elastic strain energy. An example is the use of a springy pole in pole vaulting that stores strain energy within it and helps to increase the height attainable by the jumper. Let us consider a spiral spring (Fig. 6.20), which is probably the simplest and best understood case. The fundamental law governing the behavior of springs is Hooke's law, which relates the extension (increase in length) of the spring to the applied force. **Hooke's law** states that the extension, x, is proportional to the applied force, F, provided that the extension is not too great (beyond the elastic limit of the spring):

$$F = -kx$$

The constant k is known as the **spring constant** or the **stiffness** of the spring and has units N/m. The extension of the spring is:

$$x = 1 - l_0$$

and is proportional to the applied force. The applied force clearly does work during the spring extension, and this energy is stored as strain energy in the spring. The spring force is clearly not constant during the extension but is of the form given by Hooke's law (Fig. 6.21).

The total work done can be worked out as the area under the F–x graph, so that:

$$\text{Work done} = \tfrac{1}{2} \times (x) \times (kx)$$

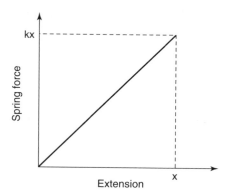

Figure 6.21 The straight-line relationship between the spring force and the extension.

This can be viewed as the elastic strain energy (SE), which is now stored in the spring, so that:

$$SE = \tfrac{1}{2} kx^2$$

Alternatively, this can be viewed as:

Average spring force × Extension

or

$$(\tfrac{1}{2} kx) \times x = \tfrac{1}{2} kx^2$$

Some springs are designed to operate in compression as well as in tension, but the same principles apply.

6.8.2 Oscillatory Motion

A mass suspended on a spring is subject to a **restoring force** that is proportional to the displacement, provided the extension is not so great as to exceed the elastic limit of the spring. If such a mass is displaced vertically and then released, it will oscillate and, provided certain conditions are met, will display simple harmonic motion (SHM). It is probably a good idea for students of mechanics and motion analysis to know about oscillatory motion because it is fundamental to the mechanics of many sports and, particularly, applied to sport equipment of various types. Some examples that may occur in sports situations are:

Vibrations and oscillations of racquets (e.g., squash, tennis)

Oscillations of membranes (e.g., trampolines)

The response of joints to sudden pulls and pushes (e.g., knee joint and ligaments)

Response of golf clubs to impact with golf balls

Although a detailed treatment of any of these examples is complex and beyond the scope of this book, it is instructive to look at a simpler example to illustrate the general nature of oscillations. Let us consider a mass m suspended on a spring of spring constant, k. Figure 6.22(a) shows the mass hanging stationary in equilibrium, and Figure 6.22(b) shows the mass displaced by an additional amount, X, by pulling or pushing. It is convenient to use a coordinate axis to describe the motion of the mass; in this case, let the origin be at the level A and the x axis point vertically down. For a general displacement x, the net restoring force on the mass m is:

$$F = - kx$$

So that, by Newton's second law, its acceleration is:

$$a = F/m = - kx/m$$

Figure 6.22 (A) Mass (_m_) hanging stationary in equilibrium at the level A. (B) Mass displaced by an amount (X) via an external agency; when released, the mass will oscillate about the level marked A.

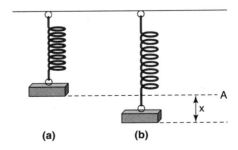

The minus sign indicates that the acceleration of the mass is upward. In terms of differential quantities, acceleration is $\dfrac{d^2x}{dt^2}$ so that we now have:

$$\frac{d^2x}{dt^2} = -\frac{k}{m}x$$

(Note that $\dfrac{d^2x}{dt^2}$ is the derivative of the velocity dx/dt; see Appendix 1 for more information on differentiation.)

If we put $\omega^2 = \dfrac{k}{m}$ this equation becomes:

$$\frac{d^2x}{dt^2} = -\omega^2 x$$

which has solutions of the following form:

$$x = A \cos(\omega t) + B \sin(\omega t)$$

If we assume that $x = X$ at $t = 0$, this will determine the constants A and B. Then:

$$X = A \cos(0) + B \sin(0) = A$$

so that the value of A is just X. Also, by experiment, it is found that the mass returns to $x = X$ after a time of T seconds. Therefore, the value of B is 0. The solution for x is:

$$x = X \cos(\omega t)$$

where:

$$\omega = \frac{2\pi}{T} = \sqrt{\frac{k}{m}}$$

A graph of this solution is shown in Figure 6.23, where the vertical axis is marked in units of X (the initial displacement) and the horizontal axis is time in seconds. For the purposes of this figure, the value of ω was taken as 0.6π. It can be seen that the function repeats itself after a time of 3.33 s. This is known as the **periodic time** T and is given by $2\pi/\omega$. The value of ω depends on the values of the spring constant, k, and the mass, m. The **frequency** of the oscillations is $f = 1/T$. This type of motion is often referred to as **simple harmonic motion (SHM).**

It is also possible to write down an expression for the velocity of the mass as a function of time, under the same initial conditions as we used previously, as follows:

$$v = -\omega X \sin(\omega t).$$

This function is graphed in Figure 6.24 and is plotted *directly under* the displacement graph of Figure 6.23 for comparison. It can be seen that when the displacement is a maximum, the velocity is 0. Also, when the displacement is 0, the velocity is a maximum, either positive or negative.

It is also possible to write down an expression for the speed of the oscillating mass at any value of displacement, x:

$$v = \omega \sqrt{X^2 - x^2}.$$

The KE of the oscillating mass can also be written down in two ways, either as a function of time, t, or as a function of displacement, x:

$$KE = \tfrac{1}{2}mv^2 = \tfrac{1}{2}m\omega^2 X^2 \sin^2(\omega t)$$

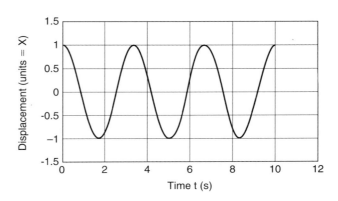

Figure 6.23
Displacement of a mass undergoing simple harmonic oscillations with a period of 3.33 s. This oscillation would continue forever in the absence of any friction forces.

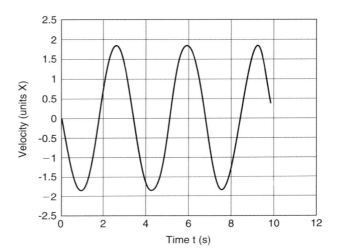

Figure 6.24 Velocity versus time for a mass undergoing simple harmonic motion. This figure uses the same mass, spring constant, and initial conditions as Figure 6.23.

or

$$K.E. = \tfrac{1}{2}mv^2 = \tfrac{1}{2}m\omega^2 \left(X^2 - x^2\right)$$

The gravitational PE of the oscillating mass can be written down simply as:

$$PE = -mgx$$

taking the level A as the reference level for measuring PE. The elastic strain energy in the spring is:

$$SE = \tfrac{1}{2}kx^2$$

As seen in Section 6.5, mechanical energy is conserved in isolated systems so that for a mass oscillating on a spring in the absence of friction or other types of energy loss, we can write that:

$$KE + PE + SE = \text{Constant}$$

or

$$\tfrac{1}{2}m\omega^2 \left(X^2 - x^2\right) - mgx + \tfrac{1}{2}kx^2 = \text{Constant}$$

6.8.3 DAMPED OSCILLATIONS

In real systems, friction always plays a part in determining the time for which oscillations persist. Sometimes friction is deliberately introduced to modify the dynamic

Figure 6.25 An oscillatory spring and mass system that is also subject to damping. The damping is shown as "friction force bv," and the spring force is shown as "−kx". The mass is assumed to be moving downward at a displacement (x) measured from the equilibrium position.

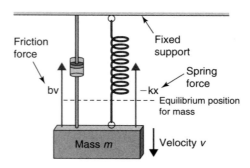

behavior of oscillatory systems; in these cases, the friction is usually referred to as **damping**. Figure 6.25 shows a spring supporting a mass that is subject to damping.

Applying Newton's second law for the net acceleration of the mass:

$$\frac{d^2x}{dt^2} = \frac{1}{m}\left(-b\frac{dx}{dt} - kx\right)$$

where b is a friction coefficient, thus introducing a frictional force proportional to the velocity of the mass. So, rearranging:

$$m\frac{d^2x}{dt^2} + b\frac{dx}{dt} + kx = 0$$

These equations will have three classes of solutions, depending on the relative magnitudes of k, m, and b. The three classes are:

(a) If $\left[\left(\frac{b}{m}\right)^2 - \frac{4k}{m}\right] < 0$, then the solution to the equation is of the form:

$$x = e(-\text{bt}/2\text{m}) \times \left[A\cos(\omega't) + B\sin(\omega't)\right]$$

where $\omega' = \sqrt{\dfrac{k}{m} - \dfrac{b^2}{4m^2}}$

This has the property of being a sinusoidal-type oscillation but having an amplitude that dies away to zero exponentially. This is called light damping or **underdamping**.

(b) If $\left[\left(\frac{b}{m}\right)^2 - \frac{4k}{m}\right] = 0$, then the solution exhibits the property of returning to zero displacement in the shortest possible time and with no oscillations. This is called **critical damping**.

(c) If $\left[\left(\frac{b}{m}\right)^2 - \frac{4k}{m}\right] > 0$, then the solution exhibits the property of returning to zero displacement in a longer time than for case (b) and with no oscillations. When $b^2 \gg 4mk$, the case is described as **overdamping**.

In the case of most oscillators moving through air as the damping medium, the damping is underdamping with several (or many) oscillations occurring before dying away completely. The time taken for oscillations to die down can be estimated from the time $t_1 = 2m/b$, which is the time taken for the oscillations to die down

$m = 0.2, k = 0.1, b1 = 0.1, b2 = 0.282,$
$b3 = $ larger value

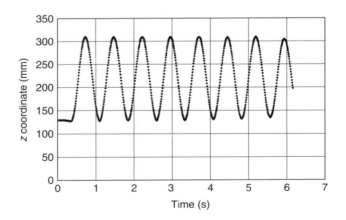

Figure 6.26 Three cases of damping. The value of the mass was 0.2 kg, and the value of the spring constant was 0.1 N/kg. In the case of the critical damped curve, the value of *b* used was 0.282. In the underdamped case, $b = 0.1$. Initial displacement = 10 U in all cases.

to $1/e$ of its value (e is a natural constant equal to about 2.7). Figure 6.26 shows the type of responses to be expected for examples of each of the three cases of damping.

CASE *Study 6.2*   **Calculation of the Friction Coefficient b in a Simple Mass–Spring Oscillator**

A mass of 320 g is suspended on a spring attached securely to a fixed support. The mass is pulled down and released from rest. The displacement of the mass in the vertical direction after release is shown in the following graph.

In this graph, the z coordinate is measured from an origin located some distance below the oscillating mass. The mass completes its first seven oscillations in 5.242 s, so that the periodic time is:

$$T = \frac{5.242}{7} = 0.749s$$

The small amount of damping results in the amplitude changing from 176.9 mm on the first oscillation to 169.1 mm on the seventh oscillation. To a good approximation, the effect of this small amount of damping on the period is negligible, so that the spring constant, k, can be calculated as:

$$\omega = \frac{2\pi}{T} = \sqrt{\frac{k}{m}}$$

so that

$$k = 0.32 \times \left(\frac{2\pi}{0.749}\right)^2 = 22.52 N/m$$

The friction coefficient, b, can be estimated from the initial and final amplitudes, A_1 and A_n, and the time, t, required to complete this number of cycles.

$$\log_e\left(\frac{A_n}{A_1}\right) = \frac{-bt}{2m}$$

$$b = -2 \times 0.32 \times \log_e\left(\frac{A_n}{A_1}\right)/6T = 0.0064 \text{ N s m}^{-1}$$

6.8.4 PENDULUMS

6.8.4.1 The Simple Pendulum

A **simple pendulum** consists of a small object or bob suspended from the end of a light cord attached to a rigid fixed support (Fig. 6.27). The weight, mg, can be resolved into two components; one along the direction of the cord ($mg \cos \theta$) and the other at right angles to the direction of the cord ($mg \sin \theta$).

Assuming that the cord is inextensible, the oscillating pendulum traces the arc of a circle as it moves with equal amplitude on either side of its equilibrium point. Figure 6.28 shows that the displacement, x, of the pendulum along the arc can be worked out from $x = L\theta$ where θ is the angle the cord makes with the vertical and L is the distance of the point of attachment from the center of mass of the bob.

If the restoring force is proportional to x or to θ, then the motion will be simple harmonic. The restoring force is the component of the weight tangential to the arc:

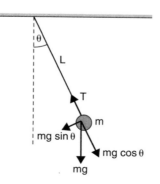

Figure 6.27 Simple pendulum of length. The weight of the bob is mg acting vertically, and the tension in the cord is T acting at an angle θ to the vertical.

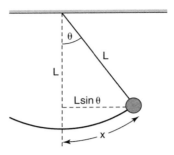

Figure 6.28 The displacement (x) of the mass measured along the circular arc is given by $x = L\theta$, where θ is measured in radians.

$$F = -mg \sin\theta$$

Because F is proportional to the sine of θ and not θ itself, the motion (in general) is not SHM. However, if θ is small, then $\sin\theta$ is very nearly equal to θ if the latter is specified in radians. Note that, from Figure 6.28, x is very nearly the same as the chord $L \sin\theta$ for small angles θ. Thus, to a very good approximation, for small angles:

$$F \sim -mg\,\theta$$

Using the fact that $x = L\theta$, we have:

$$F \sim -\frac{mg}{L}x$$

Thus, for small displacements, the motion is simple harmonic with an effective force constant given by $\frac{mg}{L}$. The period of a simple pendulum for small displacements is thus:

$$T = 2\pi\sqrt{\frac{m}{mg/l}} = 2\pi\sqrt{\frac{L}{g}}$$

It should be noted that the period of a simple pendulum does not depend on the mass.

6.8.4.2 The Physical Pendulum

This term applies to real (extended) bodies that can oscillate back and forth. Figure 6.29 shows a baseball bat suspended so that it can oscillate when disturbed from its equilibrium position. The force of gravity acts at G, the center of gravity (center of mass) of the baseball bat, which is a distance, h, from the pivot point, O. The physical pendulum is best analyzed using the equations of rotational motion. The torque on a physical pendulum, calculated about point O, is:

$$\tau = -mgh \sin\theta$$

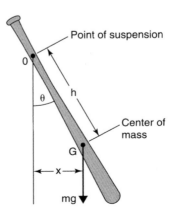

Figure 6.29 A baseball bat suspended from point O.

Newton's second law for rotational motion (see Section 8.2) gives:

$$\tau = I\alpha = I\frac{d^2\theta}{dt^2}$$

where I is the moment of inertia of the bat about an axis through the point of suspension and perpendicular to the plane of the page and $\alpha = \frac{d^2\theta}{dt^2}$ is the angular acceleration. Therefore:

$$I\frac{d^2\theta}{dt^2} = -mgh\sin\theta$$

so that:

$$\frac{d^2\theta}{dt^2} + \frac{mgh}{I}\sin\theta = 0$$

If θ is small, then $\sin\theta \approx \theta$ and

$$\frac{d^2\omega}{dt^2} + \left(\frac{mgh}{I}\right)\theta = 0$$

This is just the equation for SHM with an angular quantity replacing the usual linear displacement. For small angular displacement, the period, T, is:

$$T = 2\pi\sqrt{\frac{I}{mgh}}$$

CASE *Study 6.3* ■ **Acute Effects of Exercise on Passive Joint Stiffness**

The stiffness of a joint between body segments can be measured by the decay rate of natural oscillations of the leg–foot segment. The knee joint is modeled as a torsional spring providing a torque, $\tau = k\theta$, as shown here:

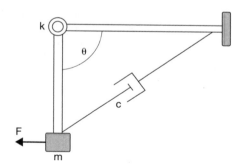

The diagram shows a spring-damper model used to describe the stiffness (k) and damping coefficient (c) of the knee (Ricard et al., 1996). The viscoelastic behavior of human joints can be modeled using a spring-damper model, as shown. A torsional spring with linear stiffness can be used to represent the elastic response of the actin–myosin filaments and connective tissue in the knee joint. The time-dependent behavior of connective tissue can be modeled using a viscous damping element, as shown. Ricard et al (1996) have reported an investigation into the variation of the knee joint stiffness as a function of exercise. The passive knee joint stiffness was measured before and after a weight training exercise bout in which knee flexion was undertaken at 75% of maximum load (0.75 RM).

Passive stiffness in a human joint is caused by muscular factors attributed to actin–myosin filaments and connective tissue factors that can be attributed to fascia, ligaments, and friction in the joint. The immediate effects of an exercise bout such as weight lifting are known to increase the stiffness of the joint involved. Lakie et al. (1988) found that joint stiffness increases after active or passive movements. However, little is known about the acute effects of exercise on joint stiffness immediately after exercise.

The Ricard (1996) study included 23 subjects with normal knees. Passive knee joint stiffness was measured before and after a weight training exercise bout. The exercise bout involved 10 sets of 10 single-knee extension/flexions at 75% of 1 RM (one repetition maximum) followed by 10 sets of 10 eccentric contractions. The stiffness of the relaxed knee was measured using an electrogoniometer. The position of the right knee was sampled for 6 s at 500 Hz. A typical result for knee joint angle versus time, a damped oscillation of the knee, is shown here:

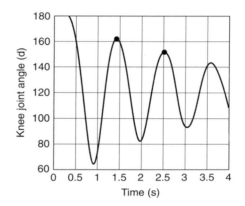

The stiffness and damping coefficients of the relaxed knee were determined with the subjects seated on a table. The lower extremity was supported by the researcher with the knee completely extended. As soon as the subject was completely relaxed, the leg–foot system was released, allowing the lower limb to freely oscillate until the lower leg came to rest in the vertical position. Five good trials were obtained before and after exercise. Stiffness was calculated from the first two complete cycles of oscillation. The logarithmic decrement (δ) of the oscillation was:

$$\delta = \log_e (A1/A2)$$

where $A1$ and $A2$ are the knee joint angles for the first two peaks in the oscillation. The viscous damping factor (ξ) was calculated as follows:

$$\xi = \sqrt{\frac{\delta}{4\pi^2 + \delta^2}}$$

where δ is the logarithmic decrement of the damped oscillation. (More information on the derivation and measurement of the viscous damping factor ξ is given in the Suggested Reading section.) The natural frequency of the oscillation (ω) was determined from the following equation:

$$\omega = \frac{\delta}{\xi \times T}$$

where δ is the logarithmic decrement, ξ is the viscous damping factor, and T is the time between oscillation peaks. The damping coefficient (c) was obtained as follows:

$$c = 2\xi\omega I$$

where ξ is the viscous damping factor, ω is the natural frequency, and I is the moment of

Table 6.5 Mean and standard deviation for joint stiffness, damping coefficient, and natural frequency of the knee joint before and after exercise

	Before Exercise	**After Exercise**
Joint stiffness (N(m/rad)	4.59 (1.23)	6.15 (2.32)
Damping coefficient (N(m/s/rad)	−0.014 (0.006)	−0.017 (0.009)
Natural frequency (Hz)	5.98 (0.33)	6.88 (0.94)

Data from Ricard, 1996.

inertia of the lower leg and foot about the knee joint. The passive stiffness (k) of the knee joint was obtained using the following equation:

$$k = I\omega^2$$

where I is the moment of inertia of the leg-foot and ω is the natural frequency. All five trials for stiffness (k) and damping coefficients (c) were averaged. Dependent t tests were used to test for significant differences in stiffness and damping after exercise.

Results

The acute effects of exercise on passive knee joint stiffness, damping coefficient, and natural frequency are shown in Table 6.5. Significant increases in passive knee joint stiffness, damping coefficient, and natural frequency were observed after exercise ($p < .05$). Mean passive knee joint stiffness increased by 1.56 N (m/rad) immediately after the exercise regimen. Single-knee extension strength decreased significantly from 37.8 (14.87 kg) before exercise to 14.28 (2.42 kg) after exercise. In conclusion, the immediate effects of exercise result in an increase in damping and passive stiffness in the human knee joint.

SUMMARY

This chapter has continued the discussion of dynamics by introducing the concepts of work, power, and momentum. The work done at the point of application of a force is discussed for constant forces and for forces that vary as a function of distance. The idea of evaluating the work done by a varying force using the method of integration is introduced as a limiting case of a sum of a series, but detailed calculus and integration methods are not covered in this book. The general concept of energy is discussed with particular reference to PE and KE, but strain energy and thermal energy are also mentioned. The conservation laws for linear momentum and energy are discussed and illustrated by a number of relevant examples. Collisions of various kinds are also considered, for example, between billiards balls or between a bat and a ball, leading to a discussion of impulses and their connection with momentum. A distinction is made between elastic and inelastic collisions. The chapter concludes by introducing spring forces and Hooke's law; this leads to a short discussion of undamped and damped oscillations. The chapter concludes with a case study in which the ideas of oscillation and damping are used to estimate the passive stiffness of the knee joint before and after exercise.

REFERENCES

Lakie M, Robson LG: Thiscotropic changes in human muscle stiffness and the effects of fatigue. Q J Exp Physiol 73(4):487–500, 1988.

Ricard M, Butterfield D, Draper D, et al: Acute Effects of Exercise on Passive Joint Stiffness. 20th Annual Meeting of American Society of Biomechanics, Atlanta, Georgia, Oct 17–19, 1996.

SUGGESTED READINGS

Meriam JL, Kraige LG: *Engineering Mechanics, vol 2: Dynamics*, edn. 5. New York: John Wiley & Sons; 2003.

STUDY QUESTIONS

1. In rugby, a player pushes a teammate forward through a total distance of 2.8 m. The pushing force used is 560 N directed horizontally. Calculate the work done by this force.

2. In a strong-man competition, a competitor attempts to pull a train along a track. The force applied is constant at 4575 N, but the connecting rope is at an angle of 10° with respect to the track. What is the work done on the train if the distance moved by the train is 15 m along the track?

3. The force applied to a discus by the hand as a function of distance during a throw is as shown in the following diagram:

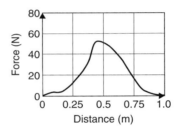

Estimate the work done on the discus using the approximate method explained in Section 6.2. Hint: Divide the horizontal axis up into a number of sections between six and 10.

4. A ball falls to the floor from a height of 2 m, hitting the floor with a velocity of 6.3 m/s. As the ball leaves the floor, its upward velocity is 5 m/s. Calculate the coefficient of restitution.

5. A tennis ball traveling at 25 m/s meets a racquet traveling in the opposite direction at 35 m/s. After the impact, the racquet and ball travel in the same direction with velocities of 10 m/s and 30 m/s, respectively. Calculate the coefficient of restitution.

6. The U.S. Tennis Association says that balls must bounce between 135 and 147 cm when dropped from 254 cm upon a concrete floor. What are the maximum and minimum values of the coefficient of restitution?

7. A basketball is dropped from a height of 2 m onto a gymnasium floor. If the coefficient of restitution between ball and floor is 0.9, how high will the ball bounce?

8. A basketball dropped from 1.83 m measured from the bottom of the ball bounces to between 1.24 and 1.37 m measured from the top of the ball. The ball is 0.25 m in diameter. Calculate the range within which the coefficient of restitution must lie.

9. Name five factors that influence the velocity and direction of a ball as it leaves a soccer player's sneaker.

10. A ball falls onto a surface from a height of 2 m, hitting the floor with a velocity of 6.3 m/s. As the ball leaves the floor, its upward velocity is 4 m/s. Calculate the coefficient of restitution between the ball and surface. What height will the ball bounce to?

11. Explain what is meant by the terms "angle of incidence" and "angle of reflection" when applied to an oblique impact.

    (a) Why is it that the two angles are not normally equal?

    (b) What conditions would give an angle of incidence greater than the corresponding angle of reflection?

12. Two tennis balls are hit so that they leave their respective tennis racquets at the same heights, speeds, and angles of release. One is hit with topspin, and the other is hit with no spin. They land on identical court surfaces.

    (a) Which ball has the greater downward vertical velocity on impact with the court?

    (b) Which ball has the greater horizontal velocity after impact with the court?

    (c) Which ball has the greater angle of reflection?

    (d) Which ball rises to the greater height during the bounce?

    (e) Which attains its peak height further from the point at which it bounced?

    (Ignore air resistance when answering these questions.)

13. Calculate how much PE possessed by a diver of mass 70 kg at the top of a 10-m diving board.

14. A top sprinter of mass 75 kg can achieve a maximum speed of 11 m/s. What is his KE?

15. By using conservation of mechanical energy, find the speed achieved by a skydiver after falling through a distance of 10 m from the airplane. (Equate the initial PE to the final KE.)

16. In a bench press, the 100-kg bar is raised through a vertical distance of 0.7 m in a time of 0.6 s. Calculate the average power in this movement.

17. A ball of mass 0.12 kg approaches a bat with velocity 15 m/s. In the collision, the bat exerts a constant force of 1250 N for a time of 0.003 s on the ball. Calculate the impulse and hence calculate the final velocity of the ball as it rebounds from the bat.

18. The vibrations of a golf club as a function of time are shown in the following diagram: Using the graph, evaluate:

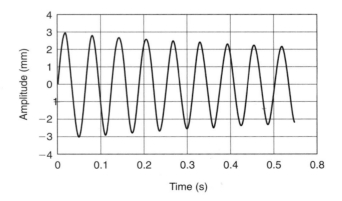

(a) The frequency of the oscillations

(b) The value of b/m (friction coefficient divided by mass)

CHAPTER *seven*

ANGULAR KINEMATICS

CHAPTER *objectives*

The objective of this chapter is to introduce the concepts of rotational kinematics.

CHAPTER *outcomes*

After reading this chapter, the reader will be able to:

- Understand the analogy between linear kinematics and rotational kinematics.
- Explain the meaning of absolute and relative angles.
- Explain what radial velocity and tangential velocity are.
- Be able to calculate centripetal and tangential accelerations for bodies moving in circular paths.
- Do calculations on angular displacements, velocities, and accelerations for the case of constant angular acceleration.
- Use spreadsheet methods to calculate angles and angular velocity from discrete $x-y$ coordinate data.

7.1 Fundamentals of Rotational Motion

7.1.1 ANGULAR DISPLACEMENT, VELOCITY, AND ACCELERATION

Chapters 4 to 6 are mainly concerned with translational movement of bodies. This chapter begins to examine rotational motion, concentrating on **angular kinematics**, that is, a description of the rotation of bodies without concern about the causes of such rotation. Although we can consider a simple system consisting of a particle moving in a circular path, in real situations, we need to consider the rotation of bodies of a finite size. Very often, we can consider such bodies to be **rigid bodies**, meaning solid bodies that do not distort or change their shape when they rotate. These rigid bodies can be thought of as being composed of particles that are fixed in position relative to each other. It is, of course, not appropriate to consider the

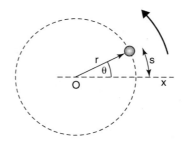

Figure 7.1 A particle moving in the path of a circle centered at O. The point is moving counterclockwise at a radius *r*.

human body as being a rigid body; instead, the human body can be considered to be an assemblage of rigid segments connected by moveable joints.

Consider a particle moving in the path of a circle (Fig. 7.1). This particle may be an isolated single particle or a constituent part of a larger body. Angles are commonly measured in degrees, but rotational motion becomes much easier to treat if angles are measured instead in radians. The angle θ specifies how far the particle has rotated during any time interval, *t*, measured from the *x* axis, which is an arbitrary reference axis. This angle, θ, is known as an **angular displacement**, which is the difference in an angle between the initial and final positions. The angle θ clearly corresponds to a distance, *s*, measured along the circumference of the circle. An angle of 1 **radian** would be turned when *s* is equal to the radius, *r*, of the circle. In general, for any angle θ:

$$\theta = \frac{s}{r}$$

where *r* is the radius of the circle and *s* is the arc length (both measured in the same units) subtended by the angle θ in radians. An angle corresponding to one full circle would be 360° or 2π radians, implying that 1 radian is 57.3°. The magnitude of the angular velocity can be evaluated simply for average and instantaneous cases. If we assume that θ_1 and θ_2 represent the angular displacements of the particle at times t_1 and t_2, respectively, then the magnitude of the **average angular velocity** is:

$$\overline{\omega} = \frac{\theta_2 - \theta_1}{t_2 - t_1} = \frac{\Delta\theta}{\Delta t}$$

The magnitude of the **instantaneous angular velocity** is the limit of this ratio as Δt approaches 0.

$$\omega = \lim_{\Delta t \to 0} \frac{\Delta\theta}{\Delta t} = \frac{d\theta}{dt}$$

and both ω and $\overline{\omega}$ are measured in radians per second (rad/s). This is the mathematical process of differentiation and is explained in Appendix 1.

Having defined the angular velocities in this way, the definition of angular acceleration follows in a natural way, following in an analogous fashion to linear velocities and accelerations. If ω_1 and ω_2 are the instantaneous angular velocities at times t_1 and t_2, respectively, then the **average angular acceleration** is:

$$\overline{\alpha} = \frac{\omega_2 - \omega_1}{t_2 - t_1} = \frac{\Delta\omega}{\Delta t}$$

and the **instantaneous angular acceleration** is defined as the limit of this quantity as Δt tends to 0:

$$\alpha = \lim_{\Delta t \to 0} \frac{\Delta\omega}{\Delta t} = \frac{d\omega}{dt}$$

with both $\overline{\alpha}$ and α being measured in radians per second squared (rad/s²).

Note that it is also possible to distinguish between angular displacement and angular distance in the same way that displacement was distinguished from distance in linear kinematics in Chapter 2. An **angular distance** is the total angle rotated over a given time interval. Perhaps the best way to distinguish between the angular displacement and the angular distance is to take an example. The ice skater shown in the diagram rotates 15.5 complete turns in a time of 5.2 seconds.

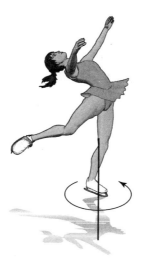

The angular distance is thus 15.5 multiplied by 2π radians, or 97.4 radians, and is a scalar quantity. However, the angular displacement is just 0.5 multiplied by 2π, or 3.14 radians, and is a vector with direction vertical. In this way, the **angular speed** is based on the angular distance and is 2.98 rad/s in this case. The angular velocity, on the other hand, is 0.6 rad/s and is regarded as a vector.

7.1.2 RELATIONSHIP BETWEEN LINEAR VELOCITY AND ANGULAR VELOCITY

The magnitude of the instantaneous angular velocity can be related to the magnitude of the instantaneous linear velocity, v, of the particle. Because:

$$v = \frac{ds}{dt}$$

and

$$s = r\theta$$

we have

$$v = \frac{d(r\theta)}{dt} = r\frac{d\theta}{dt} = r\omega$$

It should be noted that this velocity is necessarily tangential to the circle and is perpendicular to the radius.

7.1.3 TANGENTIAL AND CENTRIPETAL ACCELERATIONS

The magnitude of the instantaneous **tangential angular acceleration** a_T can also be related to ω and r. Because:

$$a_T = \frac{dv}{dt} = r\frac{d\omega}{dt}$$

then:

$$a_T = r\alpha.$$

The magnitude of the **centripetal acceleration** is:

$$a_r = \frac{v^2}{r} = \omega^2 r$$

This means that for a body moving at a varying angular velocity, a particle in the body will simultaneously experience a tangential (perpendicular to r) and a centripetal acceleration (along r directed toward the center of the circle; Fig. 7.2). In the special case of a body moving with constant angular velocity:

$$\frac{d\omega}{dt} = 0$$

so that:

$$a_T = 0$$

In this case, the only acceleration is:

$$a_r = \frac{v^2}{r} = \omega^2 r$$

acting toward the center of the circle. If the angular velocity is not constant, the resulting overall acceleration, a, can be found by adding the vectors a_r and a_T, so that:

$$a = a_r + a_T$$

Because a_r and a_T are always at right angles to each other, the magnitude of a is:

$$a = \sqrt{a_r^2 + a_T^2}$$

■ **Example 7.1**

A runner starts from rest and accelerates at a uniform rate up to a speed of 10 m/s in a time of 7.5 s, moving on a circular track of radius 30 m. Assuming constant tangential acceleration, find (a) the tangential acceleration and (b) the centripetal acceleration (radial) acceleration when the speed is 6m/s.

Solution

(a) a_T is constant of magnitude $a_T = dv/dt = (10 \text{ m/s} - 0 \text{ m/s})/(7.5 \text{ s} - 0 \text{s}) = 1.33 \text{ m/s}^2$.

(b) $a_r = v^2/r = (6 \text{ m/s})^2/30 \text{ m} = 1.2 \text{ m/s}^2$

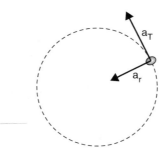

Figure 7.2 A particle moving in a circle with varying angular velocity experiences two perpendicular accelerations. The direction of the tangential acceleration (i.e., pointing clockwise or counterclockwise) depends on whether the angular velocity is increasing or decreasing. The overall acceleration can be obtained by combining a_r and a_T vectorially.

■ **EXAMPLE 7.2**   An individual's arm segment is 0.32 m long and has an angular velocity of 123°/s. What is the tangential velocity of the wrist?

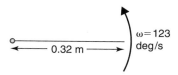

The tangential velocity is given by $v = r\omega$ so that:

$$v = (0.32 \text{ m}) \times (123/57.3 \text{ rad/s}) = 0.687 \text{ m/s}$$

Note that in this example, the angular velocity was given in degrees per second so that a conversion to radians per second was necessary.

■ **EXAMPLE 7.3**   A runner is running around a bend with a 12-m radius at a running speed of 5 m/s. What is the runner's centripetal acceleration?

Solution   The centripetal (radial) acceleration is given by

$$a_r = r\omega^2 = \frac{v^2}{r}$$

so that, in this case

$$a_r = \frac{5^2}{12} = 0.833 m/s^2$$

■ **EXAMPLE 7.4**   A hammer thrower rotates at 14.7 rad/s with an angular acceleration of 6.28 rad/s² prior to releasing the hammer. Given a radius (length of the arm of the athlete plus the length of the chain of the hammer) of 1.5m, what are the magnitudes of:

(a) The tangential acceleration
(b) The centripetal acceleration
(c) The resultant acceleration

Solution   (a) For angular motion

$$v = r\omega$$

so that:

$$\frac{dv}{dt} = r\frac{d\omega}{dt}$$
$$a_T = r\alpha$$

where a_T = tangential acceleration

α = angular acceleration
$$a_T = (1.5 \text{ m}) \times (6.28 \text{ rad/sec}^2)$$
$$= 9.42 \text{ m/s}^2$$

(b) $a_r = r\omega^2 = \dfrac{v^2}{r}$

so that:

$$a_r = (1.5 \text{ m}) \times (14.7 \text{ rad/s})^2$$
$$a_r = 324.14 \text{ m/s}^2$$

(c) The resultant acceleration is:

$$a = \sqrt{a_T^2 + a_r^2} = 324.27 m/s^2$$

7.2   Absolute and Relative Angles

An angle is composed of two lines that intersect at a point called the vertex. In many mechanical devices, one arm rotates about a fixed joint center. In the case of a nutcracker (Fig. 7.3), the joint center is located at the center of a hinge joint at the intersection of the two arms (the vertex).

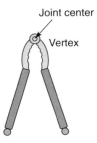

Joint center

Vertex

Figure 7.3 A nutcracker with a fixed joint center.

In the case of joints in the human body, the joint center of rotation is often not fixed and may change with time because of the shape of the bone surfaces. The **instantaneous joint center** (Fig. 7.4) is the center of rotation at an instant in time. There are two types of angle regularly encountered in biomechanics. **Relative angles** are the included angles between longitudinal axes of two segments, and

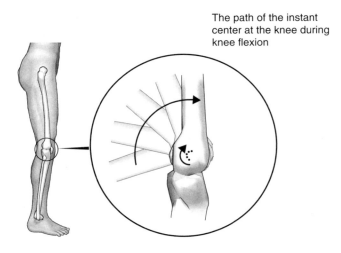

The path of the instant center at the knee during knee flexion

Figure 7.4 Knee joint center and its variation with knee flexion angle.

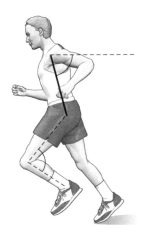

Figure 7.5 Relative and absolute angles.

absolute angles are the angles of inclination of body segments with reference to a fixed axis. There are two possible measurements (Fig. 7.5):

1. Place a coordinate system at the proximal end point of the segment and measure the angle counterclockwise from the right horizontal.
2. Place a coordinate system at the distal endpoint of the segment and measure the angle counterclockwise from the right horizontal.

7.3   Calculation of Angular Information from (*x,y*) Coordinate Data

7.3.1 CALCULATION OF ANGULAR DISPLACEMENTS

It is convenient sometimes to calculate absolute angles from (*x,y*) coordinate data. Let us assume that the positions of knee and ankle points have been ascertained from video data with reference to *x* and *y* coordinate axes, representing the endpoints of the lower leg. The vertical side of the triangle (Fig. 7.6) has a length of:

$$a = 0.51 - 0.09 = 0.42$$

The horizontal side of the triangle has a length of:

$$b = 1.22 - 1.09 = 0.13$$

The angle θ can be found from:

$$\tan \theta = a/b$$
$$= 0.42/0.13$$
$$= 3.23$$

Figure 7.6 Positions of knee and ankle. Points refer to the *x* and *y* axes; not to scale.

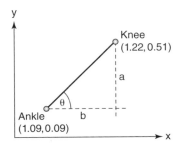

so that

$$\theta = \tan^{-1}(3.23)$$
$$= 72.8°$$

EXAMPLE 7.5

Calculate the absolute leg angle from the following (x,y) coordinate data for the end points of the upper leg segment.

Hip (1.14, 0.80)
Knee (1.22, 0.51)

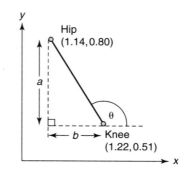

$$a = 0.80 - 0.51$$
$$a = 0.29$$
$$b = 1.22 - 1.14$$
$$b = 0.08$$
$$\tan(180 - \theta) = a/b = 0.29/0.08$$
$$\tan(180 - \theta) = 3.625$$
$$180 - \theta = \tan^{-1}(3.625)$$
$$180 - \theta = 74.6$$
$$\theta = 180 - 74.6$$
$$\theta = 105.4°$$

7.3.2 CALCULATION OF ANGULAR VELOCITY FROM ANGULAR DISPLACEMENT

Following on from such calculations, it may be necessary to calculate angular velocities from a series of absolute angles measured at regular time intervals. This can easily happen during analysis of a series of frames from a video recording, for example. Consider Table 7.1, which includes data taken from a person video

Table 7.1	Absolute angles for upper leg segment at the knee for a series of frames in a video recording	
Frame	**Time t (s)**	**Absolute Angle at Knee (°)**
1	0.3125	140
2	0.3500	151
3	0.3875	158
4	0.4250	164

Figure 7.7 Variation of angle θ with time, t. The graph shows three measured θ values at three different times. The *thick line* shows how the instantaneous angle may be varying with time. The angular velocity can be estimated from the slope of the hypotenuse of the triangle (*solid lines*).

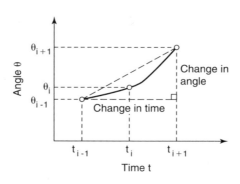

recorded while walking. Let us assume that it is required to calculate the angular velocity of this upper leg segment at frames 2 and 3. The angular velocity can be calculated by consideration of a graph of angle versus time (Fig. 7.7).

At time i, the angular velocity is the change in angle per unit time. This is the slope of the tangent to the curve at time i, not shown in Figure 7.4. It is approximately the same as the slope of the line joining the two points (t_{i-1}, θ_{i-1}) and (t_{i+1}, θ_{i+1})

$$\text{Angular velocity} = \omega_i = \frac{\Delta\theta_i}{\Delta t_i} \sim \frac{\theta_{i+1} - \theta_{i-1}}{t_{i+1} - t_{i-1}}$$

At frame 2:

$$\omega_2 = \frac{\theta_3 - \theta_1}{t_3 - t_1}$$
$$\omega_2 = \frac{158 - 140}{0.3875 - 0.3125}$$
$$\omega_2 = \frac{18}{0.0750}$$
$$\omega_2 = 240°/s \ (4.19 \text{ rad/s})$$

At frame 3:

$$\omega_3 = \frac{\theta_4 - \theta_2}{t_4 - t_2}$$
$$\omega_3 = \frac{164 - 151}{0.425 - 0.350}$$
$$\omega_3 = \frac{13}{0.075}$$
$$\omega_3 = 173°/s \ (3.03 \text{ rad/s})$$

Note again that angular velocity is given in degrees per second in this example. This was done purely on an arbitrary basis and could have been calculated in radians per second directly. However, some motion analysis systems give angular quantities in degrees, so it is sensible to be familiar with both systems and to be able to convert between them as necessary.

7.3.3 CALCULATION OF ANGULAR ACCELERATION FROM ANGULAR VELOCITY DATA

Similar calculations arise in the estimation of instantaneous angular accelerations from consecutive sequential angular velocity data. Consider the following example data in Table 7.2. Calculate the angular acceleration at frames 12 and 13

Table 7.2	Discrete angular velocity versus time data for four consecutive frames	
Frame Number	**Time t (s)**	**Angular Velocity ω (rad/s)**
11	0.6167	1.033
12	0.6333	1.511
13	0.6500	1.882
14	0.6667	2.190

A general angular velocity-versus-time curve is shown in Figure 7.8. At time i, the acceleration is the change in velocity per unit time, which is the slope of the tangent to the curve drawn at time i. It is approximately the same as the slope of the line joining the points (t_{i-1}, ω_{i-1}) and (t_{i+1}, ω_{i+1}).

$$\text{Angular acceleration } \alpha_i = \frac{\Delta\omega_i}{\Delta t_i} \sim \frac{\omega_{i+1} - \omega_{i-1}}{t_{i+1} - t_{i-1}}$$

At frame 12:

$$\alpha_{12} = \frac{\omega_{13} - \omega_{11}}{t_{13} - t_{11}}$$

$$\alpha_{12} = \frac{1.882 - 1.033}{0.6500 - 0.6167}$$

$$\alpha_{12} = \frac{0.849}{0.0333}$$

$$\alpha_{12} = 25.5 \text{ rad/s}^2$$

At frame 13:

$$\alpha_{13} = \frac{\omega_{14} - \omega_{12}}{t_{14} - t_{12}}$$

$$\alpha_{13} = \frac{2.190 - 1.511}{0.6667 - 0.6333}$$

$$\alpha_{13} = \frac{0.679}{0.0334}$$

$$\alpha_{13} = 20.3 \text{ rad/s}^2$$

7.4   Formulas for Rotation for the Case of Constant Angular Acceleration

It is useful to realize the close analogy that exists between angular kinematics and linear kinematics. The formulas for linear kinematics discussed in Section 3.2.2 and the corresponding ones for rotational motion are given in Table 7.3 without proof.

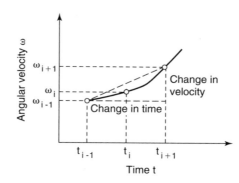

Figure 7.8 Generalized graph of angular velocity versus time. The graph shows three measured values of angular velocity at three separate times. The *thick line* shows how the instantaneous angular velocity may vary with time.

Table 7.3 Four equations relating the various quantities important in uniformly accelerated motion*

Formula	Linear Motion	Rotational Motion
Velocity in terms of acceleration and time	$v = v_0 + at$	$\omega = \omega_0 + \alpha t$
Displacement in terms of initial velocity, acceleration, and time	$s = s_0 + v_0 t + \frac{1}{2} at^2$	$\theta = \theta_0 + \omega_0 t + \frac{1}{2}\alpha t^2$
Velocity in terms of acceleration and displacement	$v^2 = (v_0)^2 + 2a(s - s_0)$	$\omega^2 = \omega_0^2 + 2\alpha (\theta - \theta_0)$
Average velocity in terms of initial and final velocities	$\bar{v} = \dfrac{v + v_0}{2}$	$\bar{\omega} = \dfrac{\omega + \omega_0}{2}$

*Both linear and rotational equations are given so the analogy between them is clear.

a, α = accelerations (constant for these equations to apply); s θ = final displacements; s_0, θ_0 = initial displacements; t = time, v ω = final velocities; v_0 ω_0 = initial velocities; $\bar{v}$, $\bar{\omega}$ are mean (average) velocities

■ **EXAMPLE 7.6**

A pitcher pitches a baseball at a waiting batter and releases the ball with an angular speed of 36 rad/s. If the ball takes 0.85 s to reach the batsman and is rotating at 25 rad/s when it arrives, calculate the angular deceleration of the ball. Through what angle has the ball turned in its flight from the pitcher to the batter? Through how many revolutions does the ball turn? (Assume the angular deceleration of the ball is constant.) Using:

$$\omega = \omega_0 + \alpha t$$
$$\omega = 25, \omega_0 = 36, t = 0.85$$
$$\alpha = \frac{\omega - \omega_0}{t} = \frac{25 - 36}{0.85}$$

so that the angular deceleration is:

$$\alpha = -12.94 \text{ rad/s}^2$$

To work out the angle turned, use:

$$\theta = \theta_0 + \omega_0 t + \tfrac{1}{2}\alpha t^2$$

so that:

$$\theta - \theta_0 = 36 \times 0.85 + \tfrac{1}{2} \times (-12.94) \times (0.85)^2$$
$$= 25.93 \text{ rad}$$

In terms of revolutions, this is:

$$25.93/(2\pi) = 4.13 \text{ revolutions}$$

CASE *Study 7.1*   **Rotation of a Football**

A motion analysis system is used to follow the rotation of a football. The football of diameter 0.25 m has two markers attached at two ends of a diameter on the "equator" of the ball.

The axis of rotation is through the "poles" of the football. The motion analysis system returns the x and y coordinates of the two markers every $1/120^{th}$ of a second with an accuracy of approximately 1 mm.

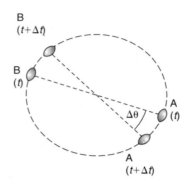

The diagram shows the positions of markers A and B at time, t, and a slightly later time, $t + \Delta t$. The rotational velocity of the football can be estimated in a number of ways from the movement of one or both of the markers. In this case study, we will estimate the angular velocity by following these steps:

1. Produce a spreadsheet containing the time data in column A, the x coordinate data in column B, and the y coordinate data in column C.
2. Calculate the x increment Δx and y increment Δy during time interval Δt.
3. From Δx and Δy, calculate the movement Δl.

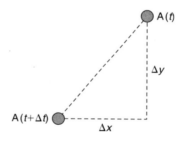

$$\Delta l = \sqrt{\Delta x^2 + \Delta y^2}$$

Δl should be identical for both markers. In the spreadsheet, Δl will be calculated for both markers and averaged to reduce errors.

4. From the movement, Δl, calculate the tangential velocity, v.
5. From the velocity, v, calculate the angular velocity.

The following diagram shows a small section of the spreadsheet near the beginning (Griffiths et al., 2003).

Column A: Time (sec), $1/120^{th}$ s = 0.01833 s

Column B: A marker x coordinate in millimeters

Column C: A marker y coordinate in millimeters

Column D: B marker x coordinate in millimeters

Column E: B marker y coordinate in millimeters

Column F: A marker x coordinate increment Δx in millimeters

Column G: A marker y coordinate increment Δy in millimeters

	A	B	C	D	E	F	G	H	I	J	K	L	M
1	time	A marker x coord	A marker y coord	B marker x coord	B marker y coord	A marker dx	A marker dy	B marker dx	B marker dy	dl	vel	angular velocity	
2	(s)	(mm)	(mm)	(mm)	(mm)	(mm)	(mm)	(mm)	(mm)	(mm)	(mm/s)	(rad/s)	
3	0.0000	1175.36	-559.29	925.76	-559.26								
4	0.0183	1175.00	-552.78	925.31	-566.16	0.36	6.51	0.45	6.90	6.72	366.48	2.932	
5	0.0367	1174.27	-545.56	926.16	-572.85	0.73	7.21	0.85	6.69	7.00	381.78	3.054	
6	0.0550	1173.84	-538.72	927.23	-580.11	0.43	6.84	1.07	7.26	7.10	387.11	3.097	
7	0.0733	1172.72	-532.72	928.44	-586.64	1.12	6.01	1.21	6.53	6.38	347.85	2.783	
8	0.0917	1170.71	-525.33	930.23	-593.13	2.01	7.39	1.79	6.49	7.19	392.37	3.139	
9	0.1100	1168.40	-518.92	932.25	-600.45	2.31	6.41	2.02	7.32	7.21	393.08	3.145	
10	0.1283	1166.53	-512.65	934.86	-606.81	1.86	6.27	2.62	6.35	6.71	365.87	2.927	
11	0.1467	1163.14	-505.97	937.85	-612.82	3.39	6.68	2.99	6.02	7.10	387.60	3.101	
12	0.1650	1160.34	-500.50	940.51	-619.04	2.80	5.47	2.66	6.21	6.45	351.93	2.815	
13													
14													
15											=J12/0.01833		
16					=ABS(C12-C11)								
17													
18						=(SQRT(F12^2+G12^2)+SQRT(H12^2+I12^2))/2					=K12*0.001*2/0.25		
19													

Column H: B marker x coordinate increment Δx in millimeters

Column I: B marker y coordinate increment Δy in millimeters

Column J: Movement of A and B markers averaged in millimeters

Column K: Velocity of markers A and B in millimeters per second

Column L: Angular velocity of ball in radians per second. A factor of 0.001 is used to convert millimeters to meters; a factor of 2 is used to convert the diameter of the ball to radius.

(Note: the units used here are millimeters because the motion analysis system uses these units for all its output; to convert to meters, multiply millimeters by 0.001 or 10^{-3}.)

The following charts show the position of the two markers in the $x-y$ plane and the angular velocity as a function of time calculated from the $x-y$ coordinate data: The angular

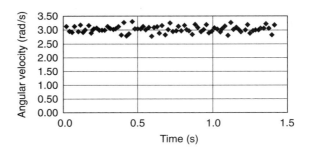

velocity data show a certain level of noise because of small uncertainties in the $x-y$ coordinate data. This is typical of data calculated from real coordinate data by finite difference methods.

CASE *Study 7.2*   **Evaluation of Centripetal and Tangential Accelerations on a Stunt Rider**

A stunt rider takes his motorcycle up the inside wall of a circular, cylindrical, enclosed track. His circular motion is filmed from above with a high-speed digital video camera for subsequent analysis. In the analysis, the origin of coordinates is taken as the center of the circular enclosure.

The x and y coordinates of his helmet, measured by a process of digitization from the video, are given in a data spreadsheet file. Here is a small section of the spreadsheet based around time $t = 0.5$ s:

time	x	y
(s)	(m)	(m)
0.495	6.663601	4.438575
0.496	6.656141	4.449467
0.497	6.650938	4.461883
0.498	6.647739	4.466777
0.499	6.636692	4.477146
0.500	6.634232	4.484579
0.501	6.625025	4.495644
0.502	6.619220	4.507084
0.503	6.612288	4.522360
0.504	6.599768	4.532888
0.505	6.598362	4.541554

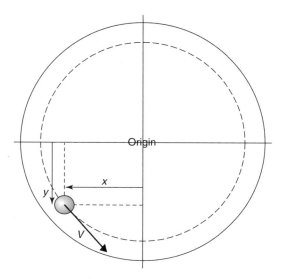

We want to calculate the centripetal and tangential accelerations for the rider at $t = 0.5$ s. Note that the rider accelerates from rest at $t = 0$ and continues to accelerate for a time of at least 1 s, but the acceleration is not constant. The discrete x–y coordinate data are used to derive the velocity of the motorcycle rider using finite difference methods. The velocity values can then be used in the spreadsheet to derive angular velocity values.

In this spreadsheet, the velocity values are affected by random noise introduced in the digitization procedure; this has a knock-on effect on the angular velocity and centripetal acceleration values, making direct reading of values from the spreadsheet difficult. It is possible to introduce some smoothing into the spreadsheet calculation to reduce the effect of digitization noise or other random noise, but this will be deferred to Chapters 9 and 10. In this case, we will continue the discussion of this case study by estimating velocity and acceleration values from the graph of velocity versus time:

The effect of noise on the velocity data is clear, but fortunately the human eye is very good at seeing "through" the noise. The velocity at a time of 0.5 s is estimated to be approximately 13.3 m/s. The line AB is drawn as the tangent to the curve at $t = 0.5$ s. The slope of this line gives the tangential acceleration of the rider at this time and is approximately 5.48 m/s^2. The centripetal acceleration is:

	A	B	C	D	E	F	G	angular velocity	centripetal acceleration a_r
1	time	x	y	dx	dy	dl	velocity		
2	(s)	(m)	(m)	(m)	(m)	(m)	(m/s)	(rad/s)	(m/s²)
3	0.495	6.664	4.439	-0.011	0.007	0.013	12.632	1.579	19.945
4	0.496	6.656	4.449	-0.007	0.011	0.013	13.202	1.650	21.788
5	0.497	6.651	4.462	-0.005	0.012	0.013	13.462	1.683	22.654
6	0.498	6.648	4.467	-0.003	0.005	0.006	5.847	0.731	4.273
7	0.499	6.637	4.477	-0.011	0.010	0.015	15.151	1.894	28.695
8	0.5	6.634	4.485	-0.002	0.007	0.008	7.829	0.979	7.661
9	0.501	6.625	4.496	-0.009	0.011	0.014	14.395	1.799	25.902
10	0.502	6.619	4.507	-0.006	0.011	0.013	12.828	1.604	20.571
11	0.503	6.612	4.522	-0.007	0.015	0.017	16.775	2.097	35.175
12	0.504	6.600	4.533	-0.013	0.011	0.016	16.358	2.045	33.449
13	0.505	6.598	4.542	-0.001	0.009	0.009	8.779	1.097	9.633

=SQRT(D8^2+E8^2)	=(F8-F7)/(A8-A7)	=G8/radius	=G8^2/radius

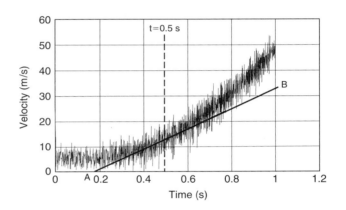

$$a_r = \frac{v^2}{r} = \frac{(13.3)^2}{8} = 22.1 \text{ m/s}^2$$

The tangential acceleration is:

$$a_T = \frac{\Delta v}{\Delta t} = 5.48 \text{ m/s}^2$$

The combined or total acceleration on the rider is:

$$a = \sqrt{a_r^2 + a_T^2} = \sqrt{22.1^2 + 5.48^2} = 22.8 \text{ m/s}^2$$

CASE Study 7.3   **The Use of Angle-to-Angle Diagrams in Comparing Sprinting Drills**

In biomechanical terms, sprinting speed is determined by stride length and stride frequency.

Speed = Stride length × Stride frequency

where the stride length is the distance measured between one heel contact and the next and the stride frequency is the number of strides in 1 s. The stride length can vary because of any of the following factors:

■ Strength
■ Flexibility
■ Injury
■ Leg length
■ Endurance
■ Biomechanical technique

Stride frequency and stride length can be improved by undertaking simple drills during training. These are called the A and B drills.

Drill A

This is a simple drill to help a sprinter achieve high knees and toes when the leg is up in front of the body during the sprint. The drill begins by walking forward slowly while staying up on the balls of the feet. As the toes leave the ground to take a step forward, the ankle is dorsiflexed and held there. The ankle is held in this position and the hamstring is flexed to pull the heel up toward the buttocks. The hips are then flexed to pull the upper leg and knee forward and upward parallel to the ground. At this point, the knee should be above and slightly in front

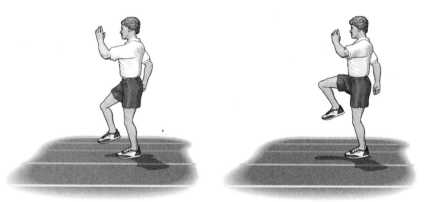

of the ankle with the toe flexed upward. The hip is then extended and the foot is put back on the ground. The A drill helps improve stride frequency and stride length.

Drill B

The B drill is performed by a continuation of the A drill. When the upper leg is parallel to the ground, the quadriceps muscles are stretched and the lower leg is swung forward and upward. When the knee is fully extended, the entire leg is pulled backward and downward toward the ground.

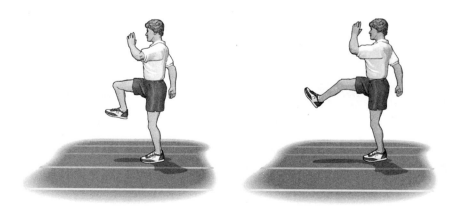

Kivi and Alexander (1998) have reported a kinematic comparison of the running A and B drills with sprinting using angle-to-angle diagrams. University-level sprinters were recorded using two genlocked cameras at a speed of 60 Hz and a shutter speed of $1/2000^{th}$ s. The subjects performed a series of running A and B drills and 60-m sprints at maximum velocity within a 7-m filming grid. The differences in the simultaneous movements of the right hip and knee during one cycle of the three skills were demonstrated using angle-to-angle diagrams. The angle-to-angle diagrams for the right hip and knee for one particular subject are shown here (courtesy of Kivi and Alexander, 1998).

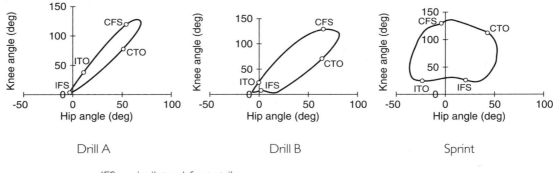

Drill A   Drill B   Sprint

IFS = ipsilateral foot strike
ITO = ipsilateral toe-off
CFS = contralateral footstrike
CTO = contralateral toe-off

The conclusion from this study was that the A and B drills are not similar to sprinting from the biomechanical point of view.

SUMMARY

This chapter has discussed angular displacement, velocity, and acceleration. The measurement of angles by means of radian measure is introduced and a distinction is made between absolute and relative angles. The discussion of rotational kinematics is continued with the relationship between the tangential velocity and acceleration and the angular velocity and acceleration for a body moving in a circular path of radius r. It is demonstrated how to calculate angular quantities from two-dimensional coordinate data. Calculation of angular quantities from three-dimensional data is not covered in this chapter, but further information on this topic is given in Chapter 12 on gait analysis. The centripetal acceleration for a body moving in a circular path is also covered. Three case studies are presented illustrating:

■ The calculation of angular velocity from x–y coordinate data
■ The evaluation of centripetal and tangential accelerations
■ The use of angle diagrams

REFERENCES

Griffiths N, Griffiths IW: Preliminary football study [unpublished data]. University of Wales Swansea; UK, 2003.

Kivi DMR, Alexander MJL: A kinematic comparison of the running A and B drills with sprinting. Paper presented at the North American Congress on Biomechanics, August 14–18, 1998, University of Waterloo, Waterloo, Ontario, Canada; 1998.

STUDY QUESTIONS

1. Given the following (*x*,*y*) data for the endpoints of the upper leg segment, calculate the following (Table 7.4):

Table 7.4	x and y coordinates for the endpoints of the lower leg segment		
Time Frame	**Time (s)**	**Hip (x, y)**	**Knee (x, y)**
1	0.025	0.16, 0.88	0.62, 0.23
2	0.050	0.34, 0.98	0.74, 0.28
3	0.075	0.62, 1.11	0.90, 0.37
4	0.100	1.04, 1.30	1.21, 0.51
5	0.125	1.68, 1.35	1.66, 0.55

  (a) The absolute leg angle, θ, at the time frames 1, 2, 3, 4, and 5

  (b) The angular velocity of the leg, ω, at time frames 2, 3, and 4

  (c) The angular acceleration, α, at time frame 3.

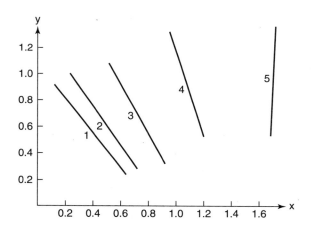

The above diagram shows the position of the segment varying in *x*–*y* space.

2. An ice skater increases his speed of rotation from 10 to 30 rad/s in a time of 1.2 s. What is his angular acceleration? Through what angle (in degrees and radians) has he turned while doing this?

3. During an elbow flexion exercise, the relative angle at the elbow was 10° at 0.5 s and 120° at 0.71 s. What was the angular velocity at the elbow?

4. A golf club is swung with the average angular acceleration of 2.5 rad/s². What is the angular velocity of the club when it strikes the ball at the end of a 0.8 s swing?

  (a) in rad/s

  (b) in °/s

5. A baseball hits a bat at a point 50 cm from the axis of rotation. If the angular velocity of the bat is 20 rad/sec at the instant the ball hits the bat, what is the linear velocity of the bat at this time?

6. A bowler bowls a ball with an overarm sweeping action through a total angle of 250°. His arm is 0.8 m long. If the average angular acceleration of the arm is 24 rad/s², what is the:

   a. angular velocity at the end of the action?

   b. velocity of the ball at the point of release?

7. The angular velocity of a cricket bat is 1 radian/s after 0.35 s and 1.5 radian/s after 0.47 s. What is the average angular acceleration over this time interval?

8. A bowler with an arm 0.75 m long bowls with an angular velocity of 2000°/s when the ball is released. Calculate the velocity of the ball.

9. A cyclist accelerates from 10 to 12.5m/s over 3 s while cycling in a curve with radius of 20 m. What are the centripetal, tangential, and overall accelerations at the end of 3 seconds?

10. A hammer is being accelerated at 15 rad/s². The radius of rotation is 1.7 m, and the angular velocity at the point of release is 14.7 rad/s. What are the tangential, centripetal, and overall accelerations at the point of release?

11. A cyclist goes around a bend with radius 30 m at a speed of 10 m/s. What is his centripetal acceleration?

12. A cyclist cycles around a bend of 20 m radius. As he does so, he slows from 10 to 8 m/s over a period of 4 s. What are his tangential and centripetal acceleration at the end of the bend? Assume that the tangential deceleration is constant and continues after the 4 s period.

13. A discus has two markers attached at opposite ends of a diameter on the rim. The x–y coordinates of the two markers (A and B) as a function of time are given in Table 7.5. The coordinates are measured with respect to a fixed origin located at a point approximately 1 m from the discus. The movement of the discus can be assumed to be purely rotational with

Table 7.5   The x-y coordinates of two markers on the rim of a discus

Time (s)	A Marker x Coordinate (mm)	A Marker y Coordinate (mm)	B Marker x Coordinate (mm)	B Marker y Coordinate (mm)
0.000000	1160.729	−559.284	940.2013	−559.590
0.018333	1158.894	−542.665	942.1615	−576.545
0.036666	1155.521	−526.225	945.8650	−593.627
0.054999	1148.832	−510.426	952.2778	−608.845
0.073332	1140.203	−495.530	961.1306	−624.072
0.091665	1129.163	−481.718	972.3432	−636.868
0.109998	1115.649	−470.823	985.3083	−648.412
0.128331	1101.069	−462.220	1000.189	−657.265
0.146664	1085.441	−454.943	1015.388	−664.043
0.164997	1069.129	−451.038	1032.267	−668.095
0.183330	1052.087	−449.333	1048.976	−669.252
0.201663	1034.353	−450.874	1066.051	−668.870
0.219996	1017.637	−454.337	1082.797	−664.250

zero translational movement. Set up a spreadsheet to find the angular velocity of the discus averaged over the first 0.22 s. Also, draw a graph of angular velocity versus time.

14. For the case study of the stunt motorcycle rider, repeat the exercise to find the centripetal and tangential accelerations at $t = 0.25$ s and $t = 0.75$ s. Can you make some estimate of the errors in your determinations?

CHAPTER eight

ROTATIONAL DYNAMICS

CHAPTER *objectives*

The objectives of this chapter are to introduce rotational kinetics and to establish the link with linear kinetics in Chapter 5. A case study is used to demonstrate how the principles can be applied in an experimental determination of the moment of inertia of the human body.

CHAPTER *outcomes*

After reading this chapter, the reader will be able to:

- Define the magnitude and direction of an angular motion vector.
- Calculate torques, moments of inertia, and angular accelerations from $\tau = I\alpha$.
- Calculate torques from lever arms and forces.
- Recognize everyday objects and link them with their moments of inertia.
- Do calculations of moments of inertia for the human body.
- Model a human performer rotating in a plane as a linked rigid-rod system.

8.1   Angular Motion Vectors

Angular velocity and angular acceleration can be treated as vectors in the same way that displacement and velocity are vectors in linear motion. Let us consider an angular displacement θ. If we take an object, say an arrow, as shown in Figure 8.1, and rotate it about an angle of 90° counterclockwise about the x axis and then rotate it 90° counterclockwise about the y axis, (Fig. 8.1a), it produces a different effect than rotating the arrow first 90° counterclockwise about the y axis and then 90° counterclockwise about the x axis (Fig. 8.1b). Shown mathematically, it is:

$$\theta_1 + \theta_2 \neq \theta_2 + \theta_1$$

so θ cannot be a vector. However, infinitesimal angles of rotation can be interpreted as vectors so that:

$$d\theta_1 + d\theta_2 = d\theta_2 + d\theta_1$$

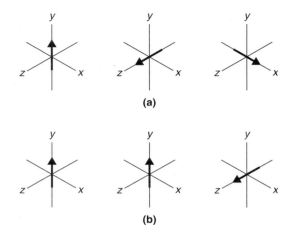

Figure 8.1 (A) Rotation of 90° about the x axis followed by 90° rotation about the y axis. (B) Rotation of 90° about the y axis followed by 90° rotation about the x axis.

The angular velocity, $\boldsymbol{\omega}$, must also be a vector because it is the product of a vector $(d\boldsymbol{\theta})$ and a scalar $(1/dt)$.

$$\boldsymbol{\omega} = \frac{d\boldsymbol{\theta}}{dt}$$

Also, the angular acceleration, $\boldsymbol{\alpha}$, is a vector because:

$$\boldsymbol{\alpha} = \frac{d\boldsymbol{\omega}}{dt}$$

Figure 8.2 shows a disc rotating counterclockwise as viewed from the top. The angular velocity vector, $\boldsymbol{\omega}$, would be shown as an arrow pointing vertically up along the axis of rotation of the disc. This direction is given by a righthand rule so that when the thumb of the right hand points along the $\boldsymbol{\omega}$ vector, the fingers of the hand curve around in the direction of rotation. If the disc rotated clockwise instead, the $\boldsymbol{\omega}$ vector would point downward. If the axis of rotation is fixed, then $\boldsymbol{\omega}$ can change only in magnitude. Thus:

$$\boldsymbol{\alpha} = \frac{d\boldsymbol{\omega}}{dt}$$

must also point along the axis of rotation. If the rotation is counterclockwise, as shown in Figure 8.2, and $\boldsymbol{\omega}$ is increasing, then the angular acceleration vector $\boldsymbol{\alpha}$ points upward. If $\boldsymbol{\omega}$ is decreasing, then $\boldsymbol{\alpha}$ points downward.

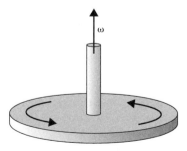

Figure 8.2 Rotating disc. The angular velocity vector $\boldsymbol{\omega}$ points straight up along the axis of rotation. To avoid any ambiguity, the direction of the vector is given by the righthand rule. Imagine curling the fingers of your right hand around the shaft of the wheel so that they point in the same direction as the rotation of the wheel. Your thumb then points in the direction of the angular velocity vector.

■ **EXAMPLE 8.1**

A baseball is delivered by the pitcher with a spin of 10 rad/s decreasing to 9 rad/s by the time the baseball reaches the batter. The baseball takes 0.42 s to travel from the pitcher to the batter. Looking from above, the spin of the baseball is about a vertical axis, in a clockwise direction.

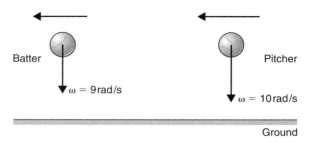

The angular velocity vector points downward. The angular acceleration vector $\boldsymbol{\alpha}$ points upward with a magnitude of:

$$\alpha = \frac{\Delta \omega}{\Delta t} = \frac{10 - 9}{0.42} = 2.38 \text{ rad/s}^2$$

(This is an angular deceleration, assumed to be constant over the flight path.)

8.2   Torque

The cause of rotational accelerations is torque, the rotational equivalent of force in linear motion. Objects are caused to start rotating by a force or forces acting at some distance from a hinge or pivot point. To take an example, consider a force, *F*, applied to a ball in which the force is off center (Fig. 8.3). The effect of the force in Figure 8.3 will start the ball rotating. (It may also cause the ball to move as a whole, but we shall ignore this movement here. We will return to it in Example 8.3.) The larger the force, the faster the ball accelerates in its rotational motion. However, the distance, *d*, is also important. If *F* is applied at a greater distance from the center of the ball (greater *d*), then the turning effect of the ball will be increased, equivalent to using a larger force at a reduced *d*. The angular acceleration is found to be proportional to the product of *F* and *d*. This product is termed the *moment of the force about the axis* and is also called **torque**. It is often abbreviated as $\boldsymbol{\tau}$. The angular acceleration, $\boldsymbol{\alpha}$, then, is found to be directly proportional to the net applied torque, $\boldsymbol{\tau}$.

$$\boldsymbol{\alpha} \propto \boldsymbol{\tau}$$

The terms *torque* and *moment of force* are used interchangeably in the literature. This means that sometimes the symbol τ is used to stand for a torque, but other authors prefer to use *M* to stand for moment. *M* is often preferred in sports science texts because moments are often applied by muscles in the body, and *M* also stands

Figure 8.3 A force, **F**, applied to a ball off center. The line of action of the force passes within a distance, *d*, of the center of the ball. The ball tends to start rotating, clockwise from this perspective.

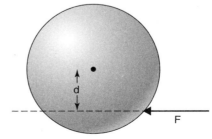

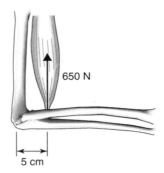

Figure 8.4 Torque applied by the biceps on the lower arm about the elbow joint. Angle of lower arm with respect to horizontal = 0°; lever arm = 5 cm.

for muscle. Unfortunately, *M* is also used to stand for mass. Both τ and *M* have the same units of Newton meters. This is the rotational analogue of Newton's second law for linear motion:

$$a \propto F.$$

The distance, *d*, is often termed the **lever arm** and is the perpendicular distance of the axis of rotation from the line of action of the force.

A similar effect can be seen when a muscle force acts on a body segment at a certain distance from the joint center. Consider for example the torque applied by the biceps on the lower arm (Fig. 8.4). This amounts to a torque of:

$$\tau = (650N) \times (0.05m) = 32.5Nm$$

If the angle at the elbow is increased so that the lower arm makes an angle of 50° with the horizontal (Fig. 8.5), the lever arm is reduced and, for the same muscle force, the torque supplied is less. In this case, the lever arm is:

$$R_{perp} = (0.05m) \times \cos(50°)$$

so that the torque is reduced to:

$$\tau = (650N) \times (0.05m) \times \cos(50°) = 20.9 \text{ Nm}$$

As a matter of convention, we assign counterclockwise torques as positive and clockwise ones as negative, so that the muscle torques on the lower arm about the elbow in the previous example were +32.5 Nm and +24.9 Nm, respectively.

8.3   Rotational Inertia

Because we have established that there is a rotational analogue of Newton's second law for translational motion, that is, $\alpha \propto \tau$, it is natural to ask what the analogous quan-

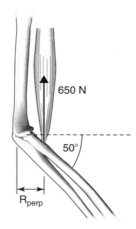

Figure 8.5 Torque applied by the biceps to the lower arm segment about the elbow joint. Angle of lower arm with respect to horizontal = 50°. Lever arm = R_{perp}.

tity is that is assuming the place of mass. It turns out that the mass is replaced by a quantity called **moment of inertia**, which is the sum of mr^2 for all particles making up the body. It is usually given the symbol I so that, for any object, I can be defined as:

$$I = \Sigma \, m_i R_i^2 = m_1 R_1^2 + m_2 R_2^2 + \ldots + m_n R_n^2$$

representing the sum of the masses of each particle in the object multiplied by the perpendicular distance of each particle from the axis of rotation. It then follows that the rotational equivalent of Newton's second law can be expressed as:

$$\tau = I\alpha$$

provided that the axis of rotation can be considered fixed. This equation is also valid when the body is accelerating uniformly, but only if I and α are calculated about the center of mass of the body and if the rotation axis through the center of mass does not change direction. Then:

$$\tau_{cm} = I_{cm}\,\alpha_{cm} \text{ (direction of axis fixed)}$$

For many bodies, the mass is distributed in an even and consistent way throughout the volume occupied by the body and, when the body also has some element of symmetry, the moment of inertia can be worked out using calculus methods. Figure 8.6 gives the moments of inertia for various objects of uniform composition.

Object	Location of Axis		Moment of Inertia	Radius of Gyration
(a) Thin hoop of radius R_0	Through center	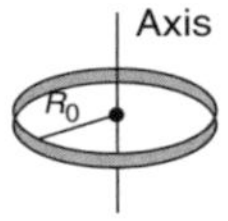	MR_0^2	R_0
(b) Thin hoop of radius R_0 and width w	Through central diameter	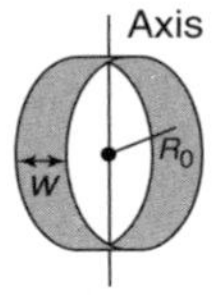	$\frac{1}{2}M R_0^2 + \frac{1}{12}Mw^2$	$\sqrt{\dfrac{R_0^2}{2} + \dfrac{w^2}{12}}$
(c) Solid cylinder of radius R_0	Through center	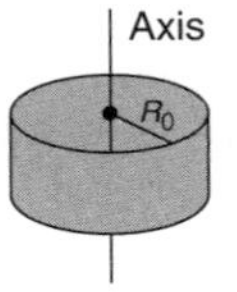	$\frac{1}{2}M R_0^2$	$\dfrac{R_0}{\sqrt{2}}$
(d) Solid sphere of radius r_0	Through center	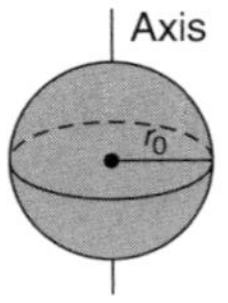	$\frac{2}{5}M r_0^2$	$\sqrt{\dfrac{2}{5}}\,r_0$
(e) Thin rod of length L	Through center	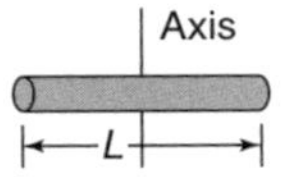	$\frac{1}{12}ML^2$	$\dfrac{L}{\sqrt{12}}$
(f) Thin rod of length L	Through end	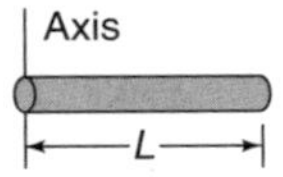	$\frac{1}{3}ML^2$	$\dfrac{L}{\sqrt{3}}$
(g) Rectangular thin plate, of length l and width w	Through center	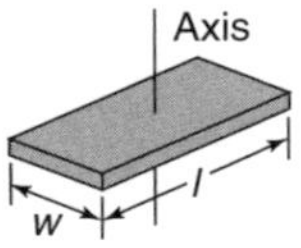	$\frac{1}{12}M(l^2 + w^2)$	$\sqrt{\dfrac{l^2 + w^2}{12}}$

Figure 8.6 Moments of inertia for various symmetrical bodies of mass M.

The **radius of gyration** is defined as the radius that if all the mass were concentrated at this distance from the axis, then it would have the same moment of inertia as the actual object. The moment of inertia of any object can be written as:

$$I = Mk^2$$

where k is the radius of gyration. The radius of gyration is often specified for unusual or irregularly shaped objects. In some biomechanical models, it is convenient to approximate segments as various symmetrical bodies for simplicity; for example, an arm might be modeled as a cylinder or a head as a sphere.

■ **EXAMPLE 8.2**

A woman of height 1.85 m and mass 70 kg is rappelling down the side of a tall building and is momentarily horizontal when she stops with her feet on a small ledge. Suddenly her support rope snaps, and she begins to fall, but her feet are still supported by the ledge. She begins a rotational movement downward about an axis approximately through her heels.

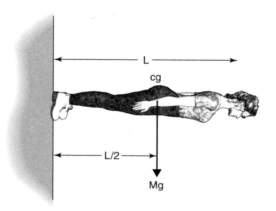

Assuming that her center of mass is at a distance $L/2$ from the wall (as shown) and that her body can be assumed to be rigid, what is her angular acceleration at the moment of release? What is the corresponding linear acceleration at the top of her head? Assume that her body can be modeled as a thin rod of length L.

Solution

The only torque acting on her body is that attributable to gravity, which acts with a force $F = Mg$ downward with a lever arm of $L/2$. The moment of inertia of a thin rod pivoted about its end is $\frac{1}{3}ML^2$ so that the initial angular acceleration is:

$$\alpha = \frac{\tau}{I} = \frac{Mg\frac{L}{2}}{\frac{1}{3}ML^2} = \frac{3g}{2L}$$

$$\alpha = \frac{3 \times 9.81}{2 \times 1.85} = 7.95 \text{ rad/s}^2$$

The linear acceleration of the top of her head is:

$$a = L\alpha = \tfrac{3}{2}g$$
$$a = 14.72 m/s^2$$

Notice that this is greater than the acceleration attributable to gravity.

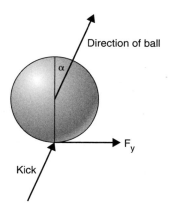

Figure 8.7 Kicking a ball off center and at an angle.

■ **EXAMPLE 8.3**   To produce a free kick in football, it is necessary to apply spin to the ball, which is achieved by striking the ball off center and at an angle (Fig. 8.7). The force applied in the kick has a sideways component, $F_y(t)$, that gives the ball a velocity component of $v_y(t)$ in the direction of F_y and a spin of $\omega(t)$. The equations for the **transfer of linear** and **angular momentum** are:

$$m\frac{dv_y}{dt} = F_y$$

$$I\frac{d\omega}{dt} = rF_y$$

where r is the radius of the ball and I is the moment of inertia about a diameter. For a hollow sphere, the moment of inertia is $\frac{2}{3}mr^2$. These equations combine to yield:

$$\frac{dv_y}{d\omega} = \frac{2}{3}r$$

so that the final values are:

$$v_y = \frac{2}{3}\omega r$$

Because the radius of a standard size 5 football is 0.11 m, this gives a relationship between v_y and ω (Fig. 8.8).

Figure 8.8 Relationship between transverse velocity and spin rate for a football kicked off center and at an angle.

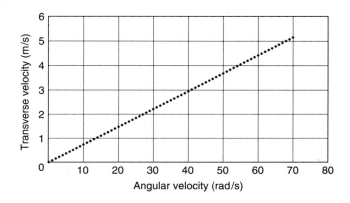

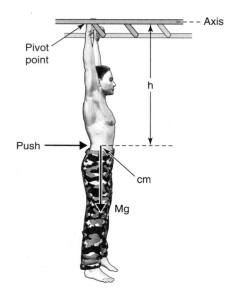

Figure 8.9 Body in a dead hang position. If the body is given a small push, it will execute small oscillations about the vertical position.

8.4 Calculating the Moment of Inertia

One easy way to find the moment of inertia of a body is to suspend the body from one end and to measure its period of oscillation. (See Section 6.8.4.2 on oscillatory motion and a physical pendulum.) Let us assume we can take a human subject and ask him to hang from a horizontal bar in a dead hang position (Fig. 8.9). We will assume that the contact at the hands is fairly low in friction so that it is possible for the subject to swing about the hands as pivot point.

It can be shown that the period of small oscillations of a physical pendulum is:

$$T = 2\pi \sqrt{\frac{I}{mgh}}$$

where h is the distance from the pivot point to the center of mass of the body and m is the mass of the body.

If we require the moment of inertia about another axis—for example, an axis parallel to the first axis but this time passing through the center of mass, or I_{cm}—then the parallel-axis theorem expresses this as:

$$I_{cm} = I - mh^2$$

Note, however, that this theorem can only be used when the axes are parallel and the moment of inertia about one axis is known or can be measured. In this example, it is essential that the subject's center of mass is known from a separate experiment with the subject's arms in a similar position to that shown in Figure 8.9.

■ **EXAMPLE 8.4**

A man hanging from a horizontal bar (see Fig. 8.9) has a body mass of 76 kg, and the value of h is 1.38 m. The period of small oscillations about the dead hang position is measured as 2.5 s. It follows that the moment of inertia about an axis through the hands is:

$$I = \frac{mghT^2}{4\pi^2}$$

$$I = \frac{76kg \times 9.81ms^{-2} \times 1.38m \times (2.5s)^2}{4 \times (3.14159)^2} = 162.9 \text{ kg.m}^2$$

The moment of inertia about the center of mass is:

$$I_{cm} = I - mh^2 = 177 - 76 \times (1.38)^2$$
$$I_{cm} = 162.9 - 144.7 = 18.2 \text{ kg.m}^2$$

(Data are fictitious.)

CASE *Study 8.1*   **Moment of Inertia of Human Body**

In an experiment to measure the moment of inertia of the human body (Griffiths et al., 2005), a platform is caused to rotate by the action of a falling mass. The weight of the falling mass causes a tension in a rope that exerts a torque on the rotatable platform. This method has been shown to be highly accurate for the measurement of the moment of inertia of a series of fixed masses and allows the errors attributable to frictional torques in the apparatus at the bearings to be virtually eliminated.

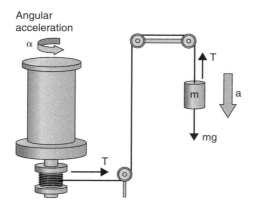

The platform incorporates a stool upon which the subject can sit, and the platform and stool are free to rotate but are subject to a small frictional force opposing the rotation. The torque exerted on the platform is determined by the tension, T, in the rope and the radius, r, of the cylindrical pulley. The resulting motion of the falling mass and rotation of the platform, can be modeled fairly easily using a combination of the equations for linear and rotational motion:

1. $a = r\alpha$

The linear acceleration of the mass is proportional to the angular acceleration of the stool. r is the radius of the bottom pulley wheel attached to the base of the stool.)

2. $mg - T = ma$

Newton's second law applied to the mass; a is its acceleration downward.)

3. $\tau = I\alpha = (I_p + I_{ch})\alpha$

(Torque is given by moment of inertia multiplied by angular acceleration of the stool. I_p is the M of I of the subject, and I_{ch} is the M of **I** of the stool plus associated parts,)

4. $\tau = rT$

Torque is given by tension force multiplied by radius, rr.)

5. $s = \frac{1}{2}at^2$

(Equation for uniformly accelerated motion, the mass falls a distance s in t seconds.)

6. $\alpha = \dfrac{\omega_{final}}{t}$

(The angular acceleration is given by the final angular velocity divided by the time, t.)

Griffiths et al. (2005) describe a series of trials on a male subject of mass 69 kg who sits on a stool with his center of mass on the axis of rotation of the stool. The rotational speed of the stool using a mass (m) of 2 kg, measured with an optoelectronic motion analysis system, is shown in the following figure:

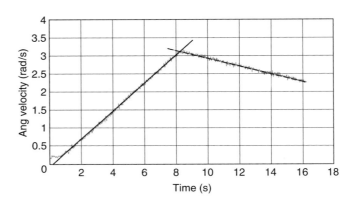

These data exhibit the linear increase of angular velocity with time that would be expected up to a time of approximately 8 seconds. At this time, the rope disengages from its pulley, and the falling mass reaches floor level, having traveled a distance of about 1 m since the start of the experiment. At times in excess of 8 s, the angular velocity decreases with time in a linear manner, indicating a small frictional force with a more or less constant magnitude. Thus, at times between 8.5 and 16.0 s, the platform is "freewheeling" and is subject only to small frictional forces. On this graph, the data between 0.5 and 8.0 s have been modeled by a trend line to model the angular acceleration as accurately as possible. The data between 8.5 and 16.0 s have been modeled as another trend line to model the frictional deceleration as accurately as possible. Both trend lines and the original angular velocity data are shown in the figure. To calculate the moment of inertia from experimental values, we can use the relationship:

$$(I_p + I_{ch}) = \frac{\tau}{\alpha}$$

so that:

$$(I_p + I_{ch}) = \frac{rTt}{\omega_{final}} = \frac{rt(mg - ma)}{\omega_{final}} = \frac{rtm(g - \dfrac{2s}{t^2})}{\omega_{final}}.$$

In this example, the radius r of the pulley wheel is 0.083 cm, and the distance fallen by the mass is 0.996 m. To evaluate the moment of inertia of the platform and stool, a separate experiment can be undertaken in which the measurements are repeated without the subject on the stool. In this case, we get a graph of angular velocity against time as follows:

Similar considerations apply to this experiment; clearly, the final angular velocity is much higher because of the smaller moment of inertia. To calculate the moments of inertia as accurately as possible, a correction can be made to allow for the friction forces acting on

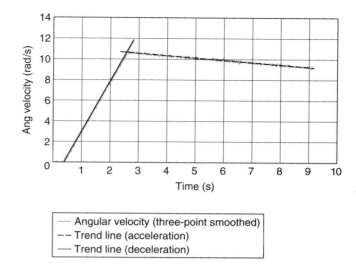

- Angular velocity (three-point smoothed)
-- Trend line (acceleration)
- Trend line (deceleration)

the platform. The effect of the friction force is to reduce the maximum angular velocity obtained, thus contributing to the experimental error. Fortunately, the linear fall-off of the angular velocity makes it easy to correct for this, resulting in improved accuracy for the moment of inertia. Some sample data obtained from the traces obtained here are as follows, with the top row for subject plus platform and bottom row for platform only:

	Platform plus subject	Platform only
Start time (s)	0.417	0.4358
Finish time (s)	16.241	9.166
Final angular speed (rad/s)	2.233	9.104
Maximum angular speed (rad/s)	3.102	10.695
Time at maximum angular speed (s)	8.266	2.591
Loss of angular speed per second (rad/s/s)	0.108	0.241
Correction to angular speed (rad/s)	0.427	0.270
Corrected final angular speed (rad/s)	3.529	10.965
Angular acceleraton (rad/s/s)	0.449	4.909
Moment of inertia (kg.m^2)	3.609	0.318

The value for the moment of inertia of the platform is 0.318 kg.m^2 and the value for the combined moment of inertia for platform plus subject is 3.610 kg.m^2. By subtraction, the moment of inertia for the subject alone is 3.29 kg/m^2.

8.5   Angular Momentum

A fundamental property of rotating bodies is that they tend to keep rotating, provided there are no torques acting to slow them down. Consider a discus, for example

Figure 8.10 A discus thrown with spin about an axis through the center of mass. The angular velocity vector usually points perpendicular to the circular face of the discus along the axis of symmetry.

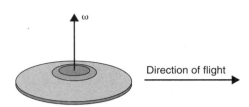

(Fig. 8.10), thrown with a certain amount of spin, usually achieved by allowing the discus to emerge from one side of the hand in the throwing action.

It is fairly easy to confirm that the spinning discus maintains an ostensibly constant angular velocity during its flight, notwithstanding small losses that may occur because of air resistance. The effect of the spin is to stabilize the orientation of the discus relative to its flight path so that it maintains its "sharp end" along its direction of motion. This avoids end-over-end tumbling, which would increase the air drag on the discus and decrease its range.

The equation $\tau = I\alpha$ (Newton's second law, with $F = ma$ for linear motion) describes the rotation of a rigid body such as a discus about a fixed axis or about an axis that moves with the discus without changing direction as long as the axis passes through the center of mass of the discus. The angular acceleration α is defined as $d\omega/dt$ so that:

$$\tau = I\alpha = I\frac{d\omega}{dt} = \frac{d(I\omega)}{dt}.$$

This equation is valid even if the moment of inertia changes, such as, for example, in the case of a diver changing from a tucked to an untucked position. The quantity $I\omega$ is called the **angular momentum**, L, of the body about its axis of rotation. It can then be seen that:

$$\tau = \frac{dL}{dt}$$

The quantity L is important because it can be shown that under certain circumstances, it is a conserved quantity. If the net torque acting on a body is 0, for example, approximately in the case of the discus, it follows that:

$$\frac{dL}{dt} = 0$$

This implies that:

$$L = I\omega = \text{constant}$$

In other words, for the discus (and all other rotating bodies that are free from net torques), the total angular momentum of the rotating body remains constant. In general, this is called the law of **conservation of angular momentum**. For bodies in which $I = $ constant (e.g., rigid bodies such as the discus), it follows that the angular velocity, ω, is constant as well.

When there is no net torque acting on a body and the body is rotating about a fixed axis or about an axis with a fixed direction passing through the center of mass, it is convenient to write:

$$I\omega = I_0\omega_0 = \text{Constant}$$

where I_0 and ω_0 are the moment of inertia and angular velocity at initial time of 0 and I and ω are the same quantities at a later time. In this latter equation, I may well be changing because the body is altering its mass distribution. Clearly, if I

increases, then ω will decrease to compensate and vice versa. The classic example of this is a skater spinning on ice about a vertical axis with her arms straight and horizontal. If she pulls in her arms close to her body, the speed of rotation increases substantially because her moment of inertia is reduced.

8.6   Angular Kinetic Energy

In linear kinetics, the kinetic energy (KE) of a body of mass m is given simply as:

$$\tfrac{1}{2}\,mv^2$$

in the case of a body rotating about a fixed axis, the **rotational kinetic energy**, by analogy, is $\tfrac{1}{2}\,I\omega^2$ where I is the moment of inertia of the body about that axis and ω is its angular velocity. The proof of this statement can be found in many textbooks on elementary physics and mechanics.

■ **EXAMPLE 8.5**

Calculate how much rotational energy is possessed by a football rotating at 3 revolutions per second. The mass of the ball is 0.42 kg, and the radius is 0.11m. If the ball is travelling at 30 mph, calculate its KE and the ratio of the ball's rotational energy to its KE.

Solution

$$E_R = \tfrac{1}{2}\,I\omega^2$$
$$I = \tfrac{2}{3}\,mr^2 = 0.666 \times 0.42kg \times (0.11m)^2$$

so that:

$$I = 0.00338kg.m^2$$
$$E_R = \tfrac{1}{2} \times 0.00338 \times (3 \times 2 \times \pi)^2$$
$$E_R = 0.6013J$$

The ball's KE is:

$$E_K = \tfrac{1}{2}\,mv^2 = 0.5 \times 0.42kg \times (13.4ms^{-1})^2$$
$$E_K = 37.71J$$

It can quite easily be shown that:

$$\frac{E_R}{E_K} = 0.32\left(\frac{f}{v}\right)^2 \quad v \text{ in } ms^{-1}$$
$$\frac{E_R}{E_K} = 0.32\left(\frac{3}{13.4}\right)^2 = 0.016$$

It can also be shown that the **work done by a torque** is the turning moment multiplied by the angle turned:

$$W = \tau \times \theta$$

and that the **power flow for a torque** τ rotating at angular velocity ω is:

$$P = \tau \times \omega$$

The power will be positive if τ and ω are in the same direction but negative if they are in opposite directions (see Chapter 2 and Appendix 1).

8.7   Combined Translation and Rotation

An object that undergoes both translation and rotation has both translational and rotational KE. Its **total kinetic energy** will be equal to the translational KE of its center of mass plus the KE of motion relative to the center of mass. The most common exam-

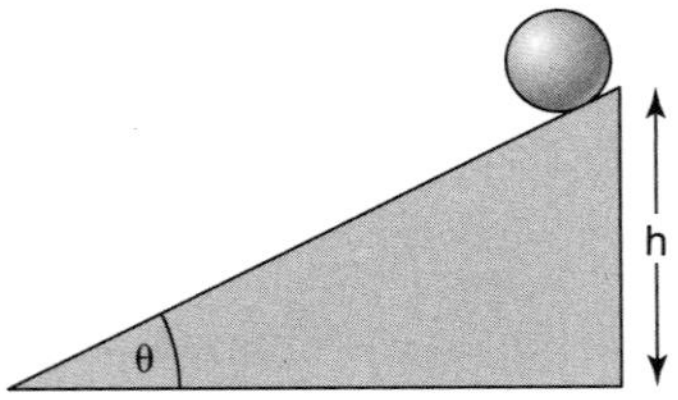

Figure 8.11   A ball of mass M rolling down a slope.

ple of an object moving both in translation and rotation in sport is a ball. Consider a ball (modeled as a solid sphere) of mass M and radius r rolling down a slope of angle θ with respect to the horizontal (Fig. 8.11). Let us assume that the ball starts at the top of the slope with zero initial speed and that it moves a vertical distance h in reaching the bottom of the slope. We can now apply conservation of momentum to this situation to find the velocity of the ball at the bottom of the slope. The total energy at a point a vertical distance y above the base of the slope is:

$$\tfrac{1}{2} Mv^2 + \tfrac{1}{2} I_{cm}\omega^2 + Mgy$$

Using conservation of energy, the total energy at the bottom of the slope must be the same as the total energy at the top of the slope so that:

$$0 + 0 + Mgh = \tfrac{1}{2} Mv^2 + \tfrac{1}{2} I_{cm}\omega^2 + 0.$$

We also know that the moment of inertia of a sphere about an axis through its center of mass is:

$$I_{cm} = \tfrac{2}{5} Mr^2$$

Assuming that the ball rolls without slipping, the speed, v, of its center of mass is:

$$\omega = v/r$$

Hence:

$$\tfrac{1}{2} Mv^2 + \tfrac{1}{2} \left(\tfrac{2}{5}Mr^2\right)\left(\tfrac{v^2}{r^2}\right) = Mgh$$

so that:

$$\left(\tfrac{1}{2} + \tfrac{1}{5}\right)v^2 = gh$$

or

$$v = \sqrt{\tfrac{10}{7}gh}$$

It is assumed that the ball is not affected by friction.

■ **EXAMPLE 8.6**

Consider a sphere of mass 0.5 kg rolling down a slope of gradient 30° with respect to the horizontal. Work out the velocity of the sphere after it has rolled a total distance of 1 m. Compare this result with the velocity of a point mass sliding down the same slope. The vertical drop is:

$$h = 1m \times \sin(30) = 0.5m$$

so that:

$$v = \sqrt{\tfrac{10}{7}gh} = \sqrt{\tfrac{10}{7} \times 9.81 \times 0.5} = 2.647ms^{-1}$$

The velocity acquired by a point mass is:

$$\sqrt{2gh} = \sqrt{2 \times 9.81 \times 0.5} = 3.132ms^{-1}$$

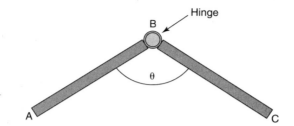

Figure 8.12 A simple body model composed of two rigid rods hinged together.

8.8   Angular Momentum in Linked Systems

Angular momentum can be transferred from one segment or group of segments to another segment or group of segments. Consider a body hinged at its midpoint and composed of two straight, rigid rod segments (Fig. 8.12). This could be used as a model for the human body performing certain simple planar movements. For example, a diver performing a piked dive could be modeled like this with AB representing the torso, arms, and head and BC representing the legs and feet. Dempster (1955) would suggest that the mass of AB would be a body fraction 0.682 approximately and the mass of BC would be a body fraction of approximately 0.318. This assumes that the body segments are perfectly rigid or at least sufficiently rigid for this to be considered a valid approximation ("quasi"-rigid). Also, of course, a diver has the ability to apply internal muscular contractions to vary the angle θ between AB and BC.

In what follows, for convenience, we will assume that the centers of mass of the segments AB and BC are both at their midpoints and that both segments are 1 m long. For more accurate data on the locations of the center of mass, refer to Dempster (1955).

As the angle between the torso and the legs varies, the location of the center of mass varies (Fig. 8.13). This diagram assumes that A (head) and B (hips) are fixed and C (feet) is free to move at a fixed distance from B. Here, the center of mass of the combined body has been calculated assuming total rigidity of the two segments.

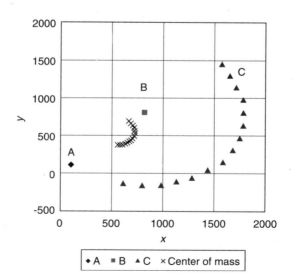

Figure 8.13 The coordinates of the points A (head), B (hips), and C (feet) for a range of body angles.

Figure 8.14 The moment of inertia of one of the segments about the common center of mass G can be worked out using the parallel axis theorem. D represents the center of mass of segment BC.

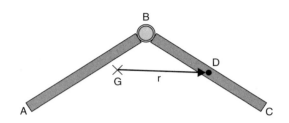

The moment of inertia of the combined body (Fig. 8.14) can be worked out by an application of the parallel axis theorem. The moment of inertia of one of the segments, say BC, about the center of mass of the combined body G is:

$$I_{com} = I_G + Mr^2$$

The moment of inertia of the other segment about the common center of mass is given in similar fashion; then the total moment of inertia of the combined body about its center of mass is given by addition. The result of this in this case is shown in Figure 8.15, where the segments AB and BC are assumed to have moments of inertia of:

$$I_G = \tfrac{1}{12} ML^2$$

about their centers of mass, and the total body mass is 90 kg.

It is clear that for a diver executing a piked dive, the angular speed about a somersault axis can be controlled to a marked extent by altering the angle between the legs and body segments. A good approximation to the angular velocity at any given instant can be calculated using:

$$I_0 \omega_0 = I_1 \omega_1$$

where I_0 and ω_0 are the initial values of the moment of inertia and angular velocity, respectively, and I_1 and ω_1 are their corresponding values at any other time.

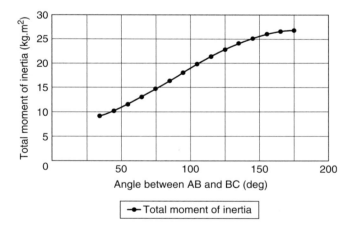

Figure 8.15 Total moment of inertia for the combined body AB–BC about its center of mass.

8.9   Manipulation of Axis of Rotation

Movement of body segments while in rotational motion can alter the axis of rotation relative to the cardinal axes of the body. For example, a diver who has

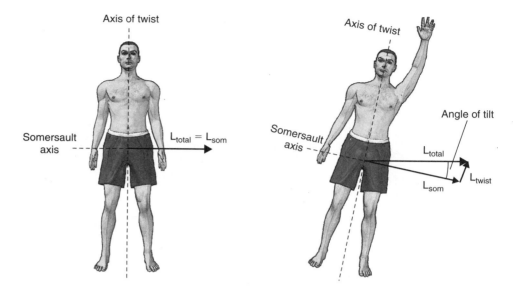

Figure 8.16 The angular momentum about a horizontal axis is constant even though arm adduction introduces twisting as well as somersaulting.

taken off with his arms at his sides and with a spin about the somersault axis can subsequently introduce a twisting motion by adducting his left arm. Because angular momentum is conserved, the rest of the diver's body rotates in the opposite sense to the arm, thus introducing an angle of tilt. The angular momentum about a horizontal axis is still the same because there has been no external torque to alter it. However, two components of angular momentum are now present, one about the somersault axis and the other about the axis of twist. This is sometimes called **angular momentum transfer**. This is illustrated in Figure 8.16, where it is clear that:

$$L_{total} = L_{som} + L_{twist}$$

CASE *Study 8.2*   **Power Flows in a Lower Leg Segment**

Consider a lower leg segment observed during normal walking gait. Energy can leave or enter the segment at muscles and across joints at the ankle and knee ends. The lefthand part of

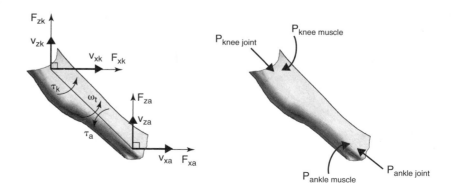

this diagram represents the state of the lower leg segment at any given time. The quantities marked on the diagram are defined thus:

	Horizontal x	Vertical z
Knee velocity (m/s)	v_{xk}	v_{zk}
Ankle velocity (m/s)	v_{xa}	v_{za}
Lower leg segment reaction force at knee (N)	F_{xk}	F_{zk}
Lower leg segment reaction force at ankle (N)	F_{xa}	F_{za}

	Ankle	Knee
Passive power flow across joint (W)	$P_{ankle\ joint}$	$P_{knee\ joint}$
Active power flow across joint (W)	$P_{ankle\ muscle}$	$P_{knee\ muscle}$
Moment across joint (Nm)	M_a	M_k

Note that the passive and active powers can be calculated as follows:

$$P_{knee\ joint} = F_{xk}v_{xk} + F_{zk}v_{zk}$$
$$P_{ankle\ joint} = F_{xa}v_{xa} + F_{za}v_{za}$$
$$P_{knee\ muscle} = \tau_k\omega_t$$
$$P_{ankle\ muscle} = \tau_a\omega_t.$$

According to the law of conservation of energy, the rate of change of energy of the segment should be equal to the sum of the four power terms:

$$\frac{dE_{lower\ leg}}{dt} = P_{knee\ joint} + P_{knee\ muscle} + P_{ankle\ joint} + P_{ankle\ muscle}$$

Here are some real values taken from a walking trial reported by Winter (1990):

Body mass $= 56.7$ kg
Knee velocity: $v_{xk} = 2.13$, $v_{zk} = 0.56$ m/s
Ankle velocity: $v_{xa} = 3.51$, $v_{za} = -0.84$ m/s
Lower leg angular velocity: $\omega_t = 4.9$ rad/s
Lower leg segment reaction forces at knee: $F_{xk} = 1.4$N, $F_{zk} = 19.1$ N
At ankle: $F_{xa} = 5.5$ N, $F_{za} = 4.8$ N
Moments at ankle: $\tau_a = 0.4$ Nm, knee: $\tau_k = -0.1$ Nm

The segment weight divided by the total body weight is 0.0465 for the lower leg (Dempster, 1955, via Miller and Nelson, 1973). The radius of gyration is given as 0.302 for rotation about the center of mass. The center of mass of the lower leg segment is located at $x = 0.624$ m, $y = 0.386$ m. The velocity of the center of mass of the lower leg segment is:

$$v_{com-x} = 2.727 m/s, \quad v_{com-y} = -0.045 m/s$$

The rotational KE is:

$$E_R = \tfrac{1}{2} I_{cm} \omega^2 = 0.5 \times 56.7 \times 0.0465 \times (0.302)^2 \times (4.9)^2 = 2.9J$$

The translational KE is:

$$E_K = \tfrac{1}{2} mv^2 = 0.5 \times 56.7 \times 0.0465 \times (2.727)^2 + (-0.045)^2 = 9.8J$$

The potential energy of the lower leg segment is:

$$mgh = 0.0465 \times 56.7 \times 9.8 \times 0.386 = 10.0J$$

Adding up all the power terms:

$$F_{xk}v_{xk} + F_{zk}v_{zk} + \tau_k \omega_s + F_{xa}v_{xa} + F_{za}v_{za} + \tau_a \, \omega_s$$

$$= 1.4 \times 2.13 + 19.1 \times 0.56 + (-0.1) \times 4.9 + 5.5 \times 3.51 + 4.8 \times (-0.84) + 0.4 \times 4.9$$

$$= 2.98 + 10.70 - 0.049 + 19.31 - 4.03 + 1.96 = 30.87\,W$$

Passive power into leg from knee joint forces

Passive power into leg from knee joint forces

Active power into leg from muscles at knee joint

Active power into leg from muscles at knee joint

To summarize, it is possible to calculate the power flows into and out of the lower leg segment from both passive and active sources. In this case, power was transferred out of the lower leg because of the muscle moment at the knee to a very slight extent ($-0.049W$). Power was transferred into the lower leg because of the muscle moment at the ankle ($1.96W$).

By a continuation of this method, it would be possible to identify the power flows into and out of neighboring body segments. Also, it is possible to link the net power flows into or out of the body segment to the total energy of the segment. For example, if the net power flow into the segment is positive, it should also be verifiable that the sum of the rotational and translational kinetic energies and potential energy of the segment should increase with time.

SUMMARY

This chapter has concentrated on the application of torque, angular acceleration, and moment of inertia to the study of rotational motion. Several topics of interest to biomechanists have been covered, including the moment of inertia of the human body and modeling a rotating body as a hinged rigid-rod system. Some of the applications of rotational dynamics to diving have been introduced.

REFERENCES

Dempster WT: *Space Requirements of the Seated Operator.* WADC-TR-55-159, Wright Patterson Air Force Base; Ohio 1955.

Griffiths IW, Watkins J, Sharpe D: Measuring the moment of inertia of the human body by a rotating platform method. *Am J Phys* 73:85–92, 2005.

Miller DI, Nelson RC: *Biomechanics of Sport.* Philadelphia: Lea and Febiger; 1973.

Winter DA: *Biomechanics and Motor Control of Human Movement*, 2nd edn. New York: John Wiley & Sons; 1990

STUDY QUESTIONS

1. A force of 130 N exerted at a distance of 0.55 m from the axis is balanced by a force of 205 N. What is the moment arm of the other force?

2. A force of 250 N exerted at a distance of 0.4 m from the axis is balanced by a force with a moment arm of 0.25 m. What is the force?

3. A therapist applies a lateral force of 95N to the forearm at a distance 35 cm from the axis of rotation at the elbow. The biceps attaches to the radius at a 90° angle and at a distance 4 cm from the elbow joint center.
   (a) How much force is required of the biceps to stabilize the arm at this position?
   (b) What is the magnitude of the reaction force exerted by the humerus on the ulna?
   (c) What is the mechanical advantage of the arm in this example?

4. A force of 110 N is exerted at a distance of 0.3 m from the axis of rotation. What is the resulting moment of force?

5. A force of 110 N is exerted at a distance of 0.34 m from the axis of rotation and is balanced by another force of 185 N. What is the moment arm of the other force?

6. A solid cricket ball is spun using the fingers to a rotation speed of 6 rev/s in a time of 0.05 s. What is the angular acceleration during this 0.05-s interval? What average torque was applied by the fingers? Assume the ball is a solid sphere with a mass of 0.156 kg and a diameter of 7.19 cm.

7. A soccer ball is kicked with a spin of 25 rad/s off center and at an angle. How much transverse velocity is given to the ball? Radius of ball = 0.11 m.

8. A man of mass 85 kg hangs from a horizontal bar in the dead hang position. The center of mass is 1.28 m below the bar. If his period of oscillation is 1.9 s, what is his moment of inertia (a) about the bar and (b) about the center of mass? Check that your figures are reasonable.

9. The rotating platform in the moment of inertia experiment described in the Case Study 8.1 is allowed to rotate freely without a subject on the platform. The rotational speed of the platform reduces from 10 to 9 rad/s in a time of 5.2 s. What is the frictional torque acting in the system?

10. Work out the velocity of a solid ball rolled down a slope with angle of 45° with respect to the horizontal after a total distance rolled of 2 m. If the mass of the ball is 0.3 kg, calculate the rotational and kinetic energies of the ball at the bottom of the slope.

11. Locate the center of mass of the diver illustrated in the following diagram: Model the upper and lower parts of the body as rigid rods. The total

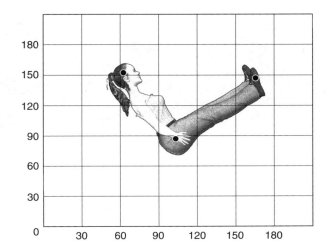

mass of the diver is 75 kg. Make some reasonable assumptions to allocate the masses of the rods in the model. Read the approximate coordinates of the distal and proximal ends of the rods from the diagram. The units are centimeters. Calculate the moment of inertia of the diver about the center of mass in kg.m^2.

12. Estimate the angle of tilt introduced when a diver adducts his arm, as in Figure 8.15. Assume the arm counts as 0.05 of the total body mass. Use the following hinged-rod model. Make any necessary assumptions to provide a realistic estimate.

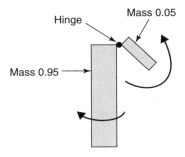

DATA FILTERING, SMOOTHING, AND TRENDS

CHAPTER *objectives*

The objectives of this chapter are to introduce the ideas of data filtering and smoothing and to examine trends in sets of data.

CHAPTER *outcomes*

After reading this chapter, the reader will be able to:

- Understand and be able to handle streams of coordinate data.
- Calculate velocities and accelerations using finite difference methods.
- Appreciate and quantify the errors arising in such calculations.
- Use polynomial and linear trend lines as best fits to sets of data.
- Understand the limitations and advantages of such trend lines.
- Use a digital filter to remove high-frequency noise from data of lower frequency.
- Understand the concept of a frequency spectrum.

9.1 Coordinate Data

Experimental investigations in biomechanics often result in streams of coordinate data for displacement, x, and time, t. Often y and z coordinate data are also produced. Inevitably, errors or uncertainties are involved in the measurement of the displacement data. These errors may be the result of systematic or random errors in the measurement process (e.g., shortcomings in the calibration process or operator error) and are usually larger than the uncertainties in the time values. Most measurements in biomechanics are taken at regularly spaced and equal time intervals; these time intervals are usually fixed by the apparatus in some sense. For example, if the

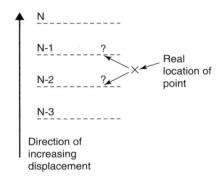

Figure 9.1   Illustration of digitization errors by a digital measurement system. The levels $N, N − 1, N − 2, N − 3$, and so on represent locations represented by consecutive digital numbers. The location of a point has to be represented by one of the digital numbers (in this case, either $N − 1$ or $N − 2$). Whereas a binary number consisting of eight digits has 256 possible levels, one of 12 bits has 4096.

recording system is a video camcorder, the frame rate is set at 50 (or 60) fields per second or a frame rate of 25 (or 30) fields per second. Although the timing is not perfect, it is usually sufficient to assume that the uncertainties arising from timing errors are quite small compared with those arising from uncertainty in the measurement of the displacement data. Even in the absence of these uncertainties, digital systems are prone to digitization errors because of the fact that the location of a point is specified as a digital number (Fig. 9.1). The error, although usually very small, can be important when it comes to calculating velocities and accelerations based on x, y, z coordinate data.

We like to think of the motion of a real object in terms of a continuum, that is, the x (or y or z) coordinate can vary smoothly and continuously to reflect the actual movement in space. In reality, we are faced with the result of a physical measurement in which the displacement data are affected by a range of uncertainties associated with the measurement. This is illustrated in Figure 9.2, where an "idealized" movement is contrasted with the result of a measurement of its movement involving errors.

Figure 9.2 illustrates the difficulty faced by researchers when faced with time-series coordinate data subject to errors. First, the shape of the curve is by no means clear because of the obscuring effect of the errors. Second, and perhaps more importantly, the calculation of velocities and accelerations from the displacement

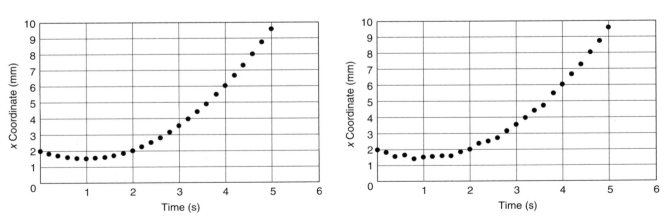

Figure 9.2   Idealized hypothetical data for displacement, x, as a function of time (*left*). Hypothetical real data based on the same data but subject to random errors (*right*).

Table 9.1 Idealized displacement data, noisy displacement data, and the differences between them

Idealized x Coordinate (mm)	Noisy x Coordinate (mm)	Difference (mm)	Idealized x Coordinate (mm)	Noisy x Coordinate (mm)	Difference (mm)
2.00	1.958	−0.042	2.78	2.720	−0.056
1.82	1.798	−0.022	3.12	3.060	−0.059
1.68	1.762	0.082	3.5	3.627	0.127
1.58	1.591	0.011	3.92	3.906	−0.014
1.52	1.458	−0.061	4.38	4.438	0.059
1.5	1.555	0.055	4.88	4.968	0.088
1.52	1.559	0.039	5.42	5.287	−0.132
1.58	1.503	−0.076	6	6.068	0.068
1.68	1.753	0.073	6.62	6.699	0.079
1.82	1.645	−0.174	7.28	7.346	0.066
2	1.854	−0.145	7.98	8.169	0.189
2.22	2.207	−0.012	8.72	8.730	0.010
2.48	2.492	0.012	9.5	9.481	−0.018

will exacerbate the problems caused by the errors. Table 9.1 shows the **idealized x coordinates**, the **noisy x coordinates**, and the differences between the two.

9.2 Calculation of Velocity and Acceleration from Displacement–Time Coordinate Data

To calculate the x component of velocity from displacement (x) and time (t) data, the most direct approach is to use the **finite-difference formula**:

$$v_x = \frac{\Delta x}{\Delta t} = \frac{x_n - x_{n-1}}{t_n - t_{n-1}}$$

where:

$x_n = x$ coordinate at time t_n

$x_{n-1} = x$ coordinate at time t_{n-1}

$t_n = $ time at reading "n"

$t_{n-1} = $ time at previous reading, "$_{n-1}$"

$v_x = $ average velocity over the time interval t_{n-1}, t_n

This calculation of velocity gives the average velocity over the time interval t_{n-1}, t_n and equates with calculating the slope of the line joining the two points in Figure 9.3. This idea is illustrated in Figure 9.4 using some hypothetical x–t data in a spreadsheet.

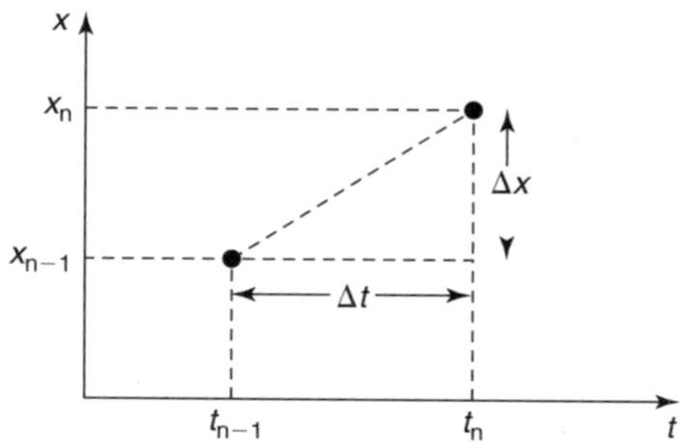

Figure 9.3 Illustration of calculation of the velocity at time t_n from the coordinates t_{n-1}, x_{n-1}, and t_n, x_n.

	A	B	C		D
1		TIME	LFHD		x-velo
2	Field #	(s)	X	"=(C4-C3)/(B4-B3)"	mm/s
3	1	0.008333	220.6673		
4	2	0.016667	220.5437		-14.8297
5	3	0.025	220.9678		50.89416
6	4	0.033333	221.0496		9.81816
7	5	0.041667	220.5612		-58.6139

Figure 9.4 Calculation of velocity using a spreadsheet calculation (hypothetical data). This formula can be copied down the D column to generate the velocity for the whole of the spreadsheet. Notice that the first cell in the D column has been left blank because the data items C2 (= X) and B2 (= (s)) would be required to complete this cell D3.

To illustrate what may happen with real data, we will return to the data in Figure 9.2. Figure 9.5 shows the calculated velocities and accelerations obtained from the idealized and "real" data using the method illustrated by Figure 9.4. Figure 9.5 shows that the noise on the data has a large impact on the calculated velocity values; the noisy data give velocity values with more **scatter**, that is, the **uncertainties** from the idealized velocity values can be positive or negative with variable magnitude. Table 9.2 quantifies the uncertainty in the velocity values in millimeter per second.

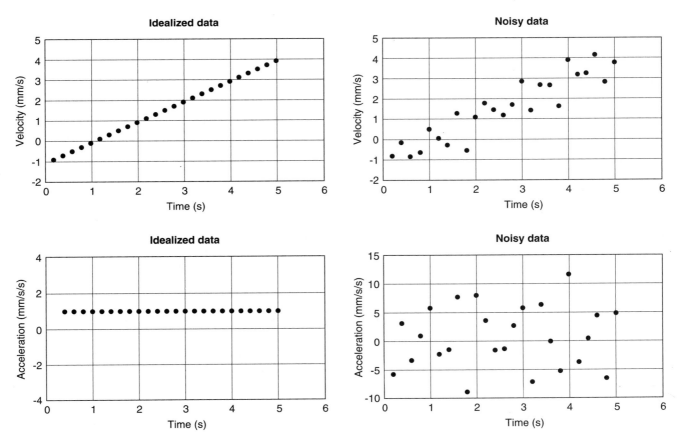

Figure 9.5 Calculated velocities (*above*) from the idealized displacement data (*left*) and the noisy displacement data (*right*). Calculated accelerations (*below*) from the calculated velocity values. Original data are shown in Figure 9.2.

Table 9.2   Idealized velocity data, noisy velocity data, and the differences between them

Idealized Velocity	Velocity (Noisy Data)	Difference (mm/s)	Idealized Velocity	Velocity (Noisy Data)	Difference (mm/s)
−0.9	−0.8	−0.1	—	—	—
−0.7	−0.2	−0.5	1.7	1.7	0.0
−0.5	−0.9	0.4	1.9	2.8	−0.9
−0.3	−0.7	0.4	2.1	1.4	0.7
−0.1	0.5	−0.6	2.3	2.7	−0.4
0.1	0.0	0.1	2.5	2.6	−0.1
0.3	−0.3	0.6	2.7	1.6	1.1
0.5	1.3	−0.8	2.9	3.9	−1.0
0.7	−0.5	1.2	3.1	3.2	−0.1
0.9	1.0	−0.1	3.3	3.2	0.1
1.1	1.8	−0.7	3.5	4.1	−0.6
1.3	1.4	−0.1	3.7	2.8	0.9
1.5	1.2	0.3	3.9	3.8	0.1

Notice that in Figure 9.5 the accelerations have been calculated from the velocities in an analogous way to the calculations of velocities from displacements. As soon as the velocity values have been calculated, the acceleration values are calculated using:

$$a_x = \frac{\Delta v_x}{\Delta t} = \frac{v_x(t_n) - v_x(t_{n-1})}{t_n - t_{n-1}}$$

where, this time, a_x represents the average acceleration between the time intervals t_n and t_{n-1}.

Again, Figure 9.6 illustrates this acceleration calculation in a spreadsheet based on hypothetical data. This calculation generates even larger errors than the velocity calculations. Figure 9.5 shows that whereas the idealized acceleration is a constant of $1mm/s^2$, the values calculated from the noisy displacement data show wild oscillations, making it difficult to make any accurate conclusions about the acceleration (Table 9.3). For ease of comparison, the standard deviations (SDs) for the differences between ideal and noisy data are given in Table 9.4 for displacement, velocity, and acceleration data.

9.3   The Problem of Noise on Signals

Example 9.1 highlights the problems associated with calculating kinematic data from experimental displacement data. It is possible to examine the same problem

Figure 9.6   The calculation of acceleration values a_x from velocity values along the x axis. Note that E3 and E4 are left blank because the velocity values required for their calculation are not available. The formula for acceleration in cell E5 can be copied down the remainder of the E column.

	A	B	C	D	E
1		TIME	LFHD	x-velo	x-accel
2	Field #	(s)	X	mm/s	mm/s/s
3	1	0.008333	220.6673		
4	2	0.016667	220.5437	-14.82972	"=(D5-D4)/(B5-B4)"
5	3	0.025	220.9678	50.89416	7886.866
6	4	0.033333	221.0496	9.81816	-4929.12
7	5	0.041667	220.5612	-58.61388	-8211.845
8					

Table 9.3   Ideal acceleration data, noisy acceleration data, and the differences between them

Ideal Acceleration (mm/s/s)	Noisy Acceleration (mm/s/s)	Difference (mm/s/s)	Ideal Acceleration (mm/s/s)	Noisy Acceleration (mm/s/s)	Difference (mm/s/s)
1	3.129	−2.129	1	5.767	−4.767
1	−3.383	4.383	1	−7.214	8.214
1	0.956	0.043	1	6.331	−5.331
1	5.741	−4.741	1	−0.058	1.058
1	−2.305	3.305	1	−5.281	6.281
1	−1.537	2.537	1	11.564	−10.564
1	7.678	−6.678	1	−3.739	4.739
1	−8.972	9.972	1	0.377	0.622
1	7.952	−6.952	1	4.427	−3.427
1	3.575	−2.575	1	−6.581	7.581
1	−1.689	2.689	1	4.761	−3.761
1	−1.338	2.338	1	5.767	−4.767
1	2.628	−1.628	1	−7.214	8.214
1	3.129	−2.129	1	6.331	−5.331
1	−3.383	4.383	1	−0.058	1.058
1	0.956	0.043	1	−5.281	6.281

from the point of view of **differentiating functions**. Consider a displacement function given by:

$$x(t) = R(t) + N(t)$$

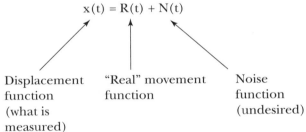

Displacement function (what is measured)   "Real" movement function   Noise function (undesired)

where the measured displacement is considered as the sum of a "real" movement and a "noise" component interfering with the measurement. The noise component can represent, for example, 50 or 60 Hz interference attributable to electrical mains or any other random errors introduced by the measurement process. The process of differentiation on the displacement variable, x, results in an instantaneous value for the velocity at time t. The idea here is to allow the time interval, Δt, to shrink to smaller and smaller values so that Δx and Δt both approach 0. A brief review of

Table 9.4   Standard deviations of the differences in displacement, velocity, and acceleration data*

Standard Deviation for Differences in Displacement Data	Standard Deviation for Differences in Velocity Data	Standard Deviation for Differences in Acceleration Data
0.086	0.61	5.35

* From data in Tables 9.1 to 9.3

calculus is given in Appendix 1. The result is a limiting value for the ratio $\Delta x / \Delta t$ equal to the **instantaneous velocity** v_x at time t.

$$v_x = \lim_{\Delta t \to 0} \frac{\Delta x}{\Delta t} = \frac{dx}{dt}$$

To calculate the velocity from this displacement function by differentiation, we obtain:

$$v_x = \frac{dx(t)}{dt} = \frac{dR(t)}{dt} + \frac{dN(t)}{dt}$$

Clearly, biomechanical investigators are interested in finding $\frac{dR(t)}{dt}$, the velocity attributable to the "real" movement, and are not particularly concerned with the noise contribution $\frac{dN(t)}{dt}$. Clearly, then, we must try to ensure that $\frac{dN(t)}{dt}$ is small compared with $\frac{dR(t)}{dt}$ ($< 10\%$) and, preferably, much smaller ($< 1\%$). The problem is that the noise component is measured along with the real component, so that it is not always possible to separate the two parts from their effects. A simple approach might be to say that $R(t)$ has to be much larger than $N(t)$. However, this does not take into account the frequency content of the components $R(t)$ and $N(t)$. When either function is differentiated, the result is proportional to the frequency of $R(t)$ or $N(t)$; hence, the higher the frequency of the noise $N(t)$ compared with the frequency of the real displacement function $R(t)$, the more the velocity will be dominated by noise.

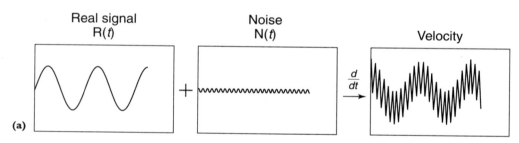

(a)

Diagram (a) shows that a slowly varying real displacement together with some high-frequency noise gives a velocity dominated by the noise after differentiation. Note that the noise effect is exaggerated because of the process of differentiation.

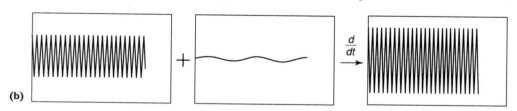

(b)

Diagram (b) shows a rapidly varying real displacement together with some low-frequency noise gives an accurate velocity after differentiation.

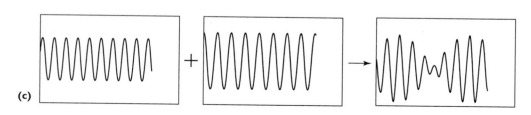

(c)

Diagram (c) shows a medium-frequency real displacement function together with a similar frequency noise gives a complex velocity function after differentiation. It would be very difficult to unscramble the real data and the noise in this situation.

The problems associated with calculating the velocity from displacement data are evident from the above figures. Even these figures do not show all the difficulties because they do not show the acceleration calculation. Calculating the acceleration requires another stage of differentiation because acceleration is the rate of change of velocity. Clearly, the calculated acceleration will be even more sensitive to noise than the velocity values.

$$x(t) \quad \overset{\frac{d}{dt}}{\Longrightarrow} \quad v_x(t) \quad \overset{\frac{d}{dt}}{\Longrightarrow} \quad a_x(t)$$

In biomechanics research, it is frequently true to say that the frequencies involved in human movements are significantly lower than the frequencies of noise or errors. For example, a golf swing is probably completed in a time of 2 s or less, but errors caused by electrical mains interference are at frequency 50 or 60 Hz; that is, they are undergoing whole cycles of change in times of the order of 0.02 s. Also, errors in measurement and noise are usually small compared with the physical quantities being measured. Even so, some movements in sports biomechanics are, by their nature, fast moving (e.g., a kicking foot in a rugby place kick or a fist in a karate punch).

In summary, it is important that high-frequency noise components are removed or reduced in magnitude in order to ensure that velocity and, in particular, acceleration calculations are reliable. In general, the noise removal takes place after reconstruction of coordinates and before calculating other data, such as joint forces and moments. This is done because the nonlinear nature of the calculations can affect the separation of signal and noise by **low-pass filtering** (Woltring, 1995).

9.4   Noise Removal by Finite Difference Smoothing

Consider the data point being smoothed and the data points nearest to it on either side. It is possible to smooth the data by taking a three-point **moving average** using:

$$x_{sm-0} = (x_{-1} + 2x_0 + x_1)/4$$

or a five-point moving average using:

$$x_{sm-0} = (x_2 + 3x_{-1} + 4x_0 + 3x_1 + x_2)/12$$

or a 7-point moving average using:

$$x_{sm-0} = (x_{-3} + 4x_{-2} + 7x_{-1} + 8x_0 + 7x_1 + 4x_2 + x_3)/32$$

These moving-average methods can be quite useful in improving the appearance of time-series coordinate data; they have the advantages of being:

■ Simple to apply
■ Easy to understand
■ Applicable more than once (with care)
■ Adequate for many but not all purposes

Their disadvantages are:

■ They do not always provide enough smoothing to enable velocities and accelerations to be calculated.

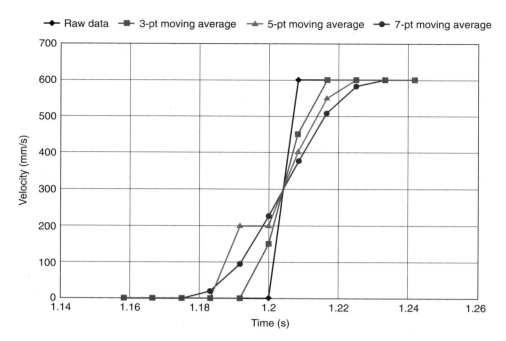

Figure 9.7 Calculated velocity after the displacement data is smoothed by varying degrees of n-point moving average. Note that whereas the raw data result in a velocity that increases from 0 to its final value in just one time interval, the three-, five-, and seven-point smoothed data require three, five, and seven time intervals to show the same increase.

■ They have a broadening effect on sharp features, especially if the number of points in the moving average is large and they are applied more than once.

The broadening effect on sharp features can be illustrated by a displacement function that is initially 0 but that then moves by 5 mm in every time interval Δt. Figure 9.7 illustrates the effect when the x data are smoothed by three-, five- and seven-point moving averages and then the velocity is calculated by the finite difference method.

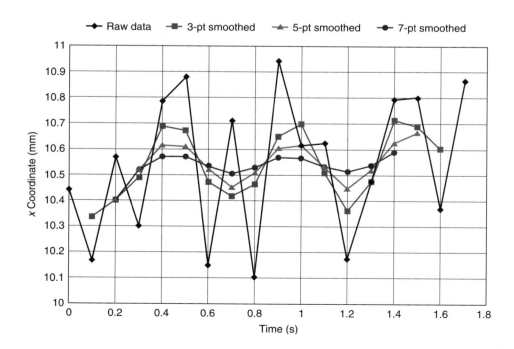

Figure 9.8 The effect of a moving average method for smoothing.

Figure 9.8 shows the effect of data smoothing on some fictitious *x* data fluctuating around a value 10.5 mm. The effect of the *N*-point smoothing is to reduce the amplitude of the fluctuations and to reduce their frequency.

9.5 Missing Data

Occasionally, a motion analysis system fails to yield the spatial coordinates of a marker for a number of possible reasons. For example, a marker or a location may have been obscured or may have moved out of the range of the recording system. In such cases, it is possible to **interpolate** between points to generate the missing data. For example, consider the following hypothetical *x–y* data where the *x, y* coordinates at times of 0.14 to 0.20 s inclusive are missing.

Time (s)	*x* (mm)	*y* (mm)
0.00	24.91	0.00
0.02	31.27	11.61
0.04	33.71	22.42
0.06	35.51	32.45
0.08	37.00	41.68
0.10	38.28	50.13
0.12	39.41	57.79
0.14	*	*
0.16	*	*
0.18	*	*
0.20	*	*
0.22	43.90	84.23
0.24	44.65	87.15
0.26	45.37	89.28
0.28	46.05	90.62
0.30	46.71	91.17
0.32	47.35	90.93
0.34	47.97	89.90
0.36	48.57	88.08
0.38	49.16	85.48
0.40	49.73	82.08
0.42	50.28	77.89
0.44	50.82	72.92
0.46	51.36	67.15
0.48	51.88	60.60
0.50	52.39	53.25
0.52	52.89	45.12
0.54	53.38	36.19
0.56	53.87	26.48

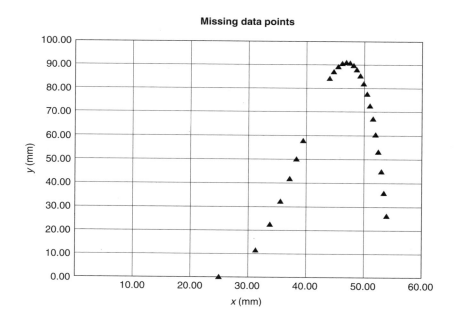

Figure 9.9 Hypothetical x–y data with four data points missing between x = 39.5 and 43.5.

Figure 9.9 shows the x and y coordinates; the four missing data points are obvious. In fact, the missing data points were:

Missing time values	Interpolated x values	Interpolated y values
0.14	40.45	64.65
0.16	41.40	70.73
0.18	42.28	76.02
0.20	43.12	80.52

but they have been deliberately cut out for this illustration. In spreadsheets, the missing data can be filled in with care by use of interpolation. In the case of interpolation functions, x and y data that are present are entered as array variables in rows or columns in a contiguous group of cells. The x and y data should be continuously increasing or decreasing.

	A	B	C	D	E	F	G
1	time (s)	x (mm)	y (mm)				
2	0.00	24.91	0.00				
3	0.02	31.27	11.61				
4	0.04	33.71	22.42				
5	0.06	35.51	32.45				
6	0.08	37.00	41.68				
7	0.10	38.28	50.13				
8	0.12	39.41	57.79	"=Interp($A$2:$A$14,$B$2:$B$14,0.14)"	missing time values	interpolated x values	interpolated y values
9	0.22	43.90	84.23		0.14	40.46	64.65
10	0.24	44.65	87.15		0.16	41.41	70.73
11	0.26	45.37	89.28		0.18	42.29	76.02
12	0.28	46.05	90.62		0.20	43.12	80.52
13	0.30	46.71	91.17				
14	0.32	47.35	90.93				
15	0.34	47.97	89.90				
16	0.36	48.57	88.08				

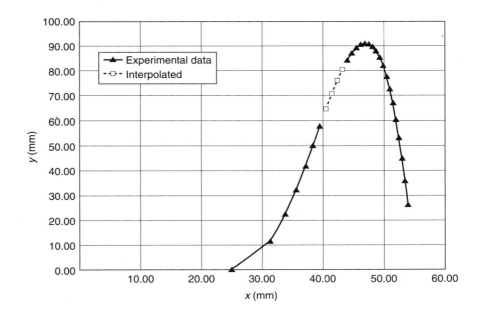

Figure 9.10 The *xy*, data including the four interpolated points.

In the case above, rows 2 to 14 were selected as the contiguous groups of cells for the array function Interp, but the four missing time values were deleted from the A column. The Interp function does a remarkably good job of generating the missing values; the *x–y* plot including the interpolated points is now shown in Figure 9.10.

Note that the four interpolated points can now be pasted back in to the data spreadsheet to complete the data set. Interpolation, although valuable, needs to be used with extreme caution if large gaps are to be filled.

9.6   Fitting Trend Lines to Data

9.6.1 FITTING CURVES TO LINEAR DATA

Spreadsheet packages allow you to fit curves to experimental data points. In general, the experimental *x–y* data is of the form:

$$x_1, y_1, x_2, y_2, x_3, \ldots\ldots\ldots x_n, y_n$$

In what follows, we will consider fitting the data by **trend lines** of the form:

$$y = cx + d \text{ (linear trend line)}$$
$$y = bx^2 + cx + d \text{ (quadratic trend line)}$$
$$y = ax^3 + bx^2 + cx + d \text{ (cubic trend line)}$$

The idea of fitting a trend line by linear regression is explained in Appendix 1. More details on the process can be found in the textbook by Vincent (2005). The general nature of these trend lines is illustrated in Figure 9.11.

Consider some hypothetical *x–y* data in which the data are nominally distributed about a straight line. Figures 9.12 to 9.14 illustrate approximately 20 data points of idealized *x–y* data. The level of the noise is 0 in these figures so that the data fall perfectly on a straight line. Figures 9.12 to 9.14 illustrate a linear trend line, quadratic trend line, and cubic trend line, respectively. The R^2 value on the figures is the **coefficient of determination**.

Figures 9.15 to 9.17 show similar data but now with random noise of magnitude

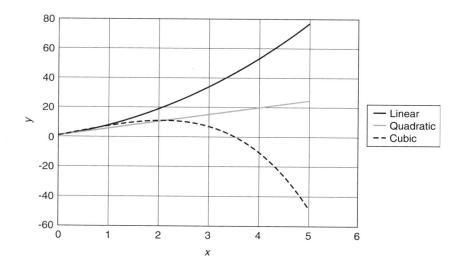

Figure 9.11 Trend lines of orders 1, 2, and 3.

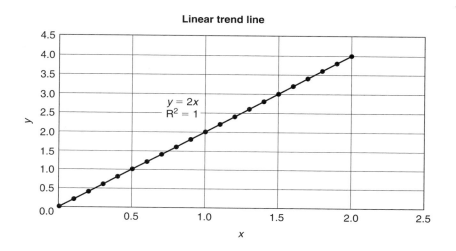

Figure 9.12 Linear data with zero noise fitted by a linear trend line. The value of c is 2, and a, b and d are all zero. The value of R^2 is 1.

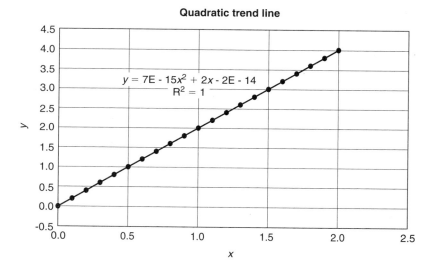

Figure 9.13 Linear data with zero noise fitted by a polynomial curve of order 2. The value of c is still 2, and b and d are extremely small. R^2 is still 1. The data are the same as in Figure 9.12.

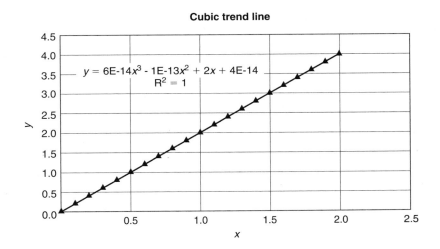

Figure 9.14 Linear data with zero noise fitted by a polynomial curve of order 3. The value of c is still 2 with extremely small values for the other coefficients, a, b, and d. The value of R^2 is still 1. The data are the same as in Figures 9.12 and 9.13. Note that a number like 6E-14 represents the number 6×10^{-14}.

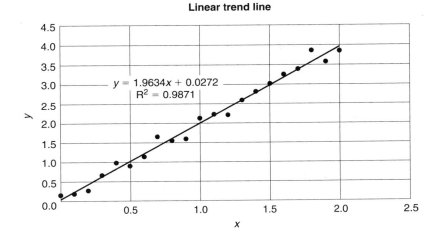

Figure 9.15 Linear data with noise $= 0.3$ fitted by a linear trend line. $c = 1.96$; $d = 0.03$; $R^2 = 0.9871$. The underlying (noise-free) data are the same as in Figures 9.12 to 9.14.

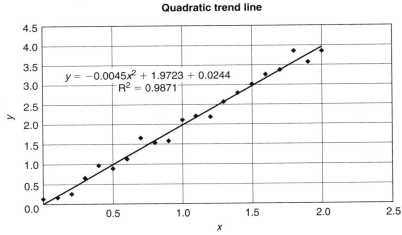

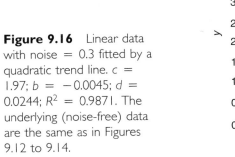

Figure 9.16 Linear data with noise $= 0.3$ fitted by a quadratic trend line. $c = 1.97$; $b = -0.0045$; $d = 0.0244$; $R^2 = 0.9871$. The underlying (noise-free) data are the same as in Figures 9.12 to 9.14.

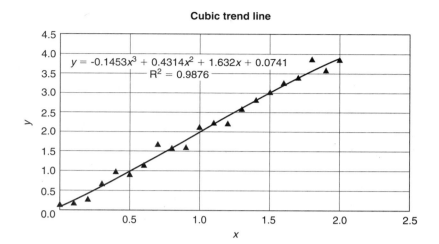

Figure 9.17 Linear data with noise $= 0.3$ fitted by a cubic trend line. $c = 1.63$; $a = -0.145$; $b = 0.431$; $d = 0.074$; $R^2 = 0.9876$. The underlying (noise-free) data are the same as in Figures 9.12 to 9.14.

0.3 added in. The same trend lines are fitted as in Figures 9.12 to 9.14 to give a comparison.

Finally, Figures 9.18 to 9.20 show similar data but now with random noise of magnitude 0.6 added in. The same trend lines are fitted as in Figures 9.12 to 9.14 to give a comparison.

In the case of the Figures 9.12 and 9.20, a simplified view is that the "real" data can be represented by the equation $y = 2x$. However, the presence of the noise within the data can sometimes mean that a quadratic or cubic fit to the data can appear to match the data better than a linear fit. The equations of the trend lines and the coefficients of determination in Figures 9.12 and 9.20 are summarized in Table 9.5.

9.6.1.1 Summary

Linear data can be fitted with linear, quadratic, or cubic curves with similar values of R^2. Increasing amounts of random noise reduce the value of R^2 for linear, quadratic, and cubic curve fits. In the presence of noise, R^2 is increased for quadratic and cubic curve fits to a slight extent. However, the conclusion that a cubic curve fit is the best is false since the increase in R^2 is far too small to be significant. In this example, the linear trend line is the most appropriate choice and yields a value for the c coefficient nearest to the ideal value of 2. Be careful about fitting polynom-

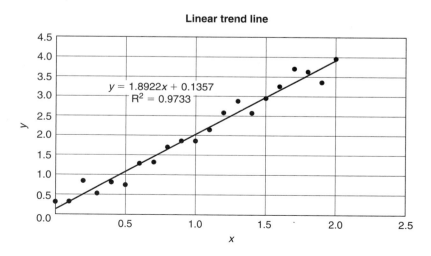

Figure 9.18 Linear data with noise $= 0.6$ fitted by a linear trend line. $c = 1.89$; $d = 0.136$; $R^2 = 0.9733$. The underlying (noise-free) data are the same as in Figures 9.12 to 9.14.

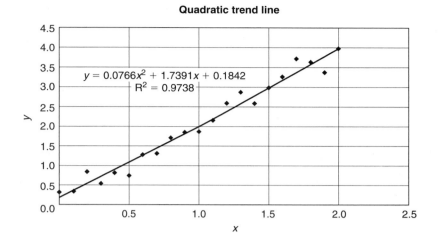

Figure 9.19 Linear data with noise = 0.6 fitted by a quadratic trend line. $c = 1.74$; $b = 0.077$; $d = 0.184$; $R^2 = 0.9738$. The underlying (noise-free) data are the same as in Figures 9.12 to 9.14.

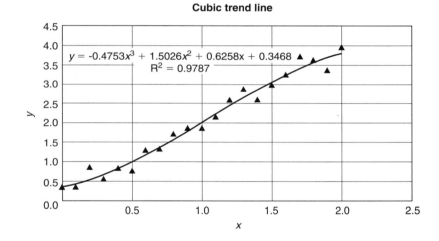

Figure 9.20 Linear data with noise = 0.6 fitted by a cubic trend line. $c = 0.626$; $a = -0.475$; $b = 1.503$; $d = -0.347$; $R^2 = 0.9787$. The underlying (noise-free) data are the same as in Figures 9.12 to 9.14.

Table 9.5	The equations of the trend lines and the values of R^2 for the curve fits of Figures 9.12 to 9.20*		
Noise	**Linear**	**Quadratic**	**Cubic**
0	$y = 2x$	$y = (7E - 15)x^2 + 2x - (2E - 14)$*	$y = (6E - 14)x^3 - (1E - 13)x^2 + 2x + (4E - 14)$
	$R^2 = 1$	$R^2 = 1$	$R^2 = 1$
0.3	$y = 1.9634x + 0.0272$	$y = -0.0045x^2 + 1.9723x + 0.0244$	$y = -0.1453x^3 + 0.4314x^2 + 1.632x + 0.0741$
	$R^2 = 0.9871$	$R^2 = 0.9871$	$R^2 = 0.9876$
0.6	$y = 1.8922x + 0.01357$	$y = 0.0766x^2 + 1.7391x + 0.1842$	$y = -0.4753x^3 + 1.5026x^2 + 0.6258x - 0.3468$
	$R^2 = 0.9733$	$R^2 = 0.9738$	$R^2 = 0.9787$

*E means 10 raised to the power of. E.g. 2E-14 is 2×10^{-14}.

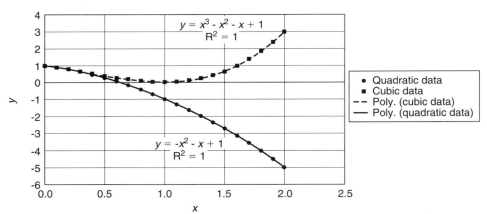

Figure 9.21 The second-order polynomial fitted to the quadratic data shows an R^2 value of 1 similar to the third-order polynomial fitted to the cubic data set.

ial curves to your data. Test a variety of curve fits, but choose the lowest order polynomial possible to give a reasonable value for R^2.

9.6.2 FITTING CURVES TO QUADRATIC AND CUBIC DATA

Section 9.6.1 examines fitting a variety of trend lines to essentially linear data. This section looks at experimental data points that follow a quadratic or cubic trend. The section then investigates the effect of curve fitting to these data sets. Here we will consider pairs of points, x_j, y_j where the values are related by the equation:

$$y_j = ax_j^3 + bx_j^2 + cx_j + d + N$$

where a, b, c, and d, are constants called **polynomial coefficients**. N represents some random noise present in the measurements and can be positive or negative.

For the purposes of illustration, we will consider the special case in which no noise is present ($N=0$) and the polynomial coefficients are:

$$a = 1, b = -1, c = -1, \text{ and } d = 1$$

Figure 9.21 shows both a quadratic data set and a cubic data set using these values for the coefficients a, b, c, and d.

Figure 9.22 shows the same two data sets in Figure 9.21, but this time with noise of 0.3 superimposed on the data. The quadratic data have been fitted with a

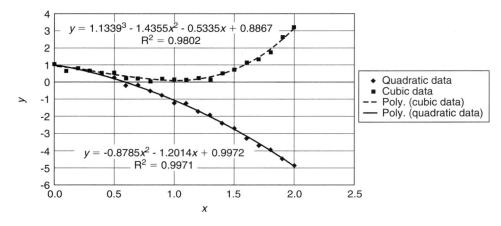

Figure 9.22 The second-order polynomial fitted to the noisy quadratic data shows a reduced R^2 value of 0.9971 similar to the third-order polynomial and the noisy cubic data set.

Figure 9.23 It is also possible to attempt to fit a second-order polynomial to a cubic data set or to fit a third-order polynomial to a quadratic data set. The top second-order curve shows a reduced fit ($R^2 = 0.9522$) but still follows the noisy cubic data quite well. The bottom third-order curve shows an excellent fit to the noisy quadratic data ($R^2 = 0.9996$).

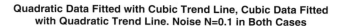

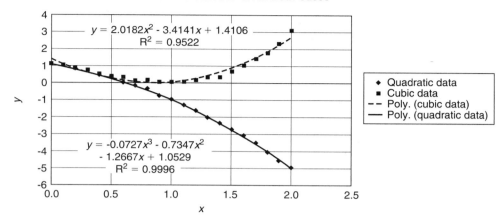

quadratic trend line, and the cubic data have been fitted with a cubic trend line; the value of R^2 is 1 for both trend lines.

Figure 9.23 shows the two data sets, this time with noise of 0.1 superimposed, with the quadratic data fitted by a cubic trend line and the cubic data fitted with a quadratic trend line. Both trend lines give reasonable fits; the value of R^2 is 0.95 for the quadratic trend line; however, the value of R^2 for the cubic trend line is greater than 0.999, indicating a near perfect fit. A reasonable interpretation of this result is that the former fit is not perfect because the trend line is not of the correct shape to fit the data *and* there is uncertainty in the data because of noise. In the latter case, the curve is of the correct shape to fit the data b, and the only reason that R^2 is slightly different from 1 is because of the uncertainty in the data.

It will be appreciated that the precise values of the polynomial coefficients obtained and the associated R^2 values depend on the noise, N, superimposed on the data. Table 9.6 shows the results of a number of simulations based on different random sets of N. The table shows the values of the coefficients a, b, c, and d and the value of R^2 for second-order polynomials fitted to quadratic data sets and for third-order polynomials fitted to cubic data sets. Remember that the "underlying" values of the coefficients are $a = 1$, $b = -1$, $c = -1$, and $d = 1$.

Table 9.7 shows the results of fitting second-order polynomials to cubic data sets and third-order polynomials to quadratic data sets.

9.7   Do My Data Fit a Trend or Not?

It is frequently required to decide if a given set of data fits a given trend or pattern. Usually, there is a given uncertainty in the measurement or a systematic or random error, and the trend might be, for example, a linear or a quadratic trend. This section examines one or two examples of how the chi-squared statistic can be used to help decide if a given data set is well represented by a given trend line or function or whether the deviations from the trend are too large for this to be concluded.

9.7.1 A Suspected Linear Trend

In this case, consider the data shown in Figure 9.24 in which the noisy displacement data, x, is plotted versus time, t. It will be assumed that whereas the displacement measurement is subject to some uncertainty, the time is exact. It will also be assumed

Table 9.6	The values of the coefficients *a, b, c,* and *d* for trend lines fitted to hypothetical data*			

a	*b*	*c*	*d*	*R²*
	1.0038	−1.000	0.9881	0.9971
0.995	−0.9535	−1.0903	1.0354	0.9979
	0.9736	−0.938	0.9647	0.9974
1.0093	−1.0012	−0.9955	0.9715	0.9975
	0.9568	−0.9129	0.9607	0.9973
1.0387	−1.1017	−0.9552	1.0286	0.9979
	0.9849	−0.9608	0.9743	0.9971
1.0531	−1.1743	−0.8531	0.9862	0.9982
	1.0078	−1.0247	1.0167	0.9952
0.9622	−0.8768	−1.0985	1.0034	0.9977
	1.011	−0.9906	0.9737	0.9978
1.1306	−1.0974	−0.9374	1.0106	0.9982
	0.9446	−0.8909	0.9679	0.9949
0.9456	−0.8278	−1.1192	0.9888	0.9977
	0.9547	−0.9335	0.9873	0.9949
1.0042	−1.0366	−0.9208	0.9404	0.9986

*These hypothetical data are based on:
(i) $y = x^3 - x^2 - x + 1 + N$ (cubic trend line)
(ii) $y = -x^2 - x + 1 + N$ (quadratic trend line)
N represents a variable uncertainty between 0.1 and −0.1. In the absence of N, the values of *a, b, c,* and *d* should be 1, −1, −1, and 1, respectively.

Table 9.7	The values of the coefficients *a, b, c,* and *d* for trend lines fitted to hypothetical data*			

a	*b*	*c*	*d*	*R²*
	1.9788	−3.2884	1.3213	0.9482
0.0072	1.0172	−1.0662	1.0329	0.9978
	2.0178	−3.3751	1.3464	0.9516
−0.0369	1.1232	−1.1208	1.0215	0.9977
	1.9784	−3.3042	1.3224	0.9454
0.0625	0.8202	−0.8584	0.9815	0.9944
	2.0032	−3.337	1.3256	0.9534
0.0373	0.8786	−0.8957	0.9795	0.9978
	1.9421	−3.233	1.3103	0.9520
−0.0965	1.3136	−1.2491	1.0474	0.9979
	2.0197	−3.3692	1.3547	0.9467
0.1135	0.6773	−0.7625	0.9573	0.9977
	1.9867	−3.3328	1.3447	0.9524
−0.0623	1.1948	−1.1647	1.0417	0.9978
	2.0315	−3.4206	1.3757	0.9507
−0.0047	1.018	−1.0111	0.9897	0.9971

*These hypothetical data are based on:
(i) $y = x^3 - x^2 - x + 1 + N$ (quadratic trend line)
(ii) $y = -x^2 - x + 1 + N$ (cubic trend line)
N represents a variable uncertainty between 0.1 and −0.1. In the absence of N, the values of *a, b, c,* and *d* should be 1, −1, −1, and 1, respectively.

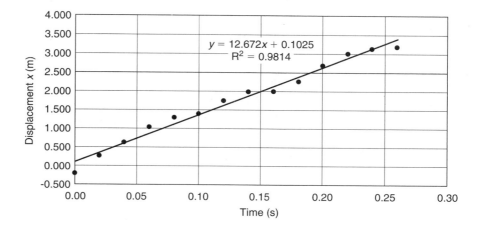

Figure 9.24
Displacement (x) versus time (t). The best fit-linear regression line is marked on the figure together with the R^2 value.

that the noise follows a Gaussian distribution and that the distribution remains the same no matter what range of t is being considered.

We can now ask the question: are the data well represented by this straight line, or would a quadratic regression line be better? The uncertainty in the displacement measurement is 0.15 m (SD), as determined from a large number of observations. To check this, we will work out the chi-squared value (χ^2) and check the value obtained against standard statistical tables. In this example, the number of data points, N, is 14, so the number of degrees of freedom is $N - 3 = 11$. In the following table, the expected value is the value obtained from the regression equation:

$$x = 12.672t + 0.1025$$

	A	B	C	D	E	F	G
1	time (s)	displacement x (m)	expected value x_2		delta-x		chi-squared χ^2
2	0.00	-0.193	0.103	"=(B2-C2)"	-0.295	=(E2/0-15)^2	3.870
3	0.02	0.276	0.356		-0.079		0.281
4	0.04	0.630	0.609		0.021		0.019
5	0.06	1.035	0.863		0.172		1.321
6	0.08	1.299	1.116		0.183		1.487
7	0.10	1.410	1.370		0.041		0.073
8	0.12	1.750	1.623		0.127		0.714
9	0.14	1.990	1.877		0.113		0.571
10	0.16	2.006	2.130		-0.124		0.685
11	0.18	2.264	2.383		-0.120		0.636
12	0.20	2.695	2.637		0.058		0.148
13	0.22	3.003	2.890		0.113		0.569
14	0.24	3.143	3.144		-0.001		0.000
15	0.26	3.189	3.397		-0.208		1.930
16							
17							
18						$\chi^2 \rightarrow$	12.304

The expected and actual x values are subtracted, divided by 0.15 (the SD of all the uncertainties), and finally squared. The values are then added together to form the final χ^2 value. The value obtained for the **chi-squared** statistic from tables is 19.68 ($df = 11$, $P = 0.05$) showing that the goodness of fit achieved is acceptable. If the χ^2 value that we obtained from the calculation was substantially larger, than this then we would have suspected that a different trend line might have fitted the data better, possibly a polynomial or exponential trend line. Note that tables of the

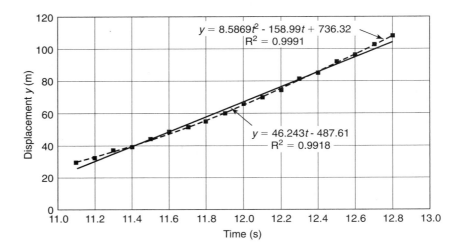

Figure 9.25 A plot of y against x with both a linear regression trend line and a quadratic trend line fitted to the data. The equations of the trend lines and the values of R^2 are shown in the figure.

chi-square statistic is given in books such as Vincent (2005) and in many statistical websites.

9.7.2 A Suspected Quadratic Trend

Consider the data shown in Figure 9.25, which shows a data set of displacement coordinates (y) versus time, t. We will assume that the noise is distributed in a similar way to that described previously in Section 9.7.1. The experimentally measured displacement data points have an uncertainty on them of ± 0.63m (SD), as determined from a large number of y measurements.

It appears in this case that the quadratic trend line has a slightly higher value of R^2. To further investigate this, we will look at the chi-squared (χ^2) values for both trend lines. In Table 9.8, y_2 is the value of y calculated from the linear trend line (linear regression line of best fit):

$$y = 46.243t - 487.61$$

and y_3 is the value calculated from the polynomial of order 2 (quadratic line of best fit):

$$y = 8.5869\,t^2 - 158.99t + 736.32$$

The details of the calculation of χ^2 follow the same pattern as those explained in Section 9.7.1. In this case, the value obtained for the χ^2 statistic for the quadratic fit is substantially smaller (23.9) than that for the linear fit (215.7) and is in line with what we would expect for 15° of freedom. (25.0, $P = 0.05$ obtained from statistical tables). The quadratic trend line is a superior fit to these data.

9.8 A Simple Method for Data Smoothing and Interpolation

Sometimes it is useful to introduce a combination of filtering and smoothing. If coordinate data are affected by random noise, it is possible to fit a quadratic curve to a small subset of the measured coordinate points and to predict interpolated or smoothed values on the basis of the value of the quadratic curve at intermediate points. For example, consider four measurements of displacement, x, at four equidistant times, t. Figure 9.26 shows four points for the special case in which the four points lie exactly on a quadratic curve. The quadratic curve of Figure 9.26 clearly has several advantages over the raw coordinates:

Table 9.8 Calculation of χ^2 for linear and quadratic fits to a displacement–time data set

Time (s)	Displace- ment y (m)	Expected Displacement y_2 (linear)	Expected Displace- ment y_3 (quadratic)	Delta y $(y - y_2)$ (linear)	Delta y $(y - y_3)$ (quadratic)	Chi- squared χ^2 (linear)	Chi- squared χ^2 (quadratic)
11.10	29.33	25.69	29.52	3.64	−0.20	33.34	0.10
11.20	32.31	30.31	32.77	2.00	−0.46	10.09	0.53
11.30	37.38	34.94	36.19	2.44	1.18	15.02	3.53
11.40	39.18	39.56	39.79	−0.38	−0.60	0.36	0.92
11.50	43.91	44.18	43.55	−0.28	0.35	0.20	0.31
11.60	48.64	48.81	47.49	−0.16	1.15	0.07	3.36
11.70	51.87	53.43	51.60	−1.56	0.27	6.14	0.19
11.80	54.64	58.06	55.88	−3.42	−1.24	29.47	3.88
11.90	59.68	62.68	60.33	−3.00	−0.65	22.66	1.06
12.00	65.92	67.31	64.95	−1.38	0.97	4.83	2.36
12.10	69.47	71.93	69.75	−2.46	−0.27	15.20	0.19
12.20	74.11	76.55	74.72	−2.45	−0.61	15.07	0.93
12.30	80.76	81.18	79.86	−0.42	0.91	0.43	2.08
12.40	84.57	85.80	85.17	−1.24	−0.60	3.85	0.91
12.50	91.73	90.43	90.65	1.30	1.08	4.27	2.94
12.60	95.99	95.05	96.30	0.94	−0.31	2.23	0.24
12.70	102.44	99.68	102.13	2.77	0.31	19.26	0.25
12.80	107.93	104.30	108.13	3.63	−0.19	33.22	0.09
					$\chi^2 \longrightarrow$	215.72	23.87

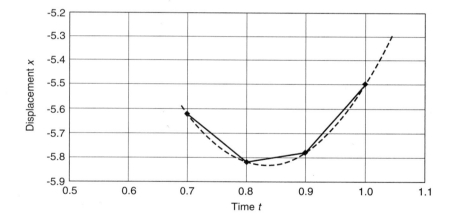

Figure 9.26 Four points lying exactly on a quadratic curve. The four points shown could form part of a much larger data set. The points are shown connected by straight-line segments and by the best fit quadratic curve through the points.

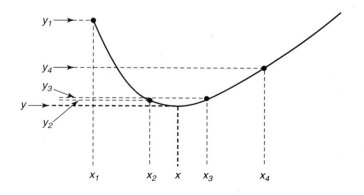

Figure 9.27 It is understood that x is midway between x_2 and x_3 and that the x_i values are equally spaced. The value of y at x can be calculated by interpolation.

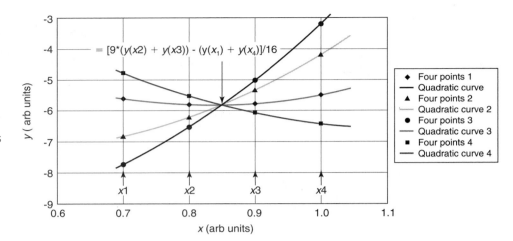

Figure 9.28 Four different sets of data points lying on four different quadratic curves. The points were especially chosen so that the curves all intersect at the same point. This point is also given by the smoothing/interpolation function shown.

(a) It can be used to predict intermediate values between the times 0.7, 0.8, 0.9, 1.0 s, and so on.

(b) The slope of the quadratic is a good estimate of the slope of the data at any time and is clearly a better estimate than that based on taking the slope of the straight lines drawn between the points also shown in Figure 9.26.

It can be shown that for any quadratic curve, the value of y can be predicted from the values of y_1, y_2, y_3, and y_4 by the relation presented here without proof. (Fig. 9.27):

$$y = (9(y_2 + y_3) - (y_1 + y_4))/16$$

If, for example, we wanted to interpolate between the data points of Figure 9.26 to find the predicted value x at $t = 0.85$, then:

$$x(t = 0.85s) = \frac{(9 \times (-5.82 - 5.78) - (-5.62 - 5.50))}{16} = -5.83$$

This principle of interpolation could be applied to every intermediate data point applicable to the original data set. It could also be applied to recalculate the

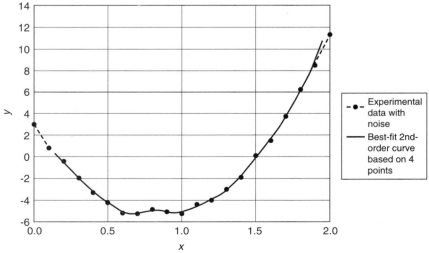

Figure 9.29 Some noisy displacement data connected by straight-line segments and by a smoothed interpolated line based on the best fit second-order polynomial fitted to successive sets of four data points.

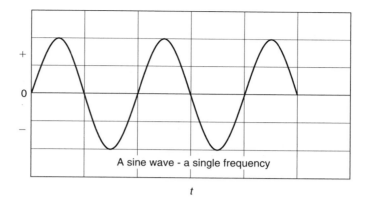

Figure 9.30 A sinusoidal waveform.

values of the original data points so that smoothing could be achieved if it was required. Before moving on to illustrating the smoothing effect, the general applicability of the principle is emphasized by calculating an interpolated point from four different sets of neighboring points. Figure 9.28 illustrates that the four-point smoothing interpolation method gives correct results in general for any set of data.

So far, we have not considered the method applied to real data with noise. To show what is possible, Figure 9.29 shows a real data set showing a displacement y in meters versus time, t, in seconds. The displacement, y, is affected by a certain amount of random noise. Figure 9.29 also shows the smoothed or interpolated data.

9.9 Fourier Analysis

A signal can be represented as a combination of sinusoidal signals with varying frequencies and a steady signal or level. The basic periodic sine wave is illustrated in Figure 9.30. The signal (displacement, acceleration, voltage, current) repeatedly changes its polarity in a smooth and predictable manner. This type of signal, if it persists for a long time, it is composed of a single frequency and can be written as:

$$x = A_1 \sin (\omega t + \phi_1)$$

where $\omega = 1/T$ and T is the **periodic time** of the sine wave. The constant A_1 represents the **amplitude** of the waveform, and ϕ_1 is the **phase** of the waveform. ω represents an **angular frequency** in radians per second and is related to **frequency** in Hz by $f = \omega/2\pi$.

Figure 9.31 shows a square wave with the same periodic time as the sine wave

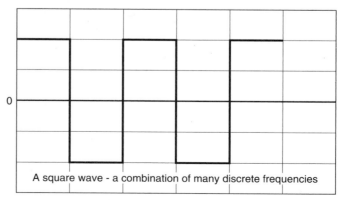

Figure 9.31 A square waveform.

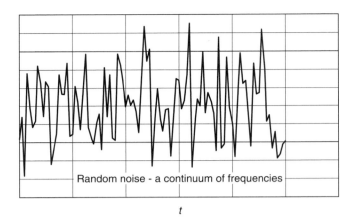

Figure 9.32 A random noise waveform.

in Figure 9.30. A square wave is one of many different types of periodic signal and can be written in terms of a **Fourier series** as:

$$x = A_1 \left[\sin (\omega t + \phi_1) + \tfrac{1}{3} \sin (3\omega t + \phi_2) + \tfrac{1}{5} \sin (5\omega t + \phi_3) + \ldots\ldots\ldots \right]$$

This means that a square wave is composed of a combination of discrete frequency sinusoidal components, including a fundamental angular frequency ω and harmonics 3ω, 5ω, 7ω up to infinitely high frequencies.

Random noise can occur in many measurement situations and is also a mixture of frequencies. But in this case, the amplitudes and phases of the components are changing unpredictably. Figure 9.32 illustrates a random noise waveform with no regular repeating pattern. Because there is no periodic time, it is impossible to define a fundamental frequency, ω. It turns out that this type of noise can be analyzed into a continuum of noise amplitudes spread over a wide range of frequencies.

A Fourier analysis of a signal gives an indication of the signal amplitude or power versus frequency. Figure 9.33 shows the Fourier transformation of the sine, square, and random noise waveforms.

In general, a signal waveform might have a steady component, a number of alternating components, and a noise component, as illustrated in Figure 9.34. Here, again, the basic repetition frequency is the same as that of the sine and square waves. This is a very brief introduction to a large subject. For more information, see Regtien (2004).

9.10 The Sampling Theorem

The **sampling theorem** states that the signal must be sampled at a frequency at least twice as high as the highest frequency present in the signal itself. Analog-to-digital

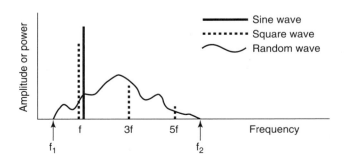

Figure 9.33 Fourier transformation of the sine, square, and noise waveforms.

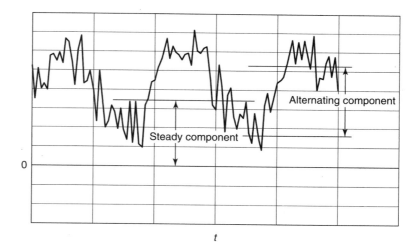

Figure 9.34 A general waveform might be composed of a steady component, alternating components, and a noise component.

conversion, digitization of video clips, and three-dimensional motion analysis are all examples of situations in which the data are obtained by sampling. In each case, the measurement is taken over a very short period, and then there is a delay before the sample is taken again. This process is usually repeated at equal intervals of time for however long is required. Figure 9.35(a) illustrates a waveform being sampled in accordance with the sampling theorem, and Figure 9.35(b) illustrates a case in which the sampling theorem is violated.

9.11   Digital Filtering

The basis of this approach is to analyze the frequency spectrum of both signal and noise. Figure 9.36 shows a diagram of a signal consisting of an equal mixture of all frequencies being filtered by a low-pass filter. The low-pass filter has a response that allows low-frequency signals to pass through unattenuated while higher frequency signals are attenuated after passing through the filter. The **characteristic frequency** associated with the filter is called the cutoff frequency, f_c. If the low-pass gain of the filter is assumed to be one, the cutoff frequency is defined as the frequency at which its gain has fallen to $\frac{1}{\sqrt{2}} = 0.707$ (Fig. 9.37)

Filtering data to remove noise works provided the frequency or the range of

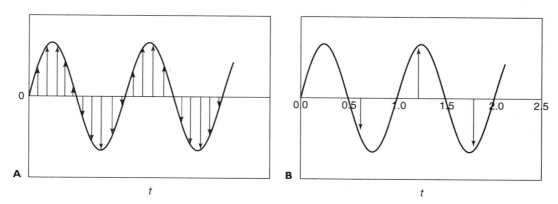

Figure 9.35   (A) A waveform being sampled at a sufficiently high frequency in accordance with the sampling theorem. (B) A waveform being sampled at too low a frequency in violation of the sampling theorem.

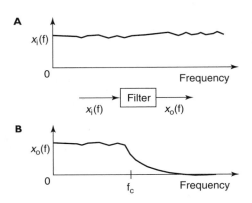

Figure 9.36 (A) Hypothetical frequency spectrum of a waveform consisting of a mixture of all frequencies before being filtered. (B) The frequency spectrum of the output from a low-pass filter.

frequencies of the data is different from the frequency or range of frequencies occupied by the noise. Therefore, filters can also be configured as high-pass filters (in which the gain is low at low frequencies and high at high frequencies) or band-pass filters (in which the gain is low at low and high frequencies and high in a band of intermediate frequencies).

For the purposes of this discussion, we will concentrate on a situation in which the signal is concentrated at lower frequency and the noise is of higher frequency. In this case, a low-pass filter is the appropriate choice of filter. Figure 9.38(a) shows a frequency spectrum of a signal together with higher frequency noise in a hypothetical case. There is some overlap of signal with noise. Figure 9.38(b) shows the corresponding **frequency spectrum** after passing through the low-pass filter. Clearly, the cutoff frequency of the filter is not perfectly sharp so that not all the signal below f_c gets through and not all of the noise above f_c is rejected.

Therefore, distortion of the signal is possible because frequencies close to the cutoff frequencies are attenuated but low-frequency signals are not attenuated at all. The value of f_c can be altered at will by changing the filter. However, setting f_c too low results in too much signal distortion, but noise is rejected very effectively. Conversely, setting f_c too high allows a lot of noise to pass, but signal distortion is reduced.

Digital filtering can be achieved easily using modern software packages. Let us assume that a displacement Y has been sampled at discrete measurement intervals, δt. A **low-pass recursive digital filter** for the filtered coordinate at time t can be set up using filter coefficients a_o, a_1, a_2, b_1, and b_2 as follows:

$$Y_f(t) = a_0 Y(t) + a_1 Y(t - \delta t) + a_2(t - 2\delta t) + b_1 Y_f(t - \delta t) + b_2 Y_f(t - 2\delta t)$$

where:

Y_f = filtered output

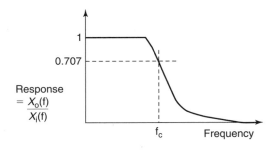

Figure 9.37 The response of a low-pass filter. The gain at frequency f_c is $1/\sqrt{2}$.

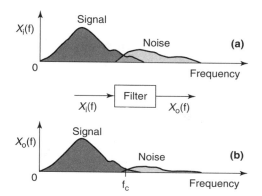

Figure 9.38 (A) Frequency spectrum of signal plus higher frequency noise. (B) Frequency spectrum of output waveform from low-pass filter.

Y = unfiltered input

t = time at the nth sample

$(t - \delta t)$ = time at $(n - 1)^{\text{th}}$ sample

$(t - 2\delta t)$ = time at $(n - 2)^{\text{th}}$ sample

It is possible to select the filter coefficients to yield different types and orders of filters with different cutoff frequencies. The order of the filter determines the sharpness of the cutoff. The higher the order, the sharper the cutoff but the larger the number of coefficients. For example, a Butterworth-type filter of second order with a cutoff frequency of 5 Hz should be used with digitized video data obtained with a frame speed of 50 Hz. The filter coefficients are determined by the ratio of frame speed to cutoff frequency. In this case, the ratio is 10, and the filter coefficients required are:

$$a_0 = 0.06746, \ a_1 = 0.13491, \ a_2 = 0.06746, \ b_1 = 1.14298, \ b_2 = -0.41280$$

Figure 9.39 shows a simple way of calculating the filter coefficients using a spreadsheet; the ratio of f_c/f_s is entered in cell A1.

9.11.1 PHASE SHIFT

In addition to amplitude attenuation, there is a **phase shift** of the output signal relative to the input. This means that the signal is shifted in time relative to where it was. For example, if the input were a sine wave, two possible outputs might appear, as shown in Figure 9.40.

For the second-order Butterworth filter, the **phase lag** is one of $90°$ ($\pi/2$ rad) at the cutoff frequency. This can introduce another form of distortion into the measurement. **Phase distortion** occurs to some extent for all frequencies entering the filter but is most severe for frequencies above the cutoff. To eliminate this phase lag, the data can be filtered a second time, but this time in the reverse direction of time (Winter et al., 1974):

	A	B	C	D	E	F	G	H	I	J	K
1	ratio f_c/f_s	ω_c	K_1	K_2	K_3	a_0	a_1	a_2	b_1	b_2	
2	0.1	0.324919403	0.459505	0.105573	1.277892	0.067455	0.13491	0.067455	1.142981	-0.4128	
3											
4											
5				"=(B2)^2"			"=2*F2"			"=1-2*F2-E2"	
6								"=F2"			
7		"=TAN(π(A2))"			"=2*F2/D2"				"=-2*F2+E2"		
8		="SQRT(2)*(B2)"			"=D2/(1+C2+D2)"						
9											

Figure 9.39 Calculation of the coefficients for a Butterworth filter using a spreadsheet.

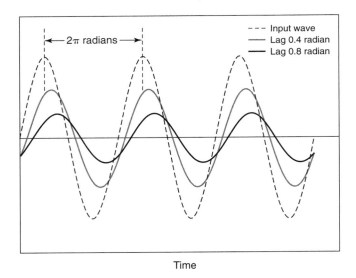

Figure 9.40 The input sine wave compared with two possible output waves. As well as reducing the amplitude, the low-pass filter introduces a phase shift.

$$Y_f(t) = a_0 Y(t) + a_1 Y(t + \delta t) + a_2 Y(t + 2\delta t) + b_1 Y_f(t + \delta t) + b_2 Y_f(t + 2\delta t)$$

This procedure introduces an equal and opposite phase lag so that the net phase shift after filtering twice is 0. Also, the attenuation is doubled so that the improved fourth-order filter has a much sharper cutoff.

Figure 9.41 illustrates a hypothetical signal composed of a low-frequency sine wave (1.5 Hz) and another higher frequency sine wave representing noise (12 Hz). The diagram also shows the output from a Butterworth second-order, low-pass digital filter and the output after filtering for the second time in the reverse time direction.

It should be noted that the 12-Hz noise component is almost completely removed after filtering twice and that the net phase shift is 0. Figure 9.42 shows a

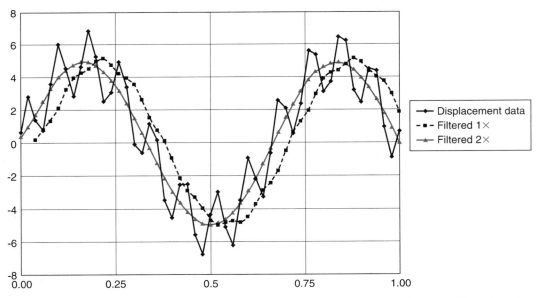

Figure 9.41 A noisy sine wave filtered once and twice by a Butterworth low-pass filter. Sampling frequency = 50 Hz; cutoff frequency = 5 Hz.

	A	B	C	D	E	F
1	time	displace ment x		filtered 1x		filtered 2x
2	(s)	(m)				
3	0.100	6.044		2.099		3.979
4	0.120	4.598		3.225		4.462
5	0.140	2.853		4.040		4.772
6	0.160	4.666	"=$B$16*B8+$B$17*B7+$B$18*B6	4.296	"=$B$16*B8+$B$17*B7+$B$18*B6	4.953
7	0.180	6.910	+$B$19*D7+$B$20*D6"	4.531	+$B$19*D7+$B$20*D6"	4.960
8	0.200	5.324		5.011		4.737
9	0.220	2.504		5.211		4.329
10	0.240	3.048		4.790		3.817
11	0.260	4.964		4.239		3.191
12	0.280	3.436		3.974		2.407
13	0.300	-0.103		3.585		1.511
14						
15						
16	a_0	0.06746	Filter			
17	a_1	0.13491	coefficients			
18	a_2	0.006746				
19	b_1	1.14298				
20	b_2	-0.4128				
21						

Figure 9.42 Implementation of low-pass second- and fourth-order Butterworth digital filters using a spreadsheet method. Only a small section of the data is shown.

section of the spreadsheet upon which Figure 9.41 was based. This type of spreadsheet can be generally applied to many situations for any value of the ratio f_s/f_c.

SUMMARY

Chapter 9 has given a thorough introduction to best-fit trend lines from linear through quadratic to higher order polynomials, smoothing of data by moving average methods, Fourier analysis of signals and noise, and digital filtration using the low-pass Butterworth method.

REFERENCES

Regtien PPL: *Electronic Instrumentation.* Delft, The Netherlands; Delft University Press; 1994.

Vincent WJ: *Statistics in Kinesiology*, edn. 3. Champaign, IL: Human Kinetics; 2005.

Winter DA, Sidwall HG, Hobson DA: Measurement and reduction of noise in kinematics of locomotion. *J Biomech* 7:157–159, 1974.

Woltring HJ: in Three-dimensional analysis of human movement: Allard P, Stokes IAF, Blanchi JP. (Eds), 79–99, Champaign, IL: Human Kinetics, 1995.

STUDY QUESTIONS

1. The data file Ch9Q1 gives the *x, y,* and *z* coordinates for the left toe of an adult male runner as he moves through the capture volume of a three-dimensional motion analysis system. The frequency of data capture is 120 Hz. The runner's direction of running is approximately the *y* direction, and the *z* axis is vertical. Open up this data file in a spreadsheet and calculate the velocity and acceleration of the runner's left toe in the

y direction (the direction of running) as a function of time *using a simple finite-difference formula* (see Section 9.2). Plot charts of the *y* coordinate, velocity, and acceleration (in the *y* direction) as a function of time for times between 0.75 and 1.45 s.

(a) What is the average velocity of the left toe in the direction of running between times 0.75 and 1.45 s?

(b) What is the maximum acceleration of the left toe between times 0.75 and 1.45 s? (Answers: Ch9Q1Ans.)

2. A golf club head is marked CLBHD and tracked during a golf swing. The data capture rate is 120 Hz. The *x*, *y*, and *z* coordinates of CLBHD are given in the data file Ch9Q2. Introduce a new column (B column) and calculate the time in seconds corresponding to each field. In this movement, displacements of CLBHD in along all three axes are important and significant, so calculate the movement, *dl*, of the club head in time, *dt*, as:

$$dl = \sqrt{(dx)^2 + (dy)^2 + (dz)^2}$$

where *dx*, *dy*, and *dz* are the displacements along the *x*, *y*, and *z* axes, respectively. Use this to calculate the velocity of CLBHD by a finite-difference method in a new column. Go on to calculate the acceleration of CLBHD by a similar method and then draw graphs of velocity and acceleration of CLBHD versus time.

(c) What are the times taken for the swing and the backswing?

(d) What are the maximum velocities on the backswing and on the swing?

(e) What is the maximum acceleration of the club head on the downward part of the swing? In terms of "*g*"?

Be sure to quote your units with all answers.

3. A gymnast is being rotated in the tucked somersault position lying on a rotatable platform. The accelerating mass is 30 kg, and the somersault axis is positioned directly over and aligned with the axis of rotation of the platform. Data file Ch9Q3 gives the coordinates of the two markers XTR1 and XTR2 on the circumference of the platform. Use the *x*, *y*, and *z* coordinates provided to calculate the angular velocity of the apparatus as a function of time. Draw a graph of this angular velocity in rad.s^{-1} versus time for the whole trial. Repeat this using a five-point moving average method to smooth the *x*, *y*, and *z* coordinates before producing the curve of angular velocity against time. Fit a linear trend line to the rising linear section using only the data between 1.4 and 3.5 s. Fit another trend line to the falling linear section using only the data between 3.75 and 9.55 s. Do this for the smoothed and unsmoothed angular velocity data. Compare the slopes of the trend lines obtained by the methods for both the rising and the falling sections. Examine the noise on the angular velocity–time graph closely between 5 and 6 s; how much noise has been removed by the smoothing? (A visual estimate will suffice.) The file Ch9Q3 gives hints on how to lay out the spreadsheet calculation.

4. A rugby player is recorded executing a place kick with his left foot. Examine the trajectories of the left hip (LASI), left knee (LKNE), and left ankle (LANK) in the *y–z* plane between frames 140 and 183 in file Ch9Q4. Try fitting a second- and a third-order polynomial to the three sets of data points. Which is the best fit to the data? A sequence of stills at the top of the back swing, at ball contact, and at the top of the follow through is shown here: the *y* direction is left to right on these diagrams and the *z* direction is vertically upward.

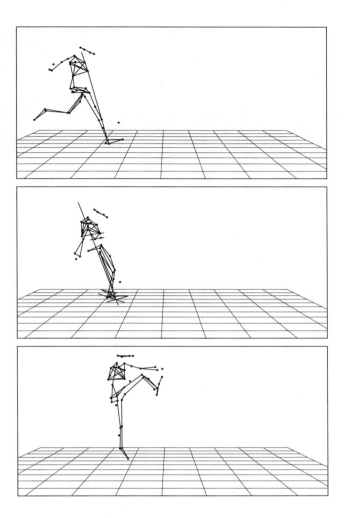

Calculate the knee angles at each of the three positions.

5. In a similar trial for a right-footed kick, the right knee marker is missing for some reason around field 165. Open up the file Ch9Q5 as a spreadsheet and use interpolation to fill the gaps in the x, y, and z coordinates. What are the coordinates of the three missing points in the RKNE trajectory? Plot graphs of the three coordinates x, y, and z versus time, including the interpolated points for $1.45 \geq t \geq 1.25$.

CHAPTER ten

EXPLORATION OF MOTION DATA USING SPREADSHEETS

CHAPTER *objectives*

The aim of this chapter is to apply some of the data treatment methods covered in Chapter 9 to some advanced topics in kinematics and kinetics.

CHAPTER *outcomes*

After reading this chapter, the reader will be able to:

- Develop proficiency in handling text and ASCII data.
- Be aware of the possibilities and limitations of moving average smoothing.
- Be able to calculate the magnitude of a velocity vector from its components.
- Develop awareness of the different types of trends present in data.
- Be able to select appropriate smoothing and interpolation methods.
- Calculate body angles from coordinate data in spreadsheets.
- Be aware of inverse dynamics as an approach to calculating joint forces and moments.
- Be able to take into account friction forces in rotational experiments.

10.1 Text or ASCII Files

It is highly convenient to obtain positional and force data from motion analysis systems in the form of **ASCII** (American Standard Code for Information Interchange) or **text files**. These can be processed quickly and easily using commercial spreadsheet packages to yield kinematic and kinetic data with a facility that could only be dreamed of in the days when digitization of video pictures was achievable only by laborious manual methods. An example of a spreadsheet output is shown in Figure 10.1, in which the *x, y, z* coordinates of a tracked point are outputted

	A	B	C	D
2	Time (s)	x coordinate (mm)	y coordinate (mm)	z coordinate (mm)
3	0.000	214.5	-34.5	1056.1
4	0.005	225.6	-22.2	1086.5
5	0.010	238.0	-10.6	1126.9
6	0.015	248.7	-1.8	1176.8
7	0.020	256.8	0.5	1236.4
8	0.025	267.3	10.4	1306.5
9	0.030	277.5	2.6	1386.1
10	0.035	288.6	-3.4	1476.4
11	0.040	295.3	-6.9	1576.1
12	0.045	304.8	-15.1	1686.7

Figure 10.1 A small section of a fictitious ASCII (text) file in which the x, y, and z coordinates of a marker point are given in time intervals of 0.005 s.

every 0.005 s. In a real motion trial, the spreadsheet of coordinate values could well be hundreds or thousands of rows and could contain many more columns with the coordinates for other marker points.

10.2   Finite-Difference Formulas

Velocities, accelerations, their angular counterparts, and many related kinetic quantities are often calculated using simple finite-difference formulas. For example, to calculate the velocity of a marker point as a function of time, the usual method is to calculate the small change in the displacement of the marker separated by a small time increment. Let us take the components of the velocity separately. To calculate the z component of the velocity of the marker or point referred to in Figure 10.1, it is natural, as an initial step, to take the time interval as the difference in the times between adjacent rows. Let us illustrate this by calculating the z component of the velocity at time 0 s as the z displacement at time 0.005 s minus the z displacement at time 0 s divided by the time interval 0.005 s. In terms of symbols, we would write:

$$v_z(t = 0) = \frac{z(t = 0.005) - z(t = 0)}{0.005}.$$

This would give us an estimate of the average z velocity over the time interval between 0 and 0.005 s. With reference to the spreadsheet, this result can be placed in, for example, cell E3 by working out (D4−D3)/(A4−A3), as shown in Figure 10.2.

The result obtained from this calculation is an average value over an interval of 0.005 s, but because this is probably a very small time interval compared with the time scale of any movements being measured, we can justifiably regard this as an instantaneous value for the z-velocity. Sometimes this assumption would not be justified, such as, for example, a case in which a ball is being hit by a bat or club and the change in the direction of the ball occurs in a time of a few milliseconds. The E column in the spreadsheet could be filled with similar z-velocity values by copying the formula down the column. We would, however, have to stop copying the formula at cell E11 in our example because we would not have the z coordinate information to calculate the z velocity in cell E12. We could then generate a z velocity column, as shown in Figure 10.3.

We can follow a similar procedure for finding the z component of the acceleration, resulting in the spreadsheet shown in Figure 10.4. In this figure, F3 would be

	A	B	C	D
2	Time (s)	x coordinate (mm)	y coordinate (mm)	z coordinate (mm)
3	0.000	214.5	-34.5	1056.1
4	0.005	225.6	-22.2	1086.5
5	0.010	238.0	-10.6	1126.9
6	0.015	248.7	-1.8	1176.8
7	0.020	256.8	0.5	1236.4
8	0.025	267.3	10.4	1306.5
9	0.030	277.5	2.6	1386.1
10	0.035	288.6	-3.4	1476.4
11	0.040	295.3	-6.9	1576.1
12	0.045	304.8	-15.1	1686.7

"=(D4-D3)/(A4-A3)"

Figure 10.2 Inserting an expression for the z component of velocity in cell E3. This expression can be copied down the E column.

	A	B	C	D	E
2	Time (s)	x coordinate (mm)	y coordinate (mm)	z coordinate (mm)	z component of velocity (mm/s)
3	0.000	214.5	-34.5	1056.1	6080
4	0.005	225.6	-22.2	1086.5	8080
5	0.010	238.0	-10.6	1126.9	9980
6	0.015	248.7	-1.8	1176.8	11,920
7	0.020	256.8	0.5	1236.4	14,020
8	0.025	267.3	10.4	1306.5	15,920
9	0.030	277.5	2.6	1386.1	18,060
10	0.035	288.6	-3.4	1476.4	19,940
11	0.040	295.3	-6.9	1576.1	22,120
12	0.045	304.8	-15.1	1686.7	N/A

Cell E12 left blank since z coord at D13 is not available

Figure 10.3 The formula calculation of z component of velocity from displacement data (column D) and time (column A). Cell E12 is left blank.

	A	B	C	D	E	F
2	Time (s)	x coordinate (mm)	y coordinate (mm)	z coordinate (mm)	z component of velocity (mm/s)	z component of acceleration (mm/s/s)
3	0.000	214.5	-34.5	1056.1	6080	400,000
4	0.005	225.6	-22.2	1086.5	8080	380,000
5	0.010	238.0	-10.6	1126.9	9980	388,000
6	0.015	248.7	-1.8	1176.8	11,920	420,000
7	0.020	256.8	0.5	1236.4	14,020	380,000
8	0.025	267.3	10.4	1306.5	15,920	428,000
9	0.030	277.5	2.6	1386.1	18,060	376,000
10	0.035	288.6	-3.4	1476.4	19,940	436,000
11	0.040	295.3	-6.9	1576.1	22,120	N/A
12	0.045	304.8	-15.1	1686.7	N/A	N/A

Figure 10.4 The calculation of the z component of the acceleration.

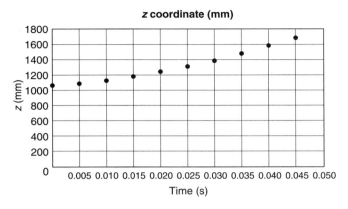

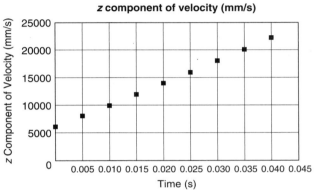

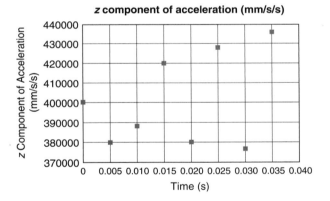

Figure 10.5 *Top:* z displacement. *Middle:* z velocity. *Bottom:* z acceleration versus time.

defined as $(E4 - E3)/(A4 - A3)$; again, the last two rows in the F column are left blank because we do not have the velocity data to fill these places.

Figure 10.5 shows the displacement, velocity, and acceleration versus time (data of Fig. 10.3) in graphical form. Figure 10.5 illustrates some of the problems associated with finding velocity and acceleration values by differentiation of coordinate data. The z values show a vertical displacement that increase smoothly with time. The z component of the velocity shows that the velocity increases very linearly with time, with the velocity points lying very close to a straight line. However, the acceleration values obtained from the velocity data show a lot of variation, with a maximum value of 428,000 mm/s² and a minimum value of 376,000 mm/s². Common sense seems to indicate that the acceleration is actually a constant value close to 400,000 mm/s²; however, the process used to calculate the acceleration values has led to uncertainties, the main one being the uncertainty in the slope of the line connecting the pair of velocity data points.

The method described for calculating the velocity from coordinate data as:

$$\Delta x / \Delta t$$

where $\Delta x = x_{i+1} - x_i$ and $\Delta t = t_{i+1} - t_i$, results in the velocity at a time midway between t_{i+1} and t_i. Sometimes this is not a significant problem because the time intervals Δt are usually small. In other situations, however, it does become problematic, especially if the velocity data are to be related to the displacement data. As an alternative method that avoids this problem, the velocity and accelerations can be calculated using a time interval $2\Delta t$ spaced Δt either side of the ith sample. So, for example:

$$v(t = t_i) = \frac{x(t = t_{i+1}) - x(t = t_{i-1})}{2\Delta t}.$$

This method is generally applicable and can be implemented in a similar way to that explained earlier in this section.

10.3   Moving-Point Averages

Sometimes it is advantageous to smooth data to reduce the obscuring effect of noise. The original data obtained is sometimes noisy because of limitations of the original experiment or if the effects measured are very small. In other examples, calculated values are noisy because of the computation methods used to generate the data. In the previous example, acceleration data were noisy because of small uncertainties in the underlying velocity data. To illustrate a simple way to reduce the effect of the noise, let us see what effect a two-point averaging strategy has. To be specific, the two-point smoothed acceleration would be calculated in cell G3 as (F2 + F3)/ 2. Figure 10.6 shows this formula being copied down the G column to complete cells in the G column down as far as G9.

The smoothed acceleration data versus time is shown in the graph of Figure 10.7. The magnitude of the fluctuations in the acceleration data is clearly reduced by the use of the two-point averaging method.

This idea of taking averages could be extended to include more data points on each average. For example, the acceleration value for cell G6 could be calculated according to any one of the following rules:

	A	B	C	D	E	F	G
2	Time (s)	x coordinate (mm)	y coordinate (mm)	z coordinate (mm)	z component of velocity (mm/s)	z component of acceleration (mm/s/s)	2-point smoothed acceleration
3	0.000	214.5	-34.5	1056.1	6080	400,000	N/A
4	0.005	225.6	-22.2	1086.5	8080	380,000	390,000
5	0.010	238.0	-10.6	1126.9	9980	388,000	384,000
6	0.015	248.7	-1.8	1176.8	11,920	420,000	404,000
7	0.020	256.8	0.5	1236.4	14,020	380,000	400,000
8	0.025	267.3	10.4	1306.5	15,920	428,000	404,000
9	0.030	277.5	2.6	1386.1	18,060	376,000	402,000
10	0.035	288.6	-3.4	1476.4	19,940	436,000	406,000
11	0.040	295.3	-6.9	1576.1	22,120	N/A	N/A
12	0.045	304.8	-15.1	1686.7	N/A	N/A	N/A

Figure 10.6   A two-point smoothing method to reduce noise (fluctuation) in the acceleration data.

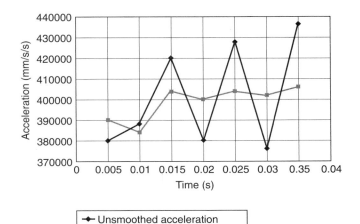

Figure 10.7 Two-point smoothed acceleration and unsmoothed acceleration data versus time. Note the smaller fluctuations on the smoothed data.

G6 = (F5 + F6 + F7)/3 (a three-point moving average)
G6 = (F4 + F5 + F6 + F7 + F8)/5 (a five-point moving average)
G6 = (F3 + F4 + F5 + F6 + F7 + F8 + F9)/7 (a seven-point moving average)

or even higher moving averages. The effect of this, in general, will be to reduce noise and fluctuations. There is, of course, a down side to this sort of procedure. The disadvantage is that the higher the number of points included in the moving average, the slower the response of the system will be to rapidly varying accelerations. To illustrate this idea, let us assume that the acceleration is of the form shown in Figure 10.8, that is, constant at 400,000 mm/s/s but jumping to 600,000 mm/s/s for a short time of 0.01 s. We will assume that the sampling rate is still once every 0.005 s.

This shows that the effect of the seven-point smoothing routine is to reduce the amplitude of acceleration changes that occur over time scales that are small compared with the averaging time (in this case, 0.035 s) and to extend their durations to approximately the same as the averaging time (0.035 s). Acceleration changes occurring over time scales that are long compared with the averaging time would be reproduced accurately.

Another method for smoothing is called **binomial smoothing**. In this method, a three-point moving average is used, but instead of taking an unweighted average

Figure 10.8 The effect of seven-point smoothing on acceleration data. The original data are fictitious, having a sharp rise by 200,000 mm/s/s between 0.105 and 0.115 s. The smoothed data show a peak that is less than half the amplitude of the original and that is much broader, extending between 0.09 and 0.13 s.

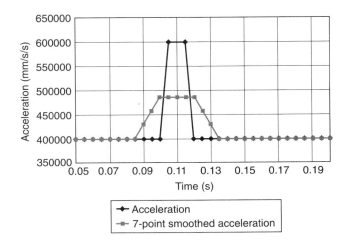

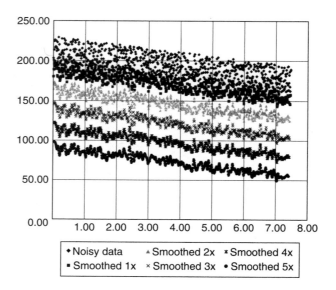

Figure 10.9 Noisy data and the same data smoothed once, twice, three times, four times, and five times using a simple binomial smoothing method. Notice that the magnitude of the fluctuations is reduced by the smoothing and that higher frequency noise is progressively removed.

of three points, a weighted average is used in the ratio of 1:2:1. This means that the contents of cell G6 (acceleration) is defined as:

$$G6 = (F5 + 2 \times F6 + F7)/4$$

and the rest of the G column could be filled in a similar way. This has a similar filtering effect and can, if required, be applied again and again, so that an H column could be defined, for example, beginning with:

$$H7 = (G6 + 2 \times G7 + G8)/4$$

To illustrate the effect of this, some arbitrary noisy data are presented in Figure 10.9 along with the same data that have been smoothed up to five times. Note that for each stage of smoothing, 25 has been subtracted from the data, so that the data and smoothed data do not overlap.

10.4   Calculating Magnitudes of Vector Quantities from the Components

In Section 10.2, we saw how to calculate the velocity components from x, y, z coordinate data. It is frequently desirable to evaluate the magnitude of the velocity, v, sometimes written as $|v|$

$$v = \sqrt{v_x^2 + v_y^2 + v_z^2}$$

(Review vectors in Chapter 2.) This can be calculated from the spreadsheet quite simply, as shown in Figure 10.10.

The resultant velocity versus time can then be plotted as a graph, as shown in Figure 10.11. Notice that the z component of the velocity showed an approximately linear relationship with time, but the overall resultant velocity shows a different relationship with time because of the x and y components of the velocity.

10.5   Drawing Smoothed and Curved Trend Lines Through Data Points

Figure 10.11 illustrates how experimental data can be fitted with a **polynomial function regression line**. In the general case, a polynomial trend line can be represented by:

$$y = a_0 + a_1x + a_2x^2 + a_3x^3 + \dots$$

S Q R T ((E3)^2 + (F3)^2 + (G3) ^2)

E	F	G			H	I
z-velocity (mm/s)	x-velocity (mm/s)	y-velocity (mm/s)			Resultant velocity (mm/s)	
6080	2220	24,580			25,417.93	
8080	2480	21,120			22,748.43	
9980	2140	15,600			18,642.42	
11,920	1620	8840			14,928.38	
14,020	2100	1000			14,211.63	
15,920	2040	-5380			16,927.86	
18,060	2220	-3580			18,544.77	
19,940	1340	-6960			21,162.25	
22,120	1900	-16,500			27,661.42	
N/A	N/A	N/A				

Figure 10.10 The calculation of the magnitude of the resultant velocity from the velocity components by the use of a formula. The velocity data in this figure are based on the displacement coordinate data shown in Figure 10.2.

where the sum can include as many terms as is thought to be beneficial. a_0, a_1, a_2 ..... are constants, called coefficients. A polynomial of order 0, including the first term only, that is:

$$y = a_0$$

represents a function that is a constant value. A polynomial of order 1, including the first two terms, is:

$$y = a_0 + a_1x$$

represents a straight line function with intercept a_0 on the y axis and slope a_1. (For a brief introduction to linear regression, see Appendix 1.)

In general, when complex functions are required, the more terms included in the polynomial, the more accurately it can reproduce the form of the data being modeled. Any function, or variation of y with x, can be reproduced to a high degree of precision using a polynomial with an appropriate number of terms. Many statistical software packages and spreadsheets offer the ability to calculate trend lines from inputted data using not only linear and polynomial fits but also exponential and other functions. In the case of regression methods, the objective is to reduce the deviations of the data points from the fitted line to a minimum. It is also sometimes advantageous to use interpolation; in this method, the line drawn passes exactly through the data points and the space between the data points is modeled using a variety of methods (e.g., quadratic **splines**, cubic splines. and higher order splines).

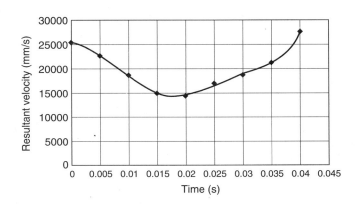

Figure 10.11 The resultant velocity–time relationship. A polynomial of order 6 has been used to fit the data using a nonlinear regression method.

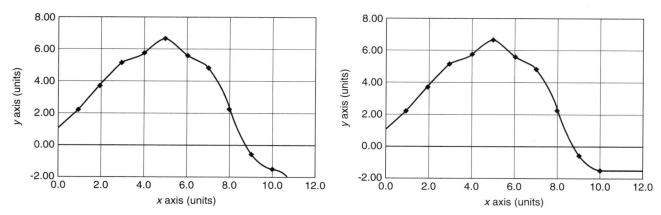

Figure 10.12   *Left:* Cubic spline interpolation. *Right:* Tension spline interpolation.

Consider, for example, some fictitious *x–y* data, as shown in Figure 10.12. The graph on the left shows the result of a cubic spline's being applied to this data, and the graph on the right shows a tension spline (tension parameter = 4) with the same data. In the case of the polynomial of order 6 shown in Figure 10.11, the function can be written:

$$v = 25401 - 2.3068 \times 10^5 t - 5.0947 \times 10^7 t^2 - 3.3097 \times 10^9 t^3 + 5.3727 \times 10^{11} t^4 - 1.7939 \times 10^{13} t^5 + 1.8712 \times 10^{14} t^6$$

The advantage of this is that data are modeled by a smooth curve. Another benefit is that polynomial functions can be differentiated and integrated to find related quantities. For example, the velocity polynomial shown in Figure 10.11 can be differentiated explicitly to give the acceleration. The result of this is shown in Figure 10.13. If you wish to review differentiation of polynomial functions, refer to Stewart (1999).

Several curve fitting routines are downloadable from the Internet. For example, a Windows-based one is CurveExpert1.3 at http://curveexpert.webhop.biz. This includes all of the regression and interpolation methods discussed here plus a lot more.

Indeed, obtaining smooth displacement coordinate data is a priority in kinematics; curve fitting, smoothing, filtering, and interpolation (see Chapter 9) can all be

Figure 10.13   Resultant acceleration obtained by differentiation of a polynomial trend curve shown in Figure 10.11.

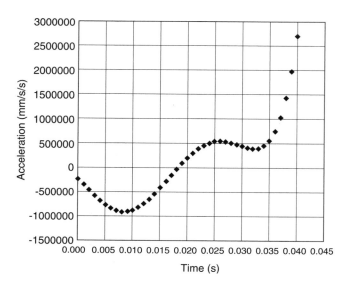

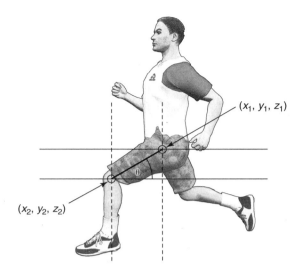

Figure 10.14 The lower leg segment marked with knee and hip markers. The z axis is assumed vertical, the x axis is into the page, and the y axis is from left to right.

applied in different circumstances depending on the nature of the noise and the requirements of the application.

10.6 Calculating Relative and Absolute Angles

Figure 10.14 shows a runner in a typical position at a given instant in time. Sometimes it is desirable to know the absolute angle θ the lower leg segment makes with the horizontal. The required absolute angle θ can then be calculated using trigonometry as:

$$\tan \theta = \frac{(z_1 - z_2)}{(y_1 - y_2)}.$$

This could be calculated from a spreadsheet containing the x, y, z coordinates of the knee and hip markers, so that obtaining the angle as a function of time is easy.

To calculate a relative angle, such as that between upper arm and arm shown in Figure 10.15, a slightly different approach is used. The relative angle E can be calculated from the x, y, z coordinates of the three points. In the triangle shown in Figure 10.15, the length of the side ELBOW–SHOULDER (w) is:

$$\sqrt{(x_1 - x_3)^2 + (y_1 - y_3)^2 + (z_1 - z_3)^2} = w$$

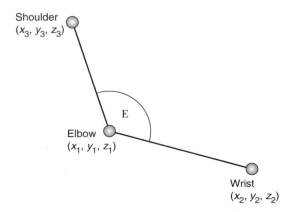

Figure 10.15 Wrist elbow and shoulder showing the relative angle E between the upper arm and arm segments.

Time	Left wrist coords			Left wrist coords			Left elbow coords							Angle
t (s)	x_2	y_2	z_2	x_1	y_1	z_1	x_3	y_3	z_3	a^2	b^2	c^2	cos E	E (deg)
0.1	4.0	6.8	0	1.8	8.5	0	0	0	0	25.09	75.49	62.24	0.8216	34.750
0.2	5.0	5.2	0	0.8	8.8	0	0	0	0	32.08	78.08	52.04	0.7690	39.735
0.3	5.6	3.6	0	0.0	8.9	0	0	0	0	42.25	79.21	44.32	0.6859	46.693
0.4	5.9	1.7	0	-0.7	8.8	0	0	0	0	51.97	77.93	37.70	0.5872	54.039
0.5	6.0	0.0	0	-1.5	8.5	0	0	0	0	62.50	74.50	36.00	0.4634	62.392
0.6	5.9	-2.0	0	-2.0	8.2	0	0	0	0	67.70	71.24	38.81	0.4027	66.253

Figure 10.16   Some x, y, z coordinate data for the left shoulder, elbow, and wrist.

ELBOW–WRIST (s) is:

$$\sqrt{(x_1 - x_2)^2 + (y_1 - y_2)^2 + (z_1 - z_2)^2} = s$$

WRIST–SHOULDER (e) is:

$$\sqrt{(x_2 - x_3)^2 + (y_2 - y_3)^2 + (z_2 - z_3)^2} = e$$

So that, by the cosine rule, the angle WRIST–E–SHOULDER (E) is:

$$\cos E = \frac{w^2 + s^2 - e^2}{2ws}$$

This angle, or any of the other angles in the triangle, can be evaluated by a spreadsheet method (Fig. 10.16). (See Appendix 1 for a reminder of basic trigonometry.)

In the data shown in Figure 10.16, the left elbow is stationary at (0, 0, 0), and the left wrist and left elbow both move in the x, y plane in an elbow extension movement. This angle E is shown graphically in Figure 10.17 using the data from Figure 10.16.

CASE Study 10.1   **Reduction of Noise on Angular Velocity–Time Graphs Using Moving-Point Average Methods**

Figure 10.18 shows the results obtained for a typical determination of angular velocity versus time in a rotating platform experiment. The top trace shows the data obtained without any averaging. Here the angular velocity is calculated using a simple finite-difference method based on the displacement of markers placed on the outside diameter of the turntable.

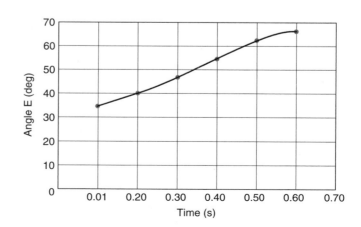

Figure 10.17   The relative angle, E, in an elbow extension movement. Data from Figure 10.16.

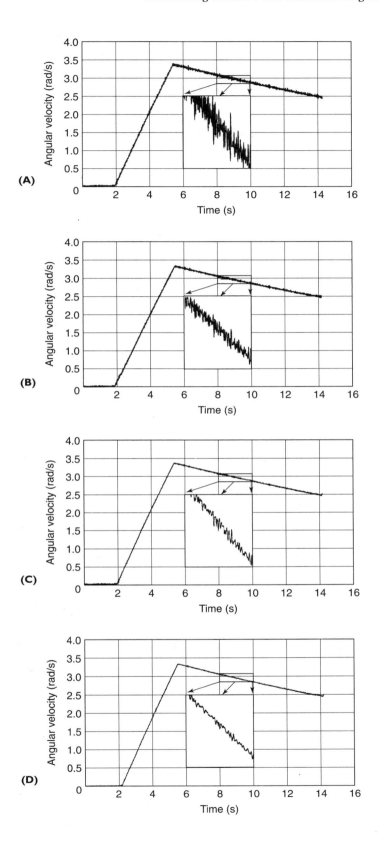

Figure 10.18 Data from the rotation experiment described in Case Study 8.1. (A) raw data, (B) three-point moving average smoothing, (C) five-point moving average smoothing, and (D) seven-point moving average smoothing. The noise level is expanded 10 times in each diagram. The simple moving average method does not change the slope of the curve in this case because the velocity changes are linear.

The three lower graphs represent the same data but with three-, five- and seven-point moving average smoothing, respectively. It is apparent that the noise level is reduced considerably and the noise is suppressed more as the number of averaged points increases. A section of the graph is shown expanded with a magnification of $10\times$ vertically so that the noise can be seen more clearly. It can be verified that the gradient of the $\omega - t$ line is not altered appreciably by the averaging.

10.7   Dynamic Analyses

A static analysis may be used to evaluate the forces on the human body when there are little significant linear or angular accelerations. When there are significant linear or angular accelerations, however, a dynamic analysis must be undertaken. A **dynamic analysis** should be used, therefore, when the accelerations are non-zero. The equations of motion are based on:

$$\Sigma F = ma \text{ for the linear case}$$
$$\Sigma \tau = I\alpha \text{ for the rotational case}$$

In a two-dimensional example, the linear acceleration may be broken down into its horizontal (x) and vertical (y) components. In a two-dimensional system, angular acceleration occurs about the z axis. If $\alpha = 0$, the motion is purely linear. If $a_x = 0$ and $a_y = 0$, the motion is purely rotational. If $\alpha = a_x = a_y = 0$, then this is a static case. There are three independent equations that are used in a dynamic two-dimensional analysis. These are:

$$\Sigma F_x = ma_x$$
$$\Sigma F_y = ma_y$$
$$\Sigma \tau_{cm} = I_{cm}\alpha$$

in which x and y represent the horizontal and vertical directions, respectively, a is the acceleration of the center of mass, m is the mass of the body, I_{cm} is the moment of inertia, about the center of mass, and α is the angular acceleration about the z axis through the center of mass. The forces acting on a body may be considered to be gravitational, muscular, contact, or inertial. The gravitational forces are the weights of each of the segments. The contact forces can be reactions or forces with another segment, the ground, or an external object. The **inertial forces** are ma_x and ma_y, and $I\alpha$ is the inertial torque. Using the equations of dynamic motion, the forces and torques acting on a segment can be calculated.

Moving from a static analysis to a dynamic analysis makes the problem somewhat more difficult. In the dynamic case, we now have linear and angular accelerations to deal with, and the body segments clearly resist these accelerations because of their inertial properties. Also, a great deal more data has to be collected in order to conduct a successful dynamic analysis. Because the forces and moments that cause the motion are determined by evaluating the resulting motion itself, a technique called an **inverse dynamics** approach is used. This approach calculates the forces and moments based on the accelerations of the object instead of measuring the forces directly.

In using the inverse dynamics approach, the system under consideration must be identified. The system is usually defined as a series of segments. The analysis on a series of segments is generally conducted beginning with the most distal segment and proceeds proximally up to the next segment and so on. Several assumptions must be made:

1. The body is considered to be a **rigid body linked system** with frictionless pin joints.

2. Each link, or segment, has a fixed mass and a center of mass located at a fixed point.

3. The moment of inertia about any axis of each segment remains constant.

Let us take a very simple example of a single segment: the foot during the swing phase of the gait cycle. Figure 10.19 shows a free-body diagram of the foot.

$$\text{Mass of foot, } m, = 1.176 \text{ kg; } I = 0.0096 \text{ kg.m}^2$$
$$\alpha = -14.66 \text{ rad/s}^2$$
$$a_x = -1.35 \text{ m/}^2, \, a_y = 7.65 \text{ m/}^2$$

The data presented here represents that taken from a single frame of video data and the appropriate inertial properties of the foot segment.

During the swing phase of the foot, no external forces other than gravity act on the foot. It can be seen that the only forces acting on the foot are those applied at the ankle joint and the weight of the foot segment acting vertically downward. The **joint reaction force** components can be calculated by using the first two equations defining the dynamic analysis. First, the horizontal joint reaction force may be defined from:

$$\Sigma F_x = ma_x$$
$$R_x = ma_x$$

If the mass of the foot is 1.16 kg and the horizontal acceleration of the center of mass of the foot is -1.35 m/^2, the horizontal reaction force is:

$$R_x = 1.16 kg \times -1.35 m/s^2$$
$$R_x = -1.57 N$$

Next, the vertical reaction force can be evaluated from:

$$\Sigma F_y = ma_y$$
$$R_y - W = ma_y$$

If the vertical acceleration of the center of mass of the foot is 7.65 m/s², then:

$$R_y = (1.16 kg \times 7.65 m/s^2) + (1.16 kg \times 9.81 m/s^2) = 20.3 N$$

To determine the **net moment** at the ankle joint, all moments acting on the system must be evaluated. If the center of mass of the foot is considered as the axis of rotation, three moments are acting on this system, two as a result of joint reaction forces and the net ankle moment itself. Thus:

$$\Sigma M_{cm} = I_{cm}\alpha$$
$$M_{ankle} + M_{Rx} + M_{Ry} = I_{cm}\alpha$$

Figure 10.19 Free-body diagram of the foot segment during the swing phase of a walking stride. Convention dictates that moments and forces at the proximal joint are positive, as indicated on the free-body diagram. Forces are shown with *thicker straight arrows*, and moments are shown as *curved arrows*. (Adapted from Hamill and Knutzen, 1995.)

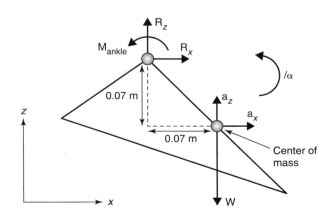

so that:

$$M_{ankle} = -M_{Rx} - M_{Ry} + I_{cm}\alpha$$

Do not forget that clockwise moments are negative. Remind yourself about the reaction force components R_x and R_y

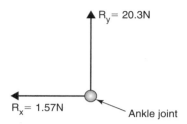

R_x is now pointing to the left because it worked out to be $-1.57N$, the minus sign indicating therefore that it points to the left. R_x constitutes a counterclockwise moment about the center of mass and so is positive. R_y, on the other hand, constitutes a clockwise moment about the center of mass, so it is negative. Bearing this in mind, therefore:

$$M_{ankle} = -M_{Rx} - M_{Ry} + I_{cm}\alpha = -(0.07m \times 1.57N) + (0.07m \times 20.3N)$$
$$+ (0.0096kg.m^2 \times -14.66rad/s^2)$$
$$M_{ankle} = -0.110Nm + 1.421Nm - 0.141Nm = 1.17Nm$$

The net moment at the ankle is thus positive, tending to result in an counterclockwise rotation. This indicates **dorsiflexor activity**, but the exact muscles acting cannot be determined from this type of analysis. Thus, it cannot be stated whether the muscle activity is dorsiflexor concentric or dorsiflexor eccentric in nature.

We have already said that a dynamic analysis proceeds from the more distal joints to the more proximal joints. The data we have produced here from the foot segment analysis would then be used in the calculations on the next segment, the leg, to calculate the net muscle moment at the knee. The calculation would then continue to the thigh to calculate the hip moment. The analysis can be conducted for each joint at each instant of time of the movement. In this way, we can create a profile of the net muscle moments for the complete movement. This analysis can be extended to a dynamic picture by using a video analysis to record the angular, horizontal, and vertical accelerations as a function of time. Figure 10.20 shows a

	A	B	C	D	E	F	G	H	I	J
1	time t	Angle θ wrt horixontal	Position of COM below ankle joint dz	Position of COM to the left of ankle joint dx	Angular acceleration α	Horizontal acceleration a_x	Vertical acceleration a_y	Horizontal ankle reaction force R_x	Vertical ankle reaction force R_y	Ankle moment M_{ank}
2	(s)	(rad)	(m)	(m)	(rad.s⁻²)	(m.s⁻²)	(m.s⁻²)	(N)	(N)	(N.m)
3	0.00	0.785	0.070	0.070	-14.66	-1.35	6.51	7.65	20.2536	1.167396
4	0.01	0.786	0.070	0.070	-14.69	-1.31	6.51	7.35	19.9056	1.144898
5	0.02	0.788	0.070	0.070	-14.72	-1.28	7.21	7.12	19.6388	1.125129
6	0.03	0.792	0.070	0.070	-14.75	-1.25	6.84	6.87	19.3488	1.101686
7	0.04	0.797	0.071	0.069	-14.78	-1.24	6.01	6.57	19.0008	1.070618
8	0.05	0.804	0.071	0.069	-14.81	-1.21	7.39	6.24	18.6180	1.036950
9	0.06	0.812	0.072	0.068	-14.76	-1.21	6.41	5.94	18.2700	1.002206
10	0.07	0.821	0.072	0.067	-14.69	-1.19	6.27	5.68	17.9684	0.970753
11	0.08	0.832	0.073	0.067	-14.65	-1.18	6.68	5.32	17.5508	0.928749
12	0.09	0.845	0.074	0.066	-14.59	-1.17	5.47	5.02	17.2028	0.890083
13	0.10	0.859	0.075	0.065	-14.57	-1.15	5.47	4.89	17.0520	0.863181

Figure 10.20 A spreadsheet calculation for the ankle reaction force and ankle moment as a function of time.

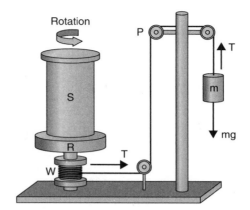

Figure 10.21 A mechanical diagram of the moment of inertia apparatus (not to scale).

spreadsheet calculation for the ankle reaction forces and ankle moment as a function of time for a small data set. Here the video capture rate was 100 Hz, and the data in the columns B to G were measured directly from the video by digitization. Columns H to J were calculated in the spreadsheet by an identical method to that already explained for the first row of data.

CASE *Study 10.2*   **Correcting for Friction in a Moment of Inertia Experiment**

In a rotating turntable experiment, shown in Figure 10.21, the experimental evidence points to a constant frictional torque, so that the angular acceleration, therefore, is given as:

$$I\alpha = \tau + \kappa$$

where τ is the constant accelerating torque and κ is the constant frictional torque (Griffiths et al., 2005).

Figure 10.22 illustrates a typical result obtained with this type of experiment. While the mass is falling, the angular velocity of the turntable increases linearly with time; after the mass has reached the floor, the angular velocity decreases linearly with time.

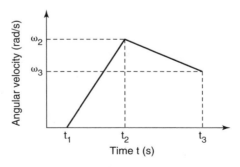

Figure 10.22 Angular velocity as a function of time graph for a typical experiment using motion analysis. The start time, or the time at which the mass (m) is released, is represented by t_1; the time at which the turntable ceases accelerating is represented by t_2; and the final time, or arbitrary end of the experiment, is represented by t_3. Note that 0 time on this graph is arbitrary and usually corresponds to when the motion analysis system was started.

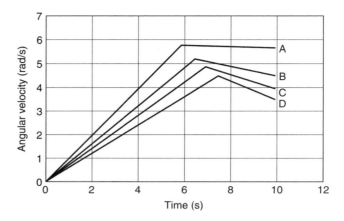

Figure 10.23 Theoretical angular velocity–time curves plotted for four different levels of frictional torque κ. After a total rotation of 17 rad, the mass disengages so that the system is then subject to friction only. Lines A, B, C, and D represent κ = 0.02, 0.2, 0.3, and 0.4, respectively.

The effect of the frictional torque is to decrease the final angular velocity, ω_2, while increasing the amount of time required to attain this angular velocity. In a hypothetical experiment, consider a system with $I = 1$ kg·m^2, torque $\tau = 1$ Nm, and various values of frictional torque κ = 0.02, 0.2, 0.3, and 0.4 Nm. Figure 10.23 shows how the angular velocity would vary as a function of time in these four cases. The results are plotted in such a way that the mass, m, disengages after an arbitrary total rotation of 17 rad. After this time, the system "free-wheels," subject only to the frictional torque. Table 10.1 shows how the value of ω_2 and t_2 are affected by the value of κ.

Linking Figure 10.20 to the experimental results, it is clear that the frictional torque is constant and does not vary with rotational speed to any marked extent. Also, the range of values of κ used here, especially the 0.2 and 0.3 Nm values and the accompanying frictional effects on the $\omega - t$ graphs, correspond fairly closely with the experimental values using masses between 50 and 100 kg on the turntable. Correcting for the effect of friction implies correcting the value of ω_2, t_2, or a combination of these two. In this case study, the correction is by means of ω_2 by a method that will now be explained.

Figure 10.24 shows measured angular velocity versus time for a typical rotation experiment. The symbols used are the same as the ones used in Figure 10.22 but also now include a corrected value for the angular velocity, ω_{final}.

In the motion analysis experiment, the measurement of time t_2 is accurate, corresponding to the time at which the rope disengages from the pulley wheel. In the correction, ω_{final} is estimated by using the measured angular velocity ω_2 and the observed loss of angular velocity occurring between t_2 and t_3.

Table 10.1	The effect of friction on the final angular velocity and the time at which the rope disengages*		
Value of Frictional Torque, κ (Nm)		**Final Angular Velocity, ω_2 (rad/s)**	**Time Rope Disengages, t_2 (s)**
0.02		5.772	5.88
0.2		5.216	6.51
0.3		4.879	6.96
0.4		4.518	7.52

* Data from Figure 10.23.

Figure 10.24
Hypothetical measured angular velocity versus time in a typical rotation experiment. If friction were absent, the angular velocity would increase further to ω_{final} during the time ($t_2 - t_1$). The *solid line* and *dashed line* indicate the $\omega - t$ relationship with and without friction, respectively.

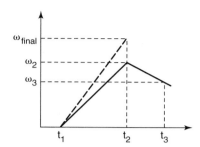

Between t_2 and t_3, the turntable decelerates uniformly because of frictional forces. t_3 can be chosen arbitrarily on a convenient part of the deceleration section or just when the motion analysis is stopped. The rate of loss of angular velocity, or angular deceleration, attributable to friction is:

$$\alpha_f = \frac{\omega_3 - \omega_2}{t_3 - t_2}$$

It can be argued that an appropriate correction to ω_2 is:

$$\alpha_f \times (t_2 - t_1).$$

The angular speed at t_2 can then be corrected to a new value:

$$\omega_{final} = \omega_2 - \alpha_f(t_2 - t_1)$$

The value of α_f is clearly negative so that $\omega_{final}\omega_2$. This new value corresponds to the angular velocity that the platform would have attained if it had accelerated without friction for the time interval between t_1 and t_2.

To check this idea, consider the theoretical friction model data presented in Figure 10.23. In this case, the values for angular velocities ω_2 and ω_3 and the times t_2 and t_3 are as shown in Table 10.2, along with the κ values. In Table 10.2, the t_3 values have been taken arbitrarily as 2 s later than t_2.

Table 10.3 shows the corresponding values for the angular acceleration for the four cases, both without using correction for friction and with correction for friction. The two columns on the right show the calculated values for moment of inertia. The true moment of inertia is 1 kg.m². Table 10.3 clearly shows the value of the friction correction because

Table 10.2 Summary of t_2, t_3, ω_2, and ω_3 values for four values of frictional torque, κ*

κ (Nm)	t_2 (s)	ω_2 (rad/s)	t_3 (s)	ω_3 (rad/s)
0.02	5.88	5.772	7.88	5.732
0.20	6.51	5.216	8.51	4.816
0.30	6.96	4.879	8.96	4.279
0.40	7.52	4.518	9.52	3.718

*Data from Figure 10.23. The time, t_1, is taken as 0 in all cases. This table is based on a theoretical model incorporating frictional torque.

Table 10.3	Angular acceleration values based on ω_2 and t_2 and ω_{final} and t_2 together with the associated moment of inertia values calculated from them			
κ (Nm)	α (based on ω_2 and t_2) (rad/s^2)	α (based on ω_{final} and t_2) (rad/s^2)	I (uncorrected for friction) (kg.m^2)	I (corrected for friction) (kg.m^2)
0.02	0.9816	1.00163	0.9816	1.00163
0.20	0.8012	1.00123	0.8012	1.00123
0.30	0.7010	1.00101	0.7010	1.00101
0.40	0.6008	1.00079	0.6008	1.00079

the corrected moments of inertia values are all within 0.1% of the known value;, without the correction, the departures from the true values can be as much as 40%.

Moment of Inertia of Turntable and Standard Masses

In a separate series of experiments using a range of falling masses, m, in the range of 2 to 3 kg and correcting for friction, the average value for the moment of inertia of the turntable together with the seat was found to be:

$$I_s = 0.313 \pm 0.01 \text{ kg.m}^2$$

When the seat was removed to leave just the turntable, this value reduced to 0.22 ± 0.01 kg·m^2. Using two diametrically opposed standard masses of 5 kg, each at a distance of 0.25 m from the axis of rotation fixed rigidly to the turntable, the moment of inertia of the turntable was increased on average by 0.63 ± 0.015 kg.m^2. This compares with a theoretical value of:

$$2 \times mr^2 = 2 \times 5 \times (0.25)^2 = 0.625 \text{ kg·m}^2$$

To emphasize the improvement obtained by correcting for friction, a series of measurements were taken using two 10-kg masses diametrically opposed to each other at various distances from the axis of rotation. These masses were rigidly fixed to the turntable of the apparatus and were used at four different distances from the center. The moment of inertia of this system can be determined theoretically using:

$$I = \sum_{i=1}^{n} m_i R_i^2$$

and can be compared directly with experimental results. The distances from the center were approximately 0.100, 0.220, 0.340, and 0.462 m. Ten trials were performed for each distance setting using three attempts with $m = 2.0$ kg, four attempts with $m = 2.5$ kg, and three attempts using $m = 3.0$ kg. Table 10.4 shows the results obtained for the theoretical moment of inertia and the moment of inertia measured both with and without a correction for friction.

Figure 10.25 shows the data of Table 10.4 plotted with theoretical moment of inertia on the horizontal axis and the measured values plotted on the vertical axis. The error bars in the vertical direction represent ± 1 standard deviation (SD).

Table 10.4 and Figure 10.25 both emphasize the improvement in accuracy and precision achieved by the friction correction. The measured values for moment of inertia including the friction correction are all within 3% of the theoretical values, with the measured values usually a little high. Also, the SD is reduced by a factor of between 3 and 10 when the friction correction is applied. The slope of the lower regression line of Figure 10.25 is 1.0062, indicating that the measurements of moment of inertia, with friction correction, are just 0.6% larger than the true ones on average. The slope of the upper regression line is 1.2019, indicating

Table 10.4	Measured and theoretical values for standard masses at various distances from the axis of rotation*			
Theoretical Moment of Inertia (kg.m^2)	**Mean Measured Moment of Inertia I_{meas}[a] (kg.m^2)**	**Standard Deviation of I_{meas}**	**Mean Measured Moment of Inertia I_{corr}[b] (kg.m^2)**	**Standard Deviation of I_{corr}**
0.000	0.00	0.016	−0.002	0.004
0.202	0.25	0.041	0.20	0.014
0.977	1.19	0.045	0.99	0.015
2.312	2.84	0.118	2.37	0.023
4.26	5.11	0.252	4.27	0.026

*The measured values are the means of 10 determinations. A value of 0.22 kg.m^2 has been subtracted away from the uncorrected measured values, and a value of 0.21 kg.m^2 has been subtracted from the corrected measured values. The theoretical values are based on ΣmR^2.
[a] Without friction correction.
[b] With friction correction.

that the measurements are 20% larger than the true ones on average. The error bars on the lower line are so small that they are invisible on the graph.

This appears to be direct confirmation that the measured moments of inertia are substantially more accurate after the friction correction has been applied. The procedure removes the single largest source of error in this type of experiment, and the calibration work reveals that any other sources of error must be extremely small in their effects. One such error might be friction in the pulley wheels, P, which transmit the tension, T, from the falling mass, m, to the turntable pulley wheel, W.

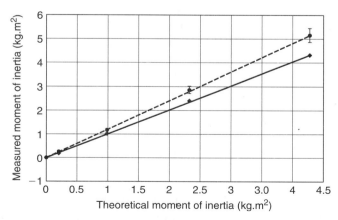

Figure 10.25   The measured moments of inertia plotted as a function of the theoretical moment of inertia. Whereas the values measured using friction correction show values just 0.6% higher than the true values on average, the values measured without any correction show values 20% higher than the true values. The *solid line* shows a linear regression line fitted to the data with friction correction (slope = 1.0062; intercept = 0.0078). The *dashed line* shows a similar regression line for the data without friction correction (slope = 1.2019; intercept = 0.0147).

SUMMARY

This chapter has introduced inverse dynamics in which joint moments and forces are inferred from measured accelerations. It has also applied careful analysis to the measurement of rotational motion whereby the obscuring effect of friction can be removed.

REFERENCES

Griffiths IW, Watkins J. Sharpe D: Measuring the moment of inertia of the human body by a rotating platform method. *Am J Phys* 73:85–92, 2005.

Hamill J, Knutzen KM: *Biomechanical Basis of Human Movement*, Baltimore: Williams and Wilkins; 1995

Stewart J: *Calculus*. Pacific Grove, CA: Brooks/Cole Pub. Co; 1999.

STUDY QUESTIONS

1. In a rotating platform experiment, a falling weight (marked MASS) is used to spin a rotating platform carrying two masses (marked XTR1 and XTR2) at equal distances from the axis of rotation. The file Ch10Q1 gives the x, y, and z coordinates of these three markers 120 times per second for a total trial time in excess of 15 s. The mass is released from rest and falls through a distance of approximately 1 m during the experiment. Use the data to plot two charts:

   (a) A graph of height of MASS versus time from row 200 to row 800 in the spreadsheet

   (b) A graph of the angular velocity versus time. The answer to Study Question 3 in Chapter 9 can be used as a model of how to lay out the solution.

   For graph a, apply a polynomial best fit curve of order 2 and apply the equation of the trend line and its R^2 value. For graph b, apply linear trend lines to the rising and falling sections of the graph. Rising section: take rows 224 to 798. Falling section: take rows 836 to 1872. Using the trend lines, give your best estimate of the downward acceleration of the mass, the angular acceleration of the turntable during the first part of its motion, and the angular deceleration during the second part of its motion.

2. Data file Ch10Q2 gives the spatial coordinates of the right wrist (RWRA) in a fast karate punch. Also given are the coordinates of two markers (RFHD) and (LFHD) attached to a target punching bag. The coordinates of these RFHD and LFHD are averaged to give the position of the center of the bag (LFHD + RFHD)/2. Calculate the velocity of RWRA and of the bag using a finite-difference method.

   Use a Butterworth fourth-order digital filter to smooth the x, y, and z coordinates of RWRA and (LFHD + RFHD)/2. Then calculate the velocity of the wrist and the punching bag again using the same finite-difference method but using the smoothed coordinates. Plot graphs of the two velocities obtained on the same chart: one chart for RWRA and one for (LFHD + RFHD)/2. Estimate the peak velocity of the wrist from your graphs. Estimate the peak velocity of the punching bag from the other set of graphs. What is the acceleration of the punching bag (given by the slope of the velocity–time graph) during fist contact?

CHAPTER eleven

BALLS IN FLIGHT AND FLUID DYNAMICS

CHAPTER *objectives*

The objectives of this chapter are to:

- Introduce the principles of aerodynamics and hydrodynamics.
- Discuss the properties of fluids, such as viscosity, density, and turbulence.
- Quantify drag and lift forces on objects moving through a fluid.

CHAPTER *outcomes*

After reading this chapter, the reader will be able to:

- Quantify dynamic fluid forces experimentally and by means of calculation.
- Have thorough understanding of the factors that influence the movement of balls through the air.

11.1   Viscosity

Objects moving through the air (e.g., golf balls, high jumpers, soccer balls) experience a resistance to their movement caused by interaction between air molecules and the surface of the object. This resistance also occurs, but to a greater extent, when objects move through water (e.g., a swimmer, the hull of a boat). In general terms, substances such as air and water are known as fluids. A fluid is known as a substance that continues to distort even when subjected to a very small **shear force** or shear stress, which tends to slide layers of the fluid past each other (Fig. 11.1).

The shear stress is the shear force divided by the area over which it acts. Solids distort only a fixed amount under the action of a shear stress. They have a fixed shape and volume, and their particles are arranged in a fixed structure. Fluids, on

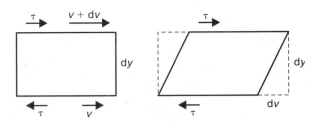

Figure 11.1 Shear stress and rate of shear on an element of fluid. The thickness of the fluid element is dy. The shear stress τ produces a velocity change dv.

the other hand, flow freely. They assume the shape of their container (if they have one), and their particles can change their positions relative to each other whenever a force acts on them. Liquids (e.g., water) have a volume that stays the same while the shape changes. Gases (e.g., air) expand to fill the whole volume available by changing density.

Although fluids have the ability to flow, this flow encounters resistance by virtue of the viscosity of the fluid. This is a property that causes shear stresses between adjacent layers of a moving fluid, leading to an irreversible loss of energy and a resistance to motion through the fluid. The relationship between **shear stress** (τ) and **rate of shear** (dv/dy) depends on the fluid. The rate of shear is dv/dy. For water, the shear stress is directly proportional to the rate of shear. The **viscosity** is formally defined as:

Coefficient of dynamic viscosity (η) = Shear stress/Rate of shear = $\tau/(dv/dy)$

which has SI (International System of Units) units of Pascal seconds (Pa.s). This coefficient depends on both the pressure and temperature of the fluid. An increase in temperature leads to a decrease in viscosity for liquids and an increase for gases. Another viscosity coefficient is defined as:

Coefficient of kinematic viscosity (ν) = Coefficient of dynamic viscosity (η)/Density of fluid

This coefficient has SI units of $m^2.s^{-1}$.

■ **EXAMPLE 11.1**   For water, the viscosity is 1.0×10^{-3} Pa.s. For air, it is 0.018×10^{-3} Pa.s at 20°C.

11.2 Buoyancy Forces

The two types of forces exerted on an object by a fluid environment are a **buoyant force** because of its immersion in the fluid and a **dynamic force** because of its relative motion in the fluid. The dynamic force is usually resolved into two components: drag and lift forces. The buoyant force always acts vertically upward.

To explain the buoyant force, let us consider the force water exerts on an immersed body. The water exerts a force on the surface of an immersed body because of all the weight of the water above the body. If you immersed yourself in a swimming pool completely in a vertical upright position, the water would be pushing down on the top of your head. It would also be pushing sideways on you around the sides of your body and vertically upward on the soles of your feet. We realize, of course, that pressure increases with depth, so that the pressure acting on your feet would be larger than the pressure acting on your head. Could this explain the buoyancy force?

Let us do a simple analysis. To make this easier, we will consider a cube being immersed in water. The cube could be made of wood, solid metal, or even water.

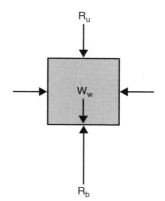

Figure 11.2 A free-body diagram of the forces acting on the cube of water. The forces acting on the top and bottom surfaces are shown as R_u and R_b respectively. W_w is the weight of the cube.

The sides of the cube are 1 m long. Figure 11.2 represents a free-body diagram of the cube showing all the forces acting on the cube.

What vertical forces act on the cube? If the top surface of the cube is 1 m below the water surface, the water exerts a pressure 9800 N/m^2 on the top of the cube. (One cubic meter of water above our other cube has a mass of 1000 kg and a weight of 9800 N.) This pressure acting on the square-meter top face of the cube creates a 9800-N resultant force acting downward on the cube. This force is shown as R_u in Figure 11.2 with "u" standing for "upper surface." The water below the cube exerts a force of 19,600 N on the bottom surface of the cube because the pressure is twice as high, and this is shown as R_b on Figure 11.2. Forces are also exerted on the sides of the cube, but these forces cancel one another out because they are directly opposed to each other in pairs. These forces amount to 14,700 N on each face and are shown as unlabeled arrows in Figure 11.2. The cube itself weighs something, and this force is shown as W_w in Figure 11.2. If it is a cube of water, it will weigh about 9800 N because of the force of gravity. If the cube is in equilibrium (not accelerating), then according to Newton's second law:

$$\Sigma F = R_b + (-R_u) + (-W_w) = 0$$
$$\Sigma F = 19600N - 9800N - 9800N = 0$$

Therefore, the cube of water is in equilibrium. This would also be the case if the cube were immersed at any other depth. Let us say the cube's top surface was at a depth of 8 m and the bottom surface was at a depth of 9 m. At 8 m, the pressure is 78,400 N/m^2; at 9 m, the pressure is 88,200 N/m^2. The cube still weighs the same so that:

$$\Sigma F = R_b + (-R_u) + (-W_w) = 0$$
$$\Sigma F = 88200N - 78400N - 9800N = 0$$

The size of the buoyant force is equal to the weight of the volume of fluid displaced by the object.

If the cube of water were to be replaced with a cube of another material (e.g., wood), the result would be different. If the density of the wood were less than that of water, say, 500 kg/m^3, then the weight of the cube would be reduced to 4900 N and the values of R_u and R_b would still be the same. There would then be a net upward force of 4900 N, and the wooden cube would float to the surface. However, the buoyancy force would still be the same, given by the weight of water displaced by the wooden cube.

11.3 Density and Specific Gravity

If a material has a density less than water, then it will float. The density of water is 1000 kg/m^3. The **density** of a material is denoted by ρ, where:

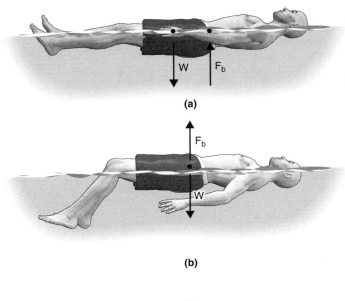

Figure 11.3 (A) When the body is floating horizontally in the water, the weight and buoyant force are not aligned, thus creating torque. (B) When the body is partially vertical, the weight and buoyant force are aligned, creating a more stable floating position. Weight of swimmer = W. Buoyant force = F_b.

$$\rho = \frac{m}{V}$$

where ρ = density, m = mass, and V = volume. The density of air is only approximately 1.2 kg/m^3 but depends on temperature and pressure.

Another way of giving the same information is to state the **specific gravity**, which is the ratio of the weight of an object to the weight of an equal volume of water. Objects with specific gravities of less than 1.0 will float.

11.3.1 BUOYANCY OF THE HUMAN BODY

Whereas muscle and bone have densities greater than 1000 kg/m^3 (specific gravities < 1.0), fat has a density less than 1000 kg/m^3 (specific gravity < 1.0). These differences are the basis for the underwater weighing techniques used to determine body composition. Someone who has low body fat can still float because the lungs and other body cavities may be filled with air or other gases that are less dense than water. Exhaling can make a lean person sink. The volume of the chest increases when you inhale and decreases when you exhale, enabling you to control your density to some extent. Most people can float if they inhale to the maximum extent. The relative positions of the center of gravity and the center of buoyancy are important for determining the stability of the body position in the water (Fig. 11.3).

■ **EXAMPLE 11.2**   A swimmer weighing 79 kg steps into an immersion tank and displaces 38 l of water. What is his apparent weight?

Density of water = 1000 kg/m^3, g = 9.81 m/s^2
Weight = 79 kg × 9.81 m/s^2 = 775N
Buoyancy force = 38 × 10^{-3}m^3 × 1000kg/m^3 × 9.81 m/s^2 = 372.8N
Apparent weight = 775 − 372.8 = 402.2 N

11.4 Dynamic Fluid Forces

When an object moves in a fluid or when a fluid moves past an object immersed in it, dynamic fluid forces are exerted on the object by the fluid. This force is proportional to:

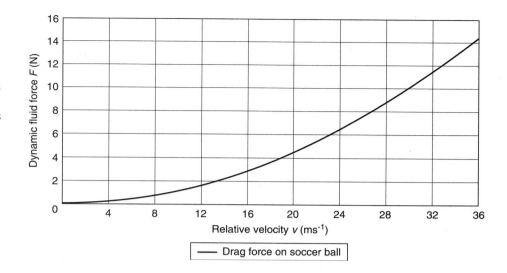

Figure 11.4 Drag force on a soccer ball as a function of relative speed in air. This model assumes that the drag force increases as v^2 and the drag coefficient is 0.2. The cross-sectional area of the ball is 0.039m², and the density of the air is 1.2 kg.m^{-3}. In reality, the drag coefficient depends on velocity, and the drag force on a soccer ball will depart from this quadratic relationship.

The density of the fluid

The surface area of the object

The square of the relative velocity of the object to the fluid

$$F \propto \rho A v^2$$

where

$\propto$ = proportional to

F = dynamic fluid force

ρ = fluid density

A = surface area of object

v = relative velocity of the object with respect to the fluid

All the terms in this equation are linear apart from the velocity term that is squared, meaning that if the velocity is doubled, the force is quadrupled. Figure 11.4 illustrates this relationship for the drag on a soccer ball. Here it is assumed that the **drag force** is:

$$F_D = \tfrac{1}{2} C_D \rho A v^2$$

where C_D is the drag coefficient, equal to approximately 0.48.

■ **EXAMPLE 11.3**

Calculate the drag force on a ball moving at 30 mph in still air at 20°C. The radius of the ball is 0.11 m. The drag coefficient is $C_D = 0.48$, and the density of air is 1.29 kg.m^{-3}.

$$F_D = \tfrac{1}{2} C_D \rho A v^2$$

30 mph = 30 × 1.609 = 48.28 kmph or 13.41 m.s^{-1}.

$$F_D = \tfrac{1}{2} \times 0.48 \times 1.29 \times \pi \times (0.11)^2 \times (13.41)^2 = 2.12N$$

11.5 Relative Velocity

The velocity of the object and the velocity of the fluid must both be considered; **relative velocity** is the difference between the object's velocity and the fluid's velocity. Suppose you throw a ball at 10 m/s (relative to the ground) into a wind that is blowing at 5 m/s (relative to the ground) in the opposite direction to that of the ball. The relative velocity would therefore be 10 + 5 = 15 m/s. If, however, the ball were thrown with the wind, the relative velocity would be 10 − 5 = 5 m/s. In this respect, it does not matter which is moving, the ball or the air around it.

11.6 Drag Force

The dynamic fluid force that results from motion within a fluid is commonly resolved into two components: the drag force and the lift force. Figure 11.5 illustrates the resolution of the dynamic fluid force into lift and drag components.

The drag force, or drag, is the component of the resultant dynamic fluid force that acts in opposition to the relative motion of the object with respect to the fluid. A drag force tends to decelerate an object if it is the only force acting on the object. The drag force is defined mathematically as:

$$F_D = \tfrac{1}{2}C_D\rho A v^2$$

Drag can be explained by remembering that air (fluid) is composed of molecules that can collide with solid objects. When a relative velocity exists between an object and fluid, fluid molecules collide with a solid surface, either head on or at an angle. This braking action tends to reduce the relative velocity between the object and the fluid. A force acts on the object because of the molecular collisions and, by Newton's third law, an equal and opposite force acts on the molecules of the fluid. The size of the drag force is proportional to the deceleration (slowing down) of the fluid molecules as they pass by the object as well as to the mass of the molecules that are slowed down. This idea is represented diagrammatically in Figure 11.6.

Drag forces can be produced in two ways: surface drag and form drag. Surface drag (Fig. 11.7) may be thought of as equivalent to the sum of the friction forces acting between the fluid molecules and the surface of the object (or between the fluid molecules themselves). Form drag (Fig. 11.8) may be thought of as equivalent to the sum of the impact forces resulting from collisions between the fluid molecules and the object.

Surface drag is also known as viscous drag and skin drag. As a fluid molecule

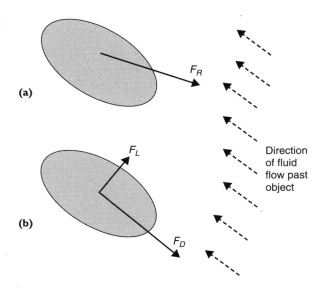

Figure 11.5 (A) The resultant dynamic fluid force (F_R) acting on an object. (B) The drag (F_D) and lift (F_L) components of this force.

Direction of fluid flow past object

Figure 11.6 Fluid molecules (*circles*) colliding with solid surface and experiencing a force (*arrows pointing to the left*). The solid experiences an equal and opposite force (*arrows pointing to the right*).

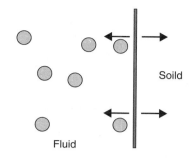

Soild

Fluid

Figure 11.7 Surface drag. Molecules (*circles*) sliding past the surface of an object and being decelerated. (Vector showing velocity is decreasing in length.) This will also slow down nearby molecules.

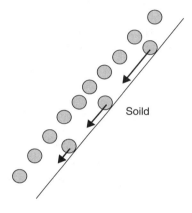

Soild

Figure 11.8 Form drag. A fluid molecule (*dark circle*) strikes the surface of an object moving through it, bounces off and then strikes other fluid molecules (*series of lighter grey circles*), and is pushed back toward the solid surface.

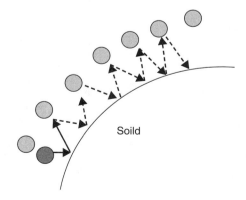

Soild

slides past the surface of a solid object, the friction between the surface and the molecule slows down the molecule. On the opposite side of this molecule are other fluid molecules that are now moving faster than this molecule, so these molecules are also slowed down as they slide past the molecules closest to the object. These molecules, in turn, slow down the molecules next to them. Therefore, the surface drag is proportional to the total mass of the molecules slowed down by the friction force and the average rate of change of velocity of these molecules.

The magnitude of the surface drag is affected by the coefficient of drag, the density of the fluid, the cross-sectional area of the object, and the square of the relative velocity. The coefficient of drag is determined by several other factors associated with surface drag. The roughness of the surface is one of these factors.

11.7   Lift Force

Lift force is the dynamic fluid force component that acts perpendicular to the relative motion of the object with respect to the fluid. The word *lift* implies that the force is upward, but this is not necessarily the case. The lift force must be perpendicular to the flow of the fluid (Fig. 11.9).

The **lift force** is defined by the following equation:

$$F_L = \tfrac{1}{2} C_L \rho A v^2$$

where

F_L = lift force

C_L = coefficient of lift

ρ = fluid density

A = cross-sectional area (frontal area) of the object perpendicular to the flow direction

v = relative velocity of the object with respect to the fluid

Relative velocity is the most important factor that affects the lift force. The shape and orientation of the object also affect the force; these factors are taken into account in the equation by the frontal area and the coefficient of lift. Wings on planes use the lift force to stay airborne; submerged wings use lift force to lift the hulls of boats out of the water. A rudder on a boat or plane uses lift force to change the direction of the craft. Propellers are used on boats and aircraft to actually

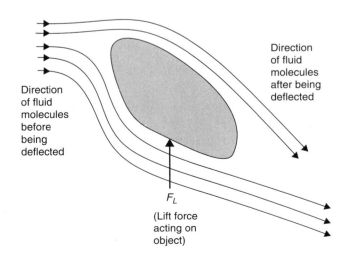

Figure 11.9 Lateral deflection of molecules passing by an object. The change in direction is a lateral acceleration caused by the force exerted by the object. The reaction to this force is the lift force acting on the object.

Direction of fluid molecules before being deflected

Direction of fluid molecules after being deflected

F_L
(Lift force acting on object)

propel the craft using the lift force. The spoilers on the rear of some racing cars use lift force to push the rear-drive wheels against the ground for better traction. Ski jumpers use long, wide skis and position themselves so that the lift force keeps them in the air longer so that they can go farther. When you tread water, you scull your hands in a horizontal plane, and the lift forces generated by your hands keep your head above water. The propulsive techniques used in various swimming strokes are a resultant of the lift and drag forces acting on the hands.

In most of these examples, the object that generates the lift force is longer in the dimension parallel to the flow and shorter in the dimension perpendicular to the flow. Also, lift is generated in these examples when the longer dimension of the object is not aligned parallel to the fluid flow. Some objects generate lift even though they are not longer in one dimension than another (e.g., a spinning ball) or even if their longest dimension appears to align with the fluid flow (e.g., a wing, a propeller blade, a rudder).

11.8   Bernoulli's Principle

Bernoulli discovered that faster moving fluids exert less pressure laterally than slower moving ones. This principle may explain why some objects are able to generate lift forces without being longer in one dimension than another or if their longest dimension is aligned with the flow.

Let us examine an airfoil to see how **Bernoulli's principle** works. An airfoil is an example of an object whose longest dimension appears to align with the fluid flow, even while it creates lift. Figure 11.10 shows an airfoil in cross-section. One surface (the upper surface in a plane wing) of the airfoil is more curved than the other surface; in fact, in this diagram, the other surface is shown flat. The curvature is gentle, and the airfoil is streamlined. When oriented with its long dimension parallel to the fluid flow, the airfoil's streamlined shape produces laminar flow and minimal drag.

Imagine two rows of four air molecules approaching the airfoil, as shown in Figure 11.10b. When they strike the leading edge of the airfoil, one row travels along the upper curved surface, and one row travels along the bottom straighter section. If the flow is laminar, each molecule on top reaches the trailing edge of the airfoil at the same time as the corresponding molecule on the bottom. The molecules on the upper surface travel farther to get to the trailing edge, but they get there at the same time as the molecules on the lower surface (Fig. 11.10c). Therefore, the velocity of the molecules moving over the upper surface is higher than that of molecules traveling over the bottom surface. According to Bernoulli's principle, the lateral pressure exerted by the faster moving molecules is less than that exerted by the slower moving molecules, and an upward lift force is generated. This is shown in Figure 11.10d, where the lower arrow represents a larger magnitude force on the lower surface of the airfoil compared with a smaller force on the upper surface.

11.9   Spin and the Magnus Effect

In 1852, the German scientist Gustav Magnus found that lift forces occur when balls are spinning. This effect is called the **Magnus effect**, and a force generated by a spin is called a Magnus force. But how can an object that does not have any broad, relatively flat surface deflect the air laterally to cause a lift force? Let us consider a ball with topspin. Figure 11.11 shows a ball moving from left to right with topspin.

The air molecules all have a backward velocity (to the left) relative to the center of the ball. When air molecules strike the lower surface of the ball, they do not

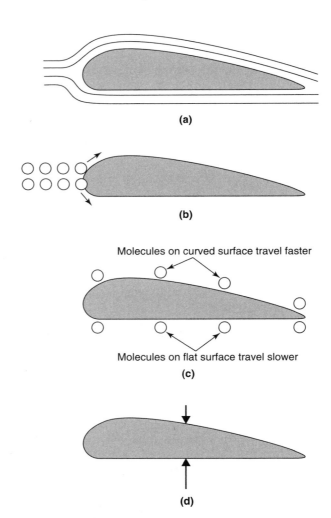

Figure 11.10 Air flow over the upper and lower surfaces of an airfoil. (A) Air molecules are moving from left to right over the airfoil. (B) The air molecules at the leading edge split, some moving over the upper surface and some moving over the lower surface. (C) The air molecules travel faster over the upper surface of the airfoil because they have to complete a longer distance in the same time. (D) A larger lift force on the lower surface compared with that on the upper surface.

slow down as much because this surface is moving in the same direction as the molecules (backward or to the left) relative to the center of the ball. The velocity of the air over the top of the ball is lower than the velocity over the bottom of the ball. According to Bernoulli's principle, less pressure will be exerted on the bottom surface and more pressure will be exerted on the top surface. This difference in pressure results in a lift force acting downward on the ball.

However, even this neat explanation is not the whole truth. It is now realized that there is a boundary layer of air surrounding all sports balls. The true explanation lies in the fact that there is a viscous drag force on the air within this boundary layer. Because of this, Bernoulli's principle does not apply. We will see later that the air

Figure 11.11 A ball with topspin spins about a horizontal axis with the top of the ball moving in the same direction as the ball is thrown or kicked. The ball with topspin experiences a lift force that acts downward on the ball.

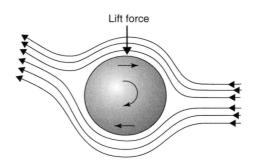

flow pattern over the surface of a ball can be quite complicated, with the airflow separating from the surface of the ball and the eddies behind the ball becoming turbulent (see Section 11.12).

The Magnus force is responsible for the curvature in flight in many ball sports; for example, whereas **backspin** causes a ball to stay aloft longer, **topspin** causes a ball to drop toward the ground sooner. **Sidespin** causes a ball to swerve to the right or to the left. This effect is used extensively in sports such as table tennis, tennis, soccer, baseball, and golf.

11.10   Center of Pressure

The resultant of the lift and drag forces that act on an object is the dynamic fluid force. This force is actually the result of pressures exerted on the surfaces of the object. The theoretical point of application of this force to the object is called the **center of pressure**. If the resultant force acting at the center of pressure is not on a line passing through the center of gravity of the object, then a torque is produced that causes the object to rotate. A Frisbee, discus, or football thrown with no spin is more likely to wobble because of this torque. The specifications adopted in 1986 by International Association of Athletic Foundations (IAAF) for men's javelin competitions essentially force the center of pressure to be behind the grip (and the center of gravity) of the javelin. The torque produced by the dynamic forces acting on the javelin during flight cause it to rotate so that the tip of the javelin tends to strike the ground first. Figure 11.12 illustrates the forces acting on a javelin.

11.11   Effects of Dynamic Fluid Forces

The dynamic fluid forces that act on an object moving through a fluid have an effect on the motion of the object. This is expressed in a general sense by Newton's second law:

$$\Sigma F = ma$$

where

ΣF = net force

m = mass of object

a = acceleration of object

The effect of a force is the acceleration that would be caused if this were the net force acting, or:

$$\frac{\Sigma F}{m} = a$$

Figure 11.12 The forces acting on a javelin in flight—its weight and the dynamic fluid force—act at different locations, thus creating a torque that causes the javelin to rotate clockwise and bringing the tip down toward the ground.
cp = center of pressure
cg = center of gravity

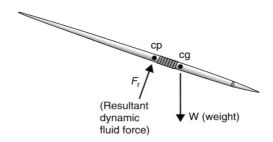

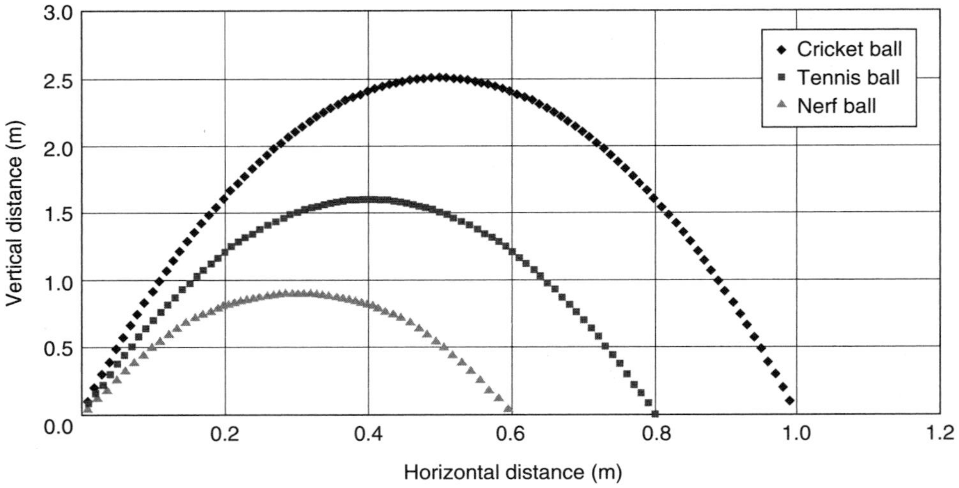

Figure 11.13 The trajectories of three balls with different masses, demonstrating that the effect of fluid forces is influenced by the mass of the object. The shapes of the trajectories are approximations to real ones.

The **dynamic fluid forces** can be determined from the equation:

$$F \propto \rho A v^2$$

$$a = \frac{\Sigma F}{m} \propto \frac{\rho A v^2}{m}$$

$$a \propto \frac{\rho A v^2}{m}$$

The symbol $\propto$ stands for "is proportional to."

The acceleration is inversely proportional to the mass of the object. This means that two objects similar in size and shape experience the same dynamic fluid forces, but the more massive object experiences less acceleration. Figure 11.13 shows the trajectories of a variety of balls. The initial velocities, angles, and heights of projection of these objects are identical, but their masses are different.

11.12 The Boundary Layer

For balls traveling at less than 0.5 ms^{-1}, the drag on the ball can be explained in terms of the Stokes viscous model. However, at higher velocities, the nature of the air flow around the ball alters, so a different model has to be used. As the velocity of the ball through the air increases, the volume of air around the ball affected by viscosity decreases in size. This can be thought of as a region of velocity gradient in the air surrounding the ball; the air in contact with the ball itself can be thought of as stationary with respect to the ball, but further away from the ball, the air flow is moving faster. This is illustrated in Figure 11.14, which shows air molecules near

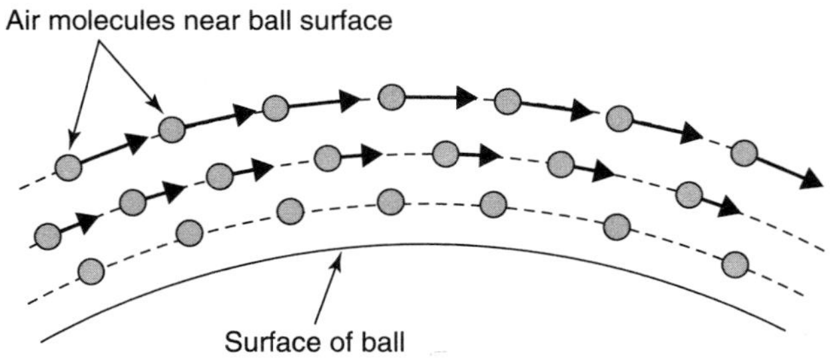

Figure 11.14 The movement of air molecules over the surface of a ball.

the surface of the ball in schematic form. The velocity gradient between the layers of air around the ball causes friction and, therefore, drag on the ball.

The narrow layer of viscous air surrounding the ball is known as a **boundary layer**. The boundary layer's behavior determines the amount of drag on the ball and, for a ball, the boundary layer is a few millimeters thick. The nature of the flow conditions around the ball can be inferred from the value of **Reynold's number**, R_e:

$$R_e = \frac{rv\rho}{\nu}$$

where

r = radius of ball (0.11 m)
v = velocity of ball through the air
ρ = density of the air (1.2 kg.m^{-3})
ν = viscosity of the air (1.8 $\times$ 10^{-5} Nsm^{-2})

Broadly speaking, the flow conditions are **laminar** for $R_e < 500$ and **turbulent** for $R_e > 500$. However, the exact values depend on the geometry of the setup and the ball's surface. If we consider a soccer ball kicked quite slowly, say 4 ms^{-1}, the value of R_e is 29,300. This is well in excess of 500, so we can say that soccer is played under turbulent air flow conditions.

At a certain point in its flow around the ball, the boundary layer separates from the surface (Fig. 11.15). The air is first accelerated from a lower speed to a higher speed as it moves around the ball. The Bernoulli effect means that the pressure exerted by the air molecules decreases as the speed increases. As the air moves around into the space behind the ball, it decelerates again, and the pressure increases. The viscosity in the boundary layer slows the air, and toward the rear of the ball, the flow is halted and the flow separates from the surface. The disruption of the air's journey around to the back of the ball means that an **eddy** can form.

Beyond the separation point, the air flow is irregular. Turbulent eddies (Fig. 11.16) are formed in a wake behind the ball. These eddies reduce the kinetic energy of the ball. The drag force increases as the square of the speed up until a certain critical speed, when things start to change again.

Many experimental studies of drag have been conducted on smooth spheres. In general, a large reduction in the drag force occurs when the relative velocity between the air and the spheres exceeds a certain **critical velocity** (Fig. 11.17). Above the critical speed, the boundary layer at the ball's surface becomes unstable and allows the faster moving air outside the boundary layer to mix with the air moving more slowly near the ball's surface. This allows the air to travel further

Figure 11.15 The viscosity slows the air in the boundary layer, causing it to separate from the ball.

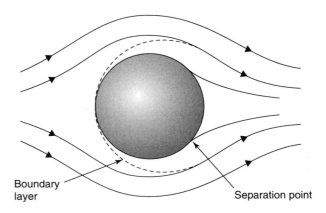

Boundary layer

Separation point

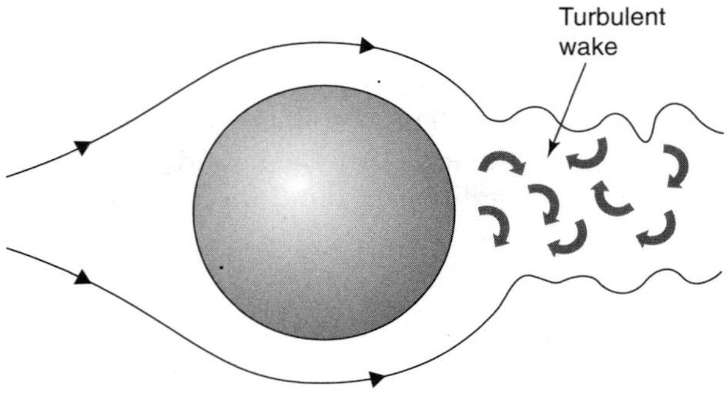

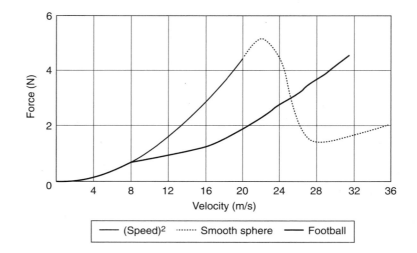

Figure 11.16 The separation leads to turbulent eddies in the wake and energy loss from the ball.

around toward the back of the ball before it separates from the surface. The delayed separation means a smaller wake and reduced drag.

The onset of the boundary layer instability around a ball depends on the roughness of the surface. For example, a rough surface produces a lower critical speed than a smooth surface. With a soccer ball, the stitching produces indentations in the surface that induce **instability** in the boundary layer. This lowers the drag force on the ball below that on a similar smooth ball at speeds in excess of 9 ms^{-1}. At speeds in excess of 25 ms^{-1}, the indentations (Fig. 11.18) increase the drag above that for a smooth sphere.

▪ **EXAMPLE 11.4**   Calculate Reynold's number for a cricket ball bowled at 90 mph. The radius of a cricket ball is 36 mm (90 mph is equivalent to 40.23 m.s^{-1}).

$$R_e = \frac{rv\rho}{\nu} = \frac{0.036m \times 40.23ms^{-1} \times 1.29kg.m^{-3}}{1.8 \times 10^{-5}Pa.s}$$
$$R_e = 103800$$

11.13   The Curling Kick

The Magnus effect can cause a spinning ball to deviate from a vertical plane in flight. Clearly, there is a sideways force on the ball, and the direction of the spin

Figure 11.17 The drag force on a soccer ball falls below that on a smooth sphere of the same size at a speed of about 9 ms^{-1}; the critical speed. At speeds higher than 25 ms^{-1}, the drag force on the soccer ball is higher than that on a smooth sphere.

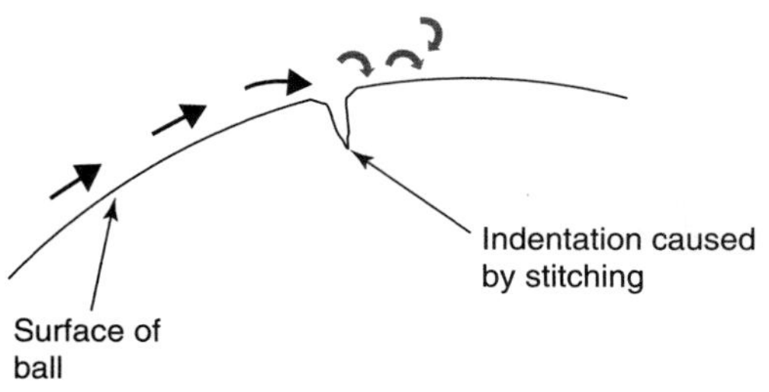

Figure 11.18 Disruption of the air flow over the surface of a soccer ball by the indentations.

Surface of ball

Indentation caused by stitching

determines the direction of the curve in flight. Figure 11.19 shows the airflow over the surface of the ball being deflected in flight giving a sideways force on the ball.

We have already seen how the boundary layer can separate from the ball. With a spinning ball, the side of the ball moving with the flow carries the flow farther around the ball before separation. On the other side of the ball, the air flow is slowed down and separates from the ball earlier. This implies that the air leaving the ball is deflected sideways.

In Figure 11.19, the air flow is directed toward the right (i.e., the ball is moving to the left). This implies that the Magnus force would deflect the ball upward in Figure 11.19 (i.e., to the right as viewed by the kicker).

The Magnus force, F_m, is perpendicular both to the spin and the velocity of the ball and is often written as:

$$F_m = \tfrac{1}{2}C_L \rho A v^2$$

In the case of a spinning ball, C_L depends on both velocity and spin. It is convenient to write:

$$C_L = \frac{\omega a}{v} C_s$$

where ω is the angular frequency of the spin and a is the radius of the ball. Then

$$F_m = \tfrac{1}{2}C_s \rho A a\, \omega v$$

Hence, for a given spin, ω, and velocity, v, the Magnus force on a ball is:

$$F_m = 2.6 \times 10^{-3} C_s\, \omega v \text{ Newtons, } v \text{ in m.s}^{-1}$$

Wesson (2002) gives the radius of curvature of the resulting flight as:

$$R = 165 \frac{v}{C_s \omega}, \ v \text{ in m.s}^{-1}$$

and the transverse deviation, D, of the ball after a longitudinal flight L as:

$$\frac{D}{L} = C_s \frac{N_{rots}}{52}$$

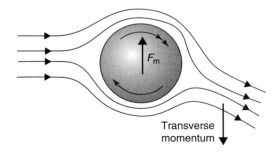

Figure 11.19 The Magnus force, F_m, on the ball is caused by the deflected air flow. View from above.

F_m

Transverse momentum

where N_{rots} is the number of rotations made by the ball during its flight. C_s is a parameter to be measured by experiment.

A Soccer Ball in Flight

A Vicon motion analysis system is used to track the linear and angular position of a soccer ball. The motion analysis system (Vicon 512, Vicon Peak Ltd., Oxford, UK) is able to record the positions of a reflective marker at intervals of $^1/_{120}$ of a second. By means of 12 cameras, it is possible to keep a marker in view for most of the time. The objective of the investigation is to determine the position and velocity of the ball, together with the magnitude and direction of its spin, and follow their variation with time. To avoid interfering with the construction or the dynamics of the ball, the markers will necessarily follow the curvature of the surface. If there are four markers, then the data recorded will consist of 12 coordinates:

$$x_1(t), y_1(t), z_1(t), \ldots x_4(t), y_4(t), z_4(t)$$

for discrete values of t, separated by $\delta t = {}^1/_{120}$ s.

A symmetrical arrangement of markers should ensure that the center of the ball has the coordinates:

$$x_c(t) = \left\{ \Sigma x_i(t) \right\}/n, \quad y_c(t) = \left\{ \Sigma y_i(t) \right\}/n, \quad z_c(t) = \left\{ \Sigma z_i(t) \right\}/n$$

From these quantities, the velocity and acceleration of the ball can be determined by suitable polynomial fitting to small groups of points. The position of the marker i relative to the center of the ball is given by a vector $r_i(t)$ with components:

$$X_i(t) = x_i(t) - x_c(t), \quad Y_i(t) = y_i(t) - y_c(t), \quad Z_i(t) = z_i(t) - z_c(t)$$

Squaring and summing these should give the square of the radius, R, of the ball. The velocity of marker i relative to the center is the vector $\dot{r}_i(t)$, with components:

$$u_i(t) = dX_i(t)/dt, \quad v_i(t) = dY_i(t)/dt, \quad w_i(t) = dZ_i(t)/dt$$

these quantities being evaluated by differentiating polynomial fits to the data. Consider the vector product for angular velocity:

$$\Omega_i(t) = \mathbf{r}_i(t) \times \dot{\mathbf{r}}_i(t)$$

If $\mathbf{r}_i$ is divided into two components, a_i parallel with the spin axis and b_i perpendicular to the axis, then both of these components are perpendicular to $\dot{\mathbf{r}}_i(t)$ so that Ω_i will have a component $a_i(t) \, \dot{\mathbf{r}}_i(t)$ perpendicular to the axis, and $b_i(t) \, \dot{\mathbf{r}}_i(t)$ parallel with it. The parallel component is equal to $b_i^2 \omega$, where ω is the spin. In practice, resolving $\mathbf{r}$ along the axis is not possible because the direction of the axis has not yet been found. If a symmetrical distribution of markers has been used, however, then in the vector sum $\Sigma\Omega_i$, the perpendicular components will cancel out, leaving only the parallel components. The value of the sum is then

$$\Sigma\Omega_i = \omega\sum b_i^2 = I\omega$$

where I is the moment of inertia of the set of markers about the axis (strictly, the moment of inertia of a set of unit masses placed at these positions).

For this to be a practical method of determining the spin, the arrangement of markers must have the property of possessing the same moment of inertia about any axis. Four points placed at the corners of a regular tetrahedron, however, should have sufficient symmetry. Checking this arrangement carefully reveals that:

$$I = {}^8/_3 R^2$$

when evaluated about *any* axis.

The design of a soccer ball makes it relatively easy to locate a tetrahedral set of points. In the design consisting of 12 pentagons and 20 hexagons, markers may be placed at the centers of four of the hexagons.

Measurement Procedure

The motion analysis system was used to track the position of a Nike Premier league size 5 soccer ball using four markers made from retro-reflective tape covering four of the hexagonal panels on the ball. These are 7.5 cm across (between opposite sides) and are arranged as shown in Figure 11.20.

In the investigation reported here (Griffiths et al., 2005), a soccer player kicked the ball toward a goal placed at one end of a motion analysis laboratory. The subject was right footed and was experienced at striking the ball with spin and launch velocity realistic of a direct free kick. No attempt was made to control the initial orientation of the seams in these experiments because the precise orientation of the spin axis could be determined in the subsequent analysis. Also, we wanted to confirm that the tetrahedral arrangement of markers would be suitable for all orientations of the ball. The experimental layout in the laboratory is illustrated in Figure 11.21.

The subject was instructed to aim the ball at an area in the top lefthand corner of the goal and to swerve the ball from right to left. A digital video camera was set up to record the final position of the ball at the target area to ensure it lay within tight limits. The capture volume was arranged to be about 2 m tall, 5.1 m long, and 1.9 m wide and was about 1 m above the floor of the laboratory so that the ball passed through the volume at a height of approximately 2.5 to 3.0 m above the floor of the laboratory en route from the origin to the target.

Results

As a result of the analysis, the following variables can be inferred as a function of time:

Spin rate
Angle of inclination of spin vector from the z axis
Angle of spin vector in the x, y plane
Coordinates of the center of the ball
Velocity of the ball

The radius of the ball was calculated as a check on the positional uncertainty of the measurement.

Results from a Typical Trial

In this trial, the average ball velocity (v_{ball}) in the capture volume was 16.9 ms^{-1} (R_e = 2.37 × 10^5), and the ball radius check was well behaved for a total of 19 data points and a time (t_{vol}) of 0.15 s. Figures 11.22 to 11.25 illustrate the spin angles (θ_z

Figure 11.20 A soccer ball with four surface markers in a tetrahedral configuration. The position vectors of the markers are measured with reference to an origin and axes fixed in the laboratory.

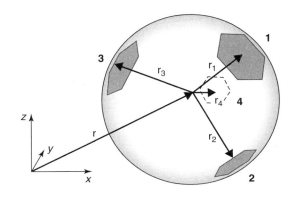

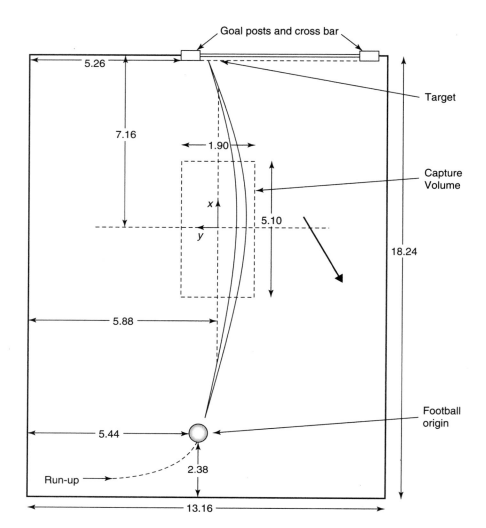

Figure 11.21
Experimental layout of laboratory in horizontal plane (not to scale). Two possible ball trajectories are represented by the two *curved lines*. Distances are in meters. The origin of the motion analysis system lies at the center of the capture volume. The *z* axis points vertically up and is at right angles to the plane of the page.

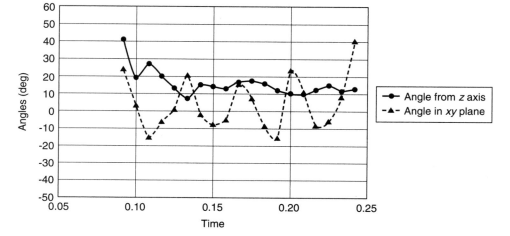

Figure 11.22 The angles of the spin axis as a function of time. Note that when the angle from the *z* axis is small, as in this case, large fluctuations may be expected in the orientation projected on to the *x*–*y* plane.

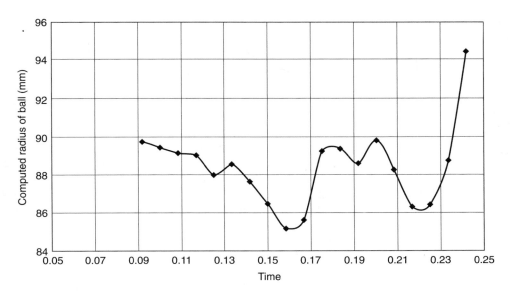

Figure 11.23 The ball radius constancy check as a function of time for 19 data points. The average ball radius calculated for the first 18 data points was 88.42 mm, and the standard deviation was 1.47 mm. The calculated radius is less than the true radius (107°mm) because of the curvature of the markers.

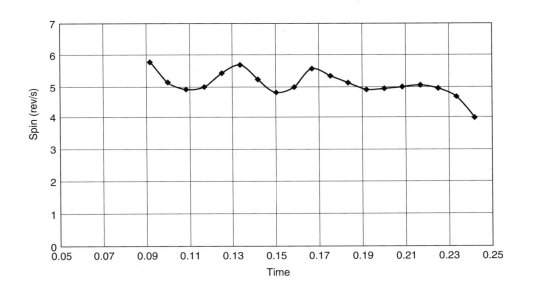

Figure 11.24 The spin rate as a function of time.

Figure 11.25 The movement of the ball in the x−y plane. (Note the magnified scale in the y-direction.) ◆ experimental data; ── best-fitting second-order polynomial;. − − − tangent to the polynomial curve at the first data point.

$y = -6.436\text{E-}06x^2 - 5.091\text{E-}02x + 4.735\text{E+}02$
$R^2 = 9.943\text{E-}01$

and θ_{xy}), the ball radius check, the spin rate (s), and the movement in the x–y plane, respectively.

The validity of the second-order polynomial fit was checked by evaluating χ^2. The motion analysis equipment is capable of 1 mm accuracy but because of the finite size and curvature of the reflectors and possible deviations of the ball from a perfectly spherical shape, the location of the center of the ball will probably not be as good as 1 mm. (For comparison, the radius-constancy check was seen to suggest that the uncertainties are of the order of 1.47 mm.) On putting the predicted uncertainties equal to 1.7 mm, χ^2 was found to be 33.9 (16 degrees of freedom), which is satisfactory. Similar values of χ^2 were found for other data sets in which deviations from a second-order polynomial appeared to be random. Occasionally, a larger-scale deviation from the second-order curve was seen, indicating a change in the transverse force, possibly attributable to the decrease in the spin rate or a change in the direction of the spin axis. Such a change would not be possible for a ball with a perfectly spherically symmetric distribution of mass. A check on the ball used in this work, however, indicated that it was imbalanced by about 10 g. If this is attributable to an additional mass on the surface (e.g., the valve), then it shifts the center of mass by about 2.5 mm and leads to differences between the principal moments of inertia amounting to about 3.6%. These differences could lead to an instability of the rotary motion.

The number of ball rotations about the z axis is:

$$N_{rots} = s_{av} \times t_{vol} \times \cos(\theta_{z.av})$$

where t_{vol} is the time spent in the capture volume, s_{av} is the average spin rate over this time interval, and $\theta_{z.av}$ is the average value of the spin inclination to the z axis. Here, the deflection, given by the difference between the polynomial and the tangent in Figure 11.25, is $D = 0.0409$ m, after a movement $L = 2.521$ m in the x direction. The average spin rate is 5.087 rev/s, and the average angle of inclination with the z axis is 16.1°. Hence, the effective number of ball rotations about the z axis is:

$$N_{rots} = 5.087 \times 0.15 \times \cos(16.1°) = 0.733$$

We can calculate the value of the constant, C_s, introduced by Wesson (2002) as:

$$C_s = \frac{52 \times 0.0409}{2.521 \times 0.733} = 1.15$$

From the deflection, D, the lift coefficient, C_L, is:

$$C_L = \frac{0.0409 \times 2 \times 0.42}{1.29 \times 0.0363 \times (0.15)^2 \times (16.91)^2} = 0.114.$$

In general, across a range of other trials, the ball velocities obtained varied from 15 to 18 m.s^{-1}. The spin rate was mainly observed to decrease as a function of time but occasionally stayed constant or even increased with time (again, possibly because of differences between the principal moments of inertia). The range of spin rates observed during these trials was from 4 to 11 rev/s. The drag on the ball, although present, was not large enough to change the velocity of the ball significantly within the capture volume.

Summary of Results

Table 11.1 shows a summary of the data obtained from 16 trials. Figures 11.26 and 11.27 show graphs of lift coefficient versus spin speed about the z axis and ball velocity, respectively. For comparison, the corresponding graphs for Wesson's C_s coefficient are shown in Figures 11.28 and 11.29.

Table 11.1 A summary of the soccer ball data obtained from 16 trials

Trial	Ball Velocity (mm/s)	Spin Inclination from z Axis (degrees)	Spin Angle in x, y Plane (degrees)	Spin Rate (s⁻¹)	Deflection of Ball in y Direction (mm)	Movement in x Direction (mm)	Number of Ball Rotations About z Axis	Wesson's Coefficient (C_s)	Lift Coefficient (C_L)	χ^2(df)
1	16,214	45.0	66.0	7.98	−111.0	−3735	1.316	1.144	0.250	49.1 (26)
2	17,730	48.7	104.1	4.04	−21.5	−2184	0.506	1.539	0.156	9.9 (13)
3	16,812	19.3	70.0	6.70	−112.0	−3877	1.422	1.060	0.242	29.1 (26)
4	16,775	24.5	76.1	5.38	−66.0	−2634	1.102	1.185	0.272	38.2 (16)
5	16,714	22.6	72.9	5.77	−111.0	−3483	1.199	1.260	0.222	42.3 (26)
6	16,573	21.3	72.7	8.96	−65.0	−2602	1.878	0.696	0.362	34.6 (16)
7	16,074	20.5	70.1	5.46	−110.0	−3704	1.151	1.340	0.238	54.0 (26)
8	16,910	16.1	4.4	5.09	−41.0	−2521	0.733	1.284	0.228	90.9 (24)
9	15,130	18.3	75.2	7.20	−114.0	−3477	1.537	1.110	0.310	48.6 (26)
10	15,970	19.8	74.5	6.52	−108.0	−3680	1.38	1.11	0.26	47.6 (26)
11	15,866	12.0	102.7	4.70	−16.5	−1703	0.513	1.003	0.20	29.9 (21)
12	16,120	35.0	91.1	5.06	−25.5	−2122	0.675	1.144	0.198	16.5 (14)
13	15,613	26.0	83.8	8.39	−111.0	−3587	1.696	0.95	0.314	34.9 (26)
14	16,848	11.1	89.4	5.00	−25.0	−2094	0.626	1.014	0.204	32.1 (13)
15	15,960	24.1	26.6	6.71	−41.0	−2379	1.05	0.925	0.254	31.7 (16)
16	17,188	23.2	70.5	9.42	−113.0	−3956	1.949	0.76	0.268	46.5 (26)

Data from Griffiths IW, Evans CJ, Griffiths NP: Tracking the flight of a spinning football in three dimensions. *Meas Sci Technol* 16,11:2005.

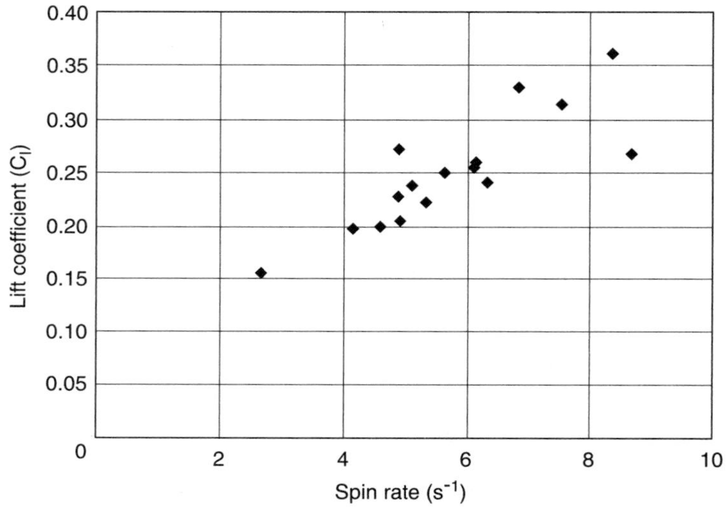

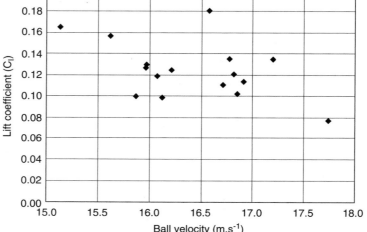

Figure 11.26 The lift coefficient versus the spin rate about the z axis. The results indicate that the lift coefficient increases with the spin rate.

Figure 11.27 The lift coefficient versus the ball velocity. A weak negative correlation exists, but the range of velocities is too small to distinguish an inverse relation from a linear one.

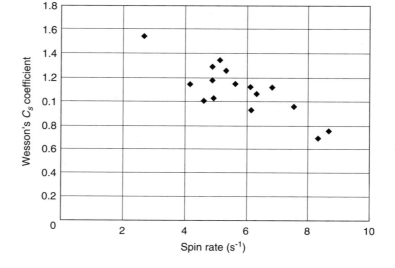

Figure 11.28 Wesson's C_s coefficient versus spin rate about the z-axis. The results show that C_s decreases with an increasing spin rate.

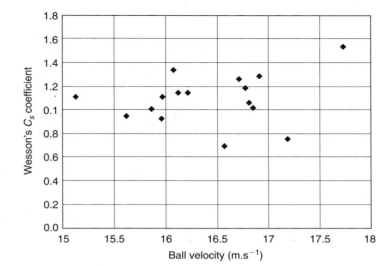

Figure 11.29 Wesson's C_s coefficient versus ball velocity. Any trend in this data is not clear.

SUMMARY

This chapter has summarized the important topics of fluid dynamics and their effects on objects in flight. Many of the basic terms (e.g., buoyancy, viscosity, density, specific gravity, center of buoyancy, and pressure) are defined and explained here. Thereafter, the effects of the dynamic fluid forces, including the phenomena of drag and lift, are examined in detail. The Magnus effect on a spinning ball is summarized, and then a case study reports some experimental work on a kick in soccer.

REFERENCES

Griffiths IW, Evans CJ, Griffiths NP: Tracking the flight of a spinning football. *Meas Sci Technol* 16,11;2005.
Wesson J: *The Science of Soccer*. Institute of Physics Publishing; 2002.

STUDY QUESTION

1. The data file Ch11Q1 contains the *x*, *y*, *z* coordinate data on four tetrahedral markers on the surface of a spinning soccer ball. A free kick has been taken, and the ball is traveling approximately in the *x* direction toward the goal. The spin makes it deviate in the *y* direction. The spreadsheet has been set up to calculate the spin rate and angles using the method described in Case Study 11.1. In Sheet 1, calculate:

   (a) The number of ball rotations about the *z* axis
   (b) The deflection in the *y* direction
   (c) The value of Wesson's C_s coefficient
   (d) The value of the lift coefficient C_L

CHAPTER twelve

GAIT ANALYSIS AND BIOMECHANICS

CHAPTER *objectives*

The objectives of this chapter are to explain how gait analysis is performed and to show some typical data obtained from normal adult subjects. The chapter also examines the link between the results from gait analysis and injuries.

CHAPTER *outcomes*

After reading this chapter, the reader will be able to:

- Recognize the different phases of the gait cycle.
- Understand the principle of marking up segments with three markers.
- Define a segmental coordinate system.
- Understand and interpret joint motions in terms of abduction, flexion, and rotation.
- Discuss the use of Euler angles to define rotations.
- Interpret foot motion in terms of pronation and supination.
- Work out the angular velocity at various joints.
- Interpret moment and power curves at the ankles, knees, and hips.
- See the connection between results from kinetic analysis and the incidence of injuries.

12.1   What is Gait Analysis?

Biomechanics is the application of Newtonian mechanics to the study of the neuro-muscular skeletal system. One branch of biomechanics is gait analysis or motion analysis of human gait. Various sources lead to a general definition of **gait** as pattern, style, or manner of walking or ambulation.

12.2 Temporal Parameters of the Gait Cycle

The **gait cycle** is defined as the period from heel contact of one foot to the next heel contact of the same foot. Figure 12.1 illustrates the walking gait cycle. The gait cycle can be divided into two parts, the **stance** phase and the **swing** phase. On average, the gait cycle is about 1 second long with 60% in stance and 40% in swing.

The stance phase can be further divided into **double stance**, followed by a period of **single stance** and then a final period of double stance. During the early part of the stance phase, the heel is in contact with the ground, progressing to flat foot during single stance and then to forefoot contact during the final double-stance phase, ending with toe-off. These are the normal contact areas of the plantar surface of the foot with the ground, but this may vary with pathological gait. For example, **equinus gait** is characterized by the forefoot's striking the ground first and then weight transferring toward the posterior, but in some cases, the heel never contacts the ground. In double stance, the weight is transferred from one foot to the other. During single stance, the center of mass (CM) of the body passes over the foot in preparation for shifting to the other limb.

12.3 Body Segments

As an approximation, human body movement can be modeled using rigid body dynamics, that is, the segments of the body are treated as objects of fixed size and shape. Gait analysis often proceeds using markers to identify anatomical positions. In the case of rigid body dynamics, three markers are sufficient to establish the location and movement of each segment. When a segment is considered as a rigid body, the distance between any two points on that body is constant. Consider a

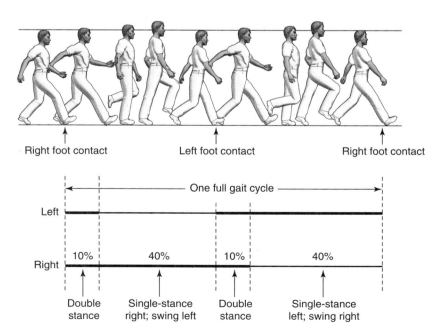

Figure 12.1 The gait cycle showing single- and double-stance phases.

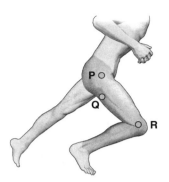

Figure 12.2 Three markers P, Q, and R defining the thigh (a rigid body segment).

body segment such as the thigh modeled as a single rigid body in Figure 12.2 using three non-collinear markers.

The markers form a triangle on the body segment, and it is assumed that the lines PQ, QR, and RP do not change in length. The position of each marker is measured by a motion analysis system, and this position is expressed as coordinates in a fixed laboratory reference system. Consider a system of rectangular axes x, y, and z. Figure 12.3 shows the x, y, and z axes and the position vectors to the three segment markers relative to these axes. The position vectors are defined as:

$$r_P = x_P(t)\,\boldsymbol{i} + y_P(t)\boldsymbol{j} + z_P(t)\boldsymbol{k} \tag{1}$$
$$r_Q = x_Q(t)\,\boldsymbol{i} + y_Q(t)\boldsymbol{j} + z_Q(t)\boldsymbol{k} \tag{2}$$
$$r_R = x_R(t)\,\boldsymbol{i} + y_R(t)\boldsymbol{j} + z_R(t)\boldsymbol{k} \tag{3}$$

where $\boldsymbol{i}$, $\boldsymbol{j}$, and $\boldsymbol{k}$ are the unit vectors in the laboratory coordinate system, that is, they are vectors of magnitude one that serve as pointers in the x, y, and z directions, respectively (Fig. 12.4). Note that the components of each position vector are the coordinates of the marker position and are shown as a function of time. The position of each marker is measured by the motion analysis system at a predetermined frequency. The coordinate system is righthanded, that is, if the thumb is aligned with the x axis and the index finger with the y axis, then the middle finger points along the z axis. For more information on unit vectors and vector components, refer to Chapter 2.

It is desirable to define a **segmental coordinate system**, which may be thought of as three mutually perpendicular lines attached to the body segment that remain at a fixed orientation with respect to the segment. For the purposes of this discussion, we will assume that the x segmental axis is in the anterior direction, the y segmental axis is in the medial–lateral direction directed to the left of the body segment, and the z segmental axis is directed in a superior direction on the body

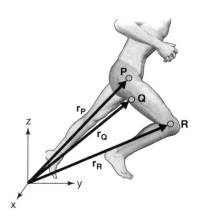

Figure 12.3 Position vectors to points P, Q, and R.

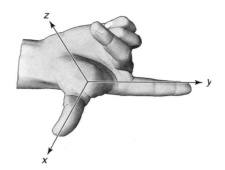

Figure 12.4 A righthanded *x, y, z* coordinate system with *z* vertical.

segment or directed distal to proximal in a lower limb segment. Although there are many ways to form the segmental coordinate system, we will assume that the three markers have been placed on the body segment in such a way that two of the markers define a segmental axis and the three markers together form a segmental anatomical plane. For example, on the thigh, markers P and R may define the **superior axis** of the thigh, and the three markers together form a **parasagittal** plane of the thigh (Fig. 12.5).

A relative position vector from R to P is designated r_{PR} (P relative to R) and is obtained by subtracting the coordinates of marker R from those of marker P.

$$r_{PR} = r_P - r_R \tag{4}$$

The length of this relative position vector does not change because we have assumed that the body segment is rigid. The relative position vector may be thought of as a pencil glued to the body segment that is oriented with the body segment but does not change its length. This length is called the magnitude of the relative position vector. A unit vector in the segmental coordinate direction *z* is obtained by dividing the relative position vector by its scalar magnitude (Fig. 12.6):

$$k = \frac{r_{PR}}{|r_{PR}|} \tag{5}$$

Similarly, r_{QR} will be:

$$r_{QR} = r_Q - r_R$$

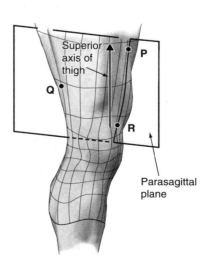

Figure 12.5 P, Q, and R define a parasagittal plane of the thigh. P and R define a superior axis of the thigh.

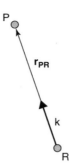

Figure 12.6 The position vector from R to P and the associated unit vector.

and the vector product of r_{QR} and r_{PR} will be perpendicular to the plane formed by the two vectors. If P, Q, and R form a parasagittal plane, then a vector at right angles to this plane in the medial–lateral direction can be obtained by taking the vector product between r_{QR} and r_{PR} giving a unit vector in the y segmental direction:

$$j = \frac{r_{QR} \times r_{PR}}{|r_{QR} \times r_{PR}|} \tag{6}$$

The unit vector in the x direction is given by the crossproduct:

$$i = j \times k \tag{7}$$

The position of the body segment can now be determined by the position vector to point R and its orientation by that of the segmental unit vectors (Fig. 12.7).

There is no widely accepted convention to determine which coordinate axis is used to specify which segment direction. However, here it is assumed that the x axis is the anterior segment direction, the z axis is the superior axis, and the y axis is the medial–lateral axis.

12.4   Joint Motions

Of particular interest are the position and orientation of one body segment relative to an adjoining one. The relative orientation of one body segment to another defines the **joint angles**. For example, the orientation of the tibia relative to the femur defines the three clinical angles of **flexion/extension**, **abduction/adduction**, and **internal/external rotation** of the tibia relative to the femur. Euler suggested that rotations should be defined by a sequence of three rotations. We will look at the knee joint angles defined by a sequence of rotations of the tibia relative to the femur using **Euler angles** (Grood and Suntay, 1983). We will represent the femoral directions by x_{fem}, y_{fem}, and z_{fem} and the tibial coordinates by x_{tib}, y_{tib}, and z_{tib}.

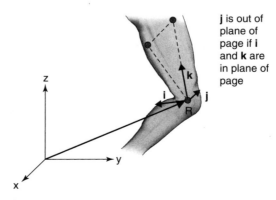

j is out of plane of page if **i** and **k** are in plane of page

Figure 12.7 Segmental coordinate system with k pointing along the superior axis.

The first rotation is about the medial–lateral axis of the femur yielding the flexion/extension angle. The tibial x and z axes will no longer be parallel with the femoral x_{fem} and z_{fem} axes and will be referred to as x' and z'. The second rotation is about the current x' axis, yielding the abduction/adduction angle. The tibial y' and z' axes have now rotated to a new position designated by y'' and z''. The third and final rotation will be about the tibial z'' axis, yielding external/internal tibial rotation.

These rotations are shown in Figure 12.8. Note that whereas the first rotation is about a femoral axis, the last rotation is about a tibial axis. The intermediate rotation is not about a current femoral or tibial axis but is about an intermediate tibial axis. This is denoted as:

$$y_{fem} - x_{tib} - z_{tib} \text{ rotation sequence (sometimes written } Yxz\text{)}.$$

A more complex example of three-dimensional motion is the shoulder joint. At the present time, only limited investigations have been conducted into this joint's motion, and most of these have been cadaveric studies. It has been proposed that the rotation sequence suitable for this joint (Zxz) is:

$$z_{tho} - x_{hum} - z_{hum}$$

1. Circumduction about the vertical axis of the thorax
2. Flexion about the current humeral axis
3. Internally or externally rotating about the distal/proximal axis of the humerus. Foot motion is frequently defined as **pronation** and **supination**, that is, a coupled motion of the ankle involving **dorsiflexion, eversion,** and **medial rotation** during pronation and **plantarflexion, inversion,** and **lateral rotation** during supination. For a summary of the anatomy of the ankle and foot, see Appendix 2. It appears that choice of joint axes should

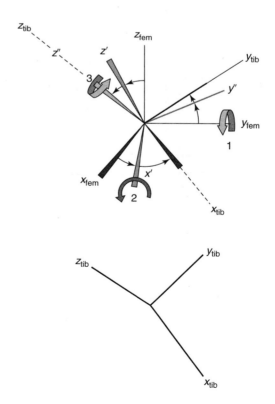

Figure 12.8 Rotation of the tibia relative to femur using a set of Euler angles.

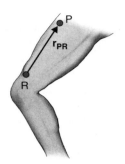

Figure 12.9 Relative position vector of P relative to R.

be made at the discretion of the researcher bearing in mind the nature of the joint and the information required.

12.5   Angular Velocity of a Body Segment

Consider two points on a body segment, as shown in Figure 12.9. The relative position vector r_{PR} can neither change in length nor move on the body segment but may change orientation in space as the body segment rotates. In fact, this is how the rotation of the body is tracked. Points P and R have absolute linear velocities in space that are not generally equal. The linear velocity of a point is defined as the time rate of change of the position vector to that point (Fig. 12.10). The velocity of point R is:

$$v_R = \lim_{\Delta t \to 0} \frac{\Delta r}{\Delta t} = \frac{dr}{dt} \tag{8}$$

The velocity of point P relative to point R is:

$$v_{PR} = v_P - v_R \tag{9}$$

Notice that if $v_P = v_R$, then there is no relative velocity between P and R. Because the length of the position vector of R relative to P cannot change, the only thing that P may do relative to R is rotate about it. This means that the **angular velocity of the body segment** can be obtained from:

$$v_{PR} = \boldsymbol{\omega} \times r_{PR} \tag{10}$$

where ω is the angular velocity of the body measured in radians per second, illustrated as a vector in Figure 12.11. The rigid body is said to have an angular velocity, ω, at this instant of time. The angular velocity is a vector with both a magnitude,

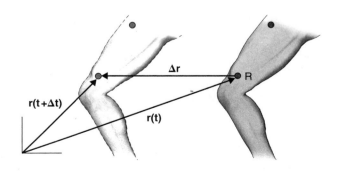

Figure 12.10 Change in position vector **r** given by **Δr**.

Figure 12.11 Velocity vector, which is the vector product of the angular velocity and position vectors.

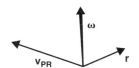

Angular velocity vector is out of plane of page if the two other vectors are in the plane of the page

measured in radians per second, and a direction, given by angles with respect to the *x*, *y*, and *z* axes. The orientation of the vector is the **axis of rotation**, and the sense of rotation is given by the righthand rule (i.e., if the thumb of the right hand is pointed in the direction of the vector, the fingers curl around the vector and designate the rotation). The angular velocity vector designates the rotation of the body segment in an absolute sense (i.e., relative to the fixed laboratory coordinates).

The **angular velocity of the joint** is the relative velocity of the body segment distal to the joint relative to the proximal segment. Therefore, the angular velocity of the knee is (Fig. 12.12):

$$\boldsymbol{\omega}_{knee} = \boldsymbol{\omega}_{tibia} - \boldsymbol{\omega}_{femur} \tag{11}$$

The angular velocity of the joint will have components in three directions, and these will be equal to the rate of flexion/extension, abduction/adduction, and internal/external rotation. A typical flexion extension curve for the knee in walking gait is shown in Figure 12.13; the knee is approximately 10° flexed at heel contact and extends for the first 100 ms (100 ms = 0.1 s). Flexion and extension then occurs in the single-stance phase and is followed by flexion through toe-off to the middle of the swing phase. In the last part of the swing phase, knee extension occurs from the maximum flexed position. Note that the angular velocity of the knee in flexion and extension is the gradient of this curve. If the gradient is positive, then the knee is flexing; if the slope is negative, the knee is extending. The largest value of knee angular velocity occurs during initial swing (flexing) and late swing (extending).

12.6 Ground Reaction Forces

During the stance phase, the foot applies a force to the ground, and a ground reaction force (GRF) is developed that is equal and opposite to the force the foot exerts on the ground. The force the foot applies to the ground can be measured with a force plate or a dynamometer that is mounted securely in the floor so that its surface is flush with the floor. The force plate shown in Figure 12.14 has an instrument center that is below the floor. The resultant force and moment about this center are measured.

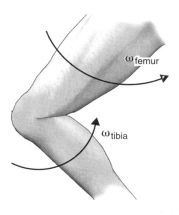

Figure 12.12 The angular velocity of the knee joint.

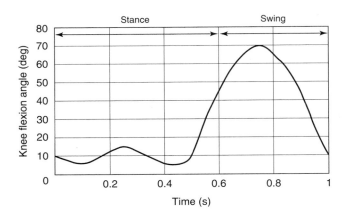

Figure 12.13 Knee flexion angle for one walking gait cycle.

The force and moment data are sampled at a set frequency (e.g., 600 Hz). The resultant force and moment data are usually expressed relative to an origin located at one of the corners of the force plate. The outputs are often quoted as F_x, F_y, and F_z for the forces and M_x, M_y, and M_z for the moments.

F_z = Vertical component
F_x and F_y = Anterior/posterior and medial/lateral (which is which depends on direction of walking)

The measurement of moments enables the center of pressure (COP) to be calculated (i.e., the location of the center of force on the force plate). The COP changes during stance, usually moving from the rear of the foot anterior toward a point between the first and second metatarsal heads.

The largest component of the GRF is the vertical one, which accounts for the acceleration of the body's CM in the vertical direction during walking and supporting the body weight (BW). A typical plot of the vertical GRF is shown in Figure 12.15, where it is plotted as a function of the BW. Heel contact occurs at time 0 in Figure 12.15. The first maximum in the vertical GRF (120% BW) curve occurs during the double-stance phase at a time of approximately 120 ms. The vertical GRF decreases to about 80% BW during the single-stance phase at a time of approximately 300 ms. Readings of less than BW during single stance can be explained by examining the vertical movement of the CM during the gait cycle. The CM is located around the pelvis, ignoring changes attributable to arm movement, and executes a sinusoidal motion rising and falling about 3.5 cm during walking (Fig. 12.16). By referring to Figure 12.16, it can be seen that the CM executes two complete oscillations vertically during every gait cycle.

The acceleration of the CM in the upward vertical direction is shown in Figure 12.17. It can be seen that this is opposite in sign at each point in the gait cycle.

Figure 12.14 The foot applied to a force plate exerts pressure over the plantar surface in contact with the plate. The "average" point of force application is known as the center of pressure (COP).

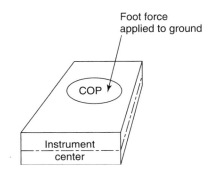

Foot force applied to ground

COP

Instrument center

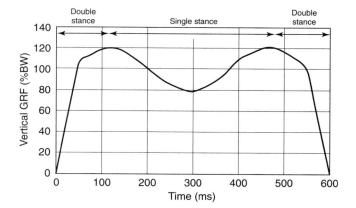

Figure 12.15 Typical vertical ground reaction force (GRF) during walking. This shows the stance phase of one foot only.

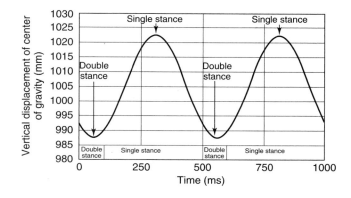

Figure 12.16 Vertical displacement of the center of gravity during one gait cycle.

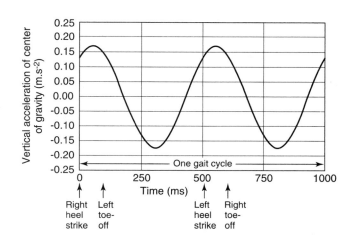

Figure 12.17 Vertical acceleration of the center of gravity during one gait cycle (approximated by a sine curve).

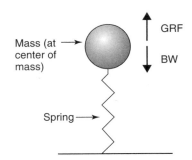

Figure 12.18 The human body's mass considered as concentrated at one point and supported by a compression spring.

If the entire body is treated as a mass on a spring, the magnitude of the GRF can be more easily understood. In Figure 12.18, the body is shown as a single mass and indicates the forces acting on the mass.

Newton's second law states that the resultant force must equal mass times acceleration. Therefore, when the acceleration is positive, the GRF must be greater than the BW. The positive acceleration occurs during double stance when the CM is at its lowest point. When the CM is at its highest point during single stance, the acceleration is negative, and the GRF must be less than the BW. It will be appreciated that the figures given for displacement and acceleration are typical values and can vary considerably between different styles and speeds of walk.

The anterior-posterior (AP) force is first a braking force and then a propulsive force. This is often approximated by a sine curve with an amplitude of roughly 20% BW (Fig. 12.19).

The area trapped between this curve and the horizontal time axis (AP GRF = 0) is the impulse of the force. The **braking impulse** (horizontal) should be approximately equal to the **propulsion impulse** for balanced gait left to right. The total impulse in the AP direction for a full gait cycle should be 0 because the impulse is equal to the change in momentum in the forward direction. There should be 0 net impulse, therefore, if the walker is doing constant speed. It may be found that, in some individuals (e.g., those who have sustained a leg injury), the propulsion impulse on one leg is greater than that on the other leg, with compensating differences in the braking impulse so that the net impulse for the whole gait cycle is still 0. In such cases, the demands placed on each leg are unequal but are necessary if walking at constant speed is to be maintained. This may result in a higher than usual incidence of stress fractures in the uninjured leg. An example of an unbalanced AP force is shown in Figure 12.20, where it is compared with a normal AP force.

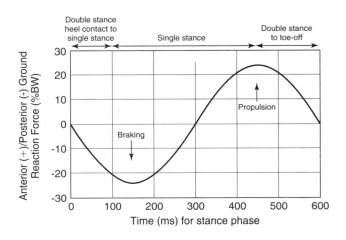

Figure 12.19 Anterior/posterior ground reaction force during the stance phase of walking.

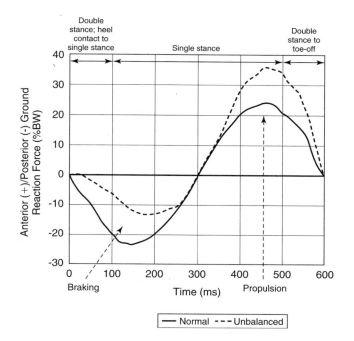

Figure 12.20 Normal and unbalanced anterior/posterior ground reaction force for the stance phase of walking.

Medial–lateral GRFs are usually around 5% of BW and relate to balance during walking. This force initially acts in the medial direction and then acts laterally for the remainder of the stance phase.

12.7   Kinetic Studies

12.7.1 OBTAINING JOINT FORCES

After the data have been filtered and differentiated, the joint forces may be obtained by solving from the most distant segment proximally. Each segment is modeled as a rigid body and isolated from the other segments. All forces acting on the segment are shown on a free-body diagram (Fig. 12.21). In this case, the GRF and the segment weight (W) are known and the ankle joint force and moment are sought. The Euler-Newton equations of motion for a rigid body are:

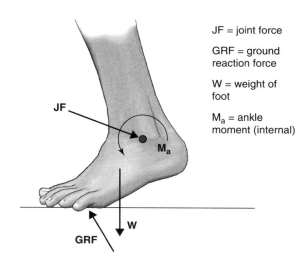

JF = joint force

GRF = ground reaction force

W = weight of foot

M_a = ankle moment (internal)

Figure 12.21 Free-body diagram of the foot.

$$\Sigma F = \frac{d\boldsymbol{p}}{dt} \tag{12}$$

$$\Sigma M_{cm} = \frac{dH_{cm}}{dt} \tag{13}$$

where $\boldsymbol{p}$ is the linear momentum of the segment and is equal to $\boldsymbol{mv}$, that is, product of mass of the segment and the velocity of the CM of the segment $\boldsymbol{M_{cm}}$ is a moment about the CM and where $\boldsymbol{H_{cm}}$ is the angular momentum of the segment about its CM. ΣF represents the sum of all the forces acting on the segment.

The angular momentum is:

$$H_{cm} = I_{xx}\omega_x i + I_{yy}\omega_y j + I_{zz}\omega_z k \tag{14}$$

where the Is are the mass moments of inertia about the segmental coordinate axes.

12.7.2 QUASI-STATIC DETERMINATION OF JOINT MOMENTS

In many cases such as during slow walking, stair ascending or descending, or mild squatting, sufficient accuracy during stance phase can be obtained by ignoring the righthand side of Equations 12 and 13. These terms are called the *inertial forces* and depend on the linear and angular acceleration of the body segments. Especially during the stance phase of gait, these terms are small compared with the GRFs, and the joint forces are calculated from the GRFs only. We may get a conceptual idea of the joint moments by examining Figure 12.22, which shows a GRF acting at the forefoot.

The concept of **sagittal plane joint moments** may be obtained from this simple figure. The GRF has been shown as two components, one acting in the anterior direction and the second acting in the vertical direction. The simplest definition of a moment is the magnitude of the force times the perpendicular distance from the joint center to the force, that is:

$$M = Fd \tag{15}$$

Examining the ankle joint represented by the ankle joint center, we can see that both the anterior GRF and the vertical reaction force produce an applied or external dorsiflexion moment. Therefore, there must be a net plantarflexion muscle moment, or the gastrocsoleus complex must produce the dominant muscle activity.

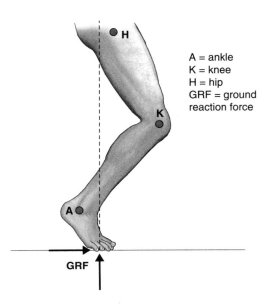

Figure 12.22 The ankle, knee, and hip joint centers and the components of the ground reaction force.

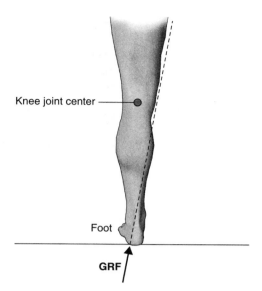

Knee joint center

Foot

GRF

Figure 12.23 The line of action of the ground reaction force and the center of the knee joint.

At the knee joint, the vertical GRF is a knee flexion force, and the anterior GRF would cause the knee to extend. It is not too obvious which of these applied moments dominates because the vertical GRF is larger but has a lower moment arm (perpendicular distance from the joint), but the lower anterior GRF has a greater moment arm.

A similar view of the moments in the **frontal plane** can be obtained by examining Figure 12.23. The net GRF passes medially to the knee center and causes an applied knee adduction moment during all of the stance phase of gait. If the individual is suffering from medial knee pain, each step aggravates this condition. If this moment is the cause of the pain, it is easy to determine by asking the patient to rotate his or her foot laterally, reducing the moment arm of the force from the joint center.

The easiest way to understand the forces produced by the muscles spanning a joint and, therefore, the loads that are applied to the joints, is to consider simple levers. The forearm provides an excellent example of this effect. Consider the forearm modeled as a simple lever (Fig. 12.24). A simple measurement on one's forearm will show that the length from the elbow to the palm of the hand is eight to 10 times longer than the length from the elbow to the tendon attachment of the biceps. This means that if 150 N is held in the palm of the hand, the muscle force must be between 1200 and 1500 N. The compression on the elbow joint, $C = F_m - W$,

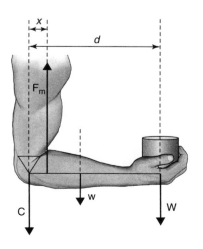

x

d

F_m

F_m = muscle force
W = weight held in hand
w = weight of forearm (ignored)
C = compression force on elbow joint
distance d is 8 or 10 times distance x

w

W

C

Figure 12.24 The forces acting on the forearm. The location of the joint is shown by the bottom vertex of the triangle.

would be between 1050 and 1350 N. Muscle attachments are close to the joint centers so that small contractions of the muscle can produce large movements at the end of the levers producing a mechanical advantage in the motion of the limbs.

12.7.3 POWER

Examination of the power expended by the muscles during a particular activity is a new tool that is being applied to gait analysis. Power is a measure of the rate of doing work, which is the product of the force being applied in a certain direction and the distance the object moves in that direction.

$$\text{Work} = \text{Force} \times \text{Distance} \tag{16}$$

The power expended is the rate at which work is performed or the product of the force applied in a certain direction and the velocity of movement in that direction.

$$\text{Power} = \text{Force} \times \text{Velocity} \tag{17}$$

Power is measured in Watts or Newton meters per second (Nm/s). A moment also does work when it rotates through an angle, and the power performed by the moment is the product of the moment and the angular velocity of the object.

Consider the power expended by the biceps when the elbow is extended or flexed, as shown in Figure 12.25. The muscle moment in both Figure 12.25(a) and (b) is a flexion moment but the arm is flexing in (a) and extending in (b). The **power expended by the muscle** in both cases is the product of the moment and the angular velocity of the forearm, but in case (a), the angular velocity, ω, is positive (in the same direction as the muscle moment) and in case (b) ω is negative (in the opposite direction to the muscle moment). The power in case (a) is positive and in case (b) is negative. When examining muscle activity, it is evident that in case (a), the muscle is doing concentric contraction, or positive work, and in case (b), the muscle is doing eccentric contraction (lengthening) or doing negative work.

Figure 12.26 shows the angle dorsiflexion and plantarflexion of the ankle joint during stance phase of gait where dorsiflexion is plotted positive, illustrating how the power can be used to understand the muscle activity. The ankle first plantarflexes as the GRF acts posterior to the ankle joint, dorsiflexes as the CM passes over the foot, and then plantarflexes until toe-off. The ankle muscle moment during stance phase is approximated by Figure 12.27.

During the initial period of stance, the tibialis anterior is active as the foot is plantarflexing to foot-flat. During the rest of the stance phase, the gastrocnemius muscles actively control the CM of the body as it passes over the foot and then provide the power to push off the body and transfer the weight to the opposite foot. The power of the muscles is shown in Figure 12.28. The initial power is negative

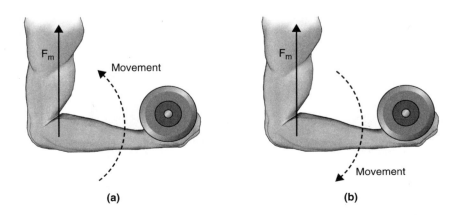

Figure 12.25 The muscle power during elbow flexing is positive (A) and elbow extending is negative (B).

(a)

(b)

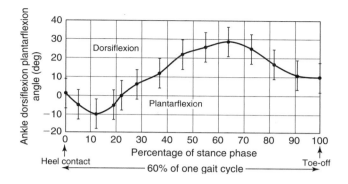

Figure 12.26 The ankle dorsiflexion/plantarflexion angle expressed as a percentage of the stance phase in walking.

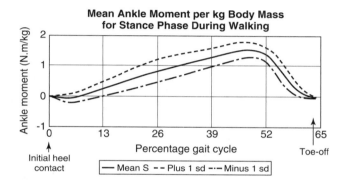

Figure 12.27 The ankle moment normalized for body mass during the stance phase of walking.

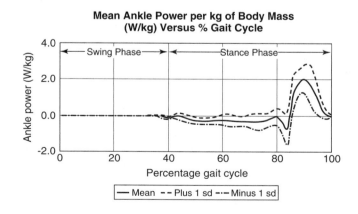

Figure 12.28 The mean ankle power per kg of body mass versus percentage of gait cycle. (Data from Winter DA: *Biomechanics and Motor Control of Human Gait.* Waterloo Ontario, Canada: Waterloo Biomechanics; 1991.)

as the tibialis anterior muscles brake the foot during foot fall, and the power is again negative as the ankle plantarflexors control the dorsiflexion of the foot. The final power is positive as the plantarflexors go into concentric contraction to power the body up and forward.

12.8 Injuries

Overuse injuries are usually associated with positive power output by the muscles (i.e., when the muscles are being used to produce positive work on the body). Examples of this are pushing off while running, jumping, rising during squatting, and other concentric contractions of the muscles. **Trauma injuries** usually occur when the power of the muscles is negative or the muscles are trying to break an external moment that is being applied. A common example of this is when a runner hits a pothole in the road and the GRF occurs on the forefoot instead of the heel. The plantarflexors are forced to try to resist a suddenly applied dorsiflexion moment, usually of a high magnitude applied at a rapid rate, and the heel cord cannot withstand the high strain rate, resulting in a partial tear or complete rupture.

SUMMARY

This chapter has given an introduction to the subject of gait analysis. Assuming no prior knowledge, the gait cycle is defined in terms of stance and support phases. It is explained what is meant by a segmental coordinate system and how this can be obtained by appropriate marking up and tracking of a body segment. The rotations that can occur at a joint are discussed in terms of Euler angles and their interpretation as flexion/extension, abduction/adduction, and internal/external rotation. Some typical results are presented for GRF, dorsiflexion, and plantarflexion of the ankle joint, ankle muscle moment, and ankle power. The link with injuries is discussed briefly.

REFERENCES

Grood ES, Suntay WJ: A joint coordinate system for the clinical description of three dimensional motions. *J Biomech Eng Trans ASME* 105:136–144, 1983.
Winter DA: *Biomechanics and Motor Control of Human Movement.* Waterloo Ontario, Canada: Waterloo Biomechanics; 1991.

SUGGESTED READINGS

Soutas-Little RW, Beavis GC, Verstraete MC, Markus TL: Analysis of foot motion during running using a joint coordinate system. Med Sci Sports Exerc 19, 285–293, 1987.
Soutas-Little RW: *Motion Analysis and Biomechanics.* Available at http://www.vard.org/mono/gait/soutas.htm
Whittle MW (ed): *Gait Analysis: An Introduction,* ed 3. Oxford, UK: Butterworth-Heinemann; 2002.

Chapter 2

1. Force-vector, torque-vector, acceleration-vector, velocity-vector, mass-scalar, volume-scalar, displacement-vector, area-scalar, length-scalar, angular velocity-vector

2.

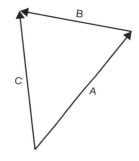

3.

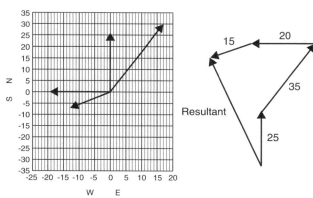

The resultant has magnitude 50.25 and makes an angle of 72° with the W axis.

4. Resultant velocity = 15.81 m/s

5.

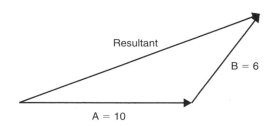

6. In (b), the wind is greater than 10 km/h and is a tail wind.
   In (c), the wind is less than 5 km/h and is a tail wind.
   In (d), the wind is greater than 10 km/h but is a head wind and also acts at an angle. Allow competition to go ahead for (c).

7. Horizontal component = 45 cos (10) = 44.3 m/s

8. Call the horizontal velocity v. Therefore:
$$40 = \sqrt{(29)^2 + v^2}$$
$$v = 27.5 \text{ m/s}$$

9.
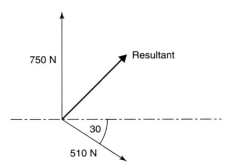

The resultant has a magnitude 663 N and acts at an angle 48° with respect to the horizontal.

10. $a_x = 13.1 \, m/s^2$ $a_y = 9.2 \, m/s^2$

11. (a) The components are 12 N, 25 N, and 0 N along the x, y, and z axes, respectively.

    (b) Total displacement = $\sqrt{2^2 + 3^2} = \sqrt{13} = 3.6 m$

    (c) Resultant velocity = (4,8,2)

12. Work done = 231.8 Nm (or Joules)

13. Work done = 150 × 0.8 + 45 × 0.75 + 0 × 0.15 = 153.75 J

14. Torque = 50 N × 0.25 m = 12.5 Nm. The effect will be to increase the angular speed of the discus.

15. The torque is $\tau = -0.5\mathbf{i} + 0.34\mathbf{j} - 0.57\mathbf{k}$. The magnitude of this torque is 0.83 Nm.

16. Magnitude of force = 30.23 N
    Radius of ball = 0.067 m

17. Speed = 10.73 m/s
    Expression for unit vector = $0.93\mathbf{i} - 0.23\mathbf{j} + 0.28\mathbf{k}$
    Drag force = 1.73 N
    Force = $1.61\mathbf{i} - 0.40\mathbf{j} + 0.48\mathbf{k}$

Chapter 3

1.
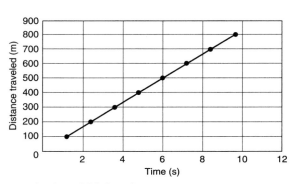

The car has a velocity of 83.3 m/s

2. $m = 9.16$, c $= 50$
3. $a = 4$ m/s^2
4. $v = 30$ m/s
5. $60/6.5 = 9.23$ m/s
6. $t_1 = 2.33$ s (Man Utd)$t_2 = 2.36$s (Liv). Answer : Man Utd
7. $a = 0.7$ m/s^2; $v = 7$ m/s
8. $a = (55 - 20)/5.3 = 6.603$ m/s^2
9. Acceleration is uniform over the period 0 to 4 s. Also, over 12 to 15 s, but this is uniform deceleration.

   Comes to a stop over the interval between 12 and 15 s.

   Between 0 and 4 s, the car is accelerating uniformly.

   The acceleration is 2.625 m/s^2.
10. $a = 2$ m/s^2
11.

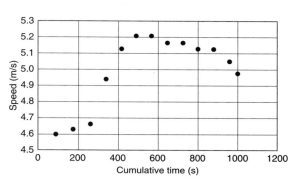

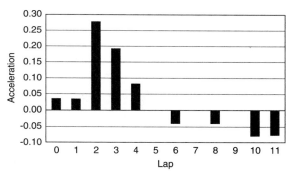

The sketch graph shows that the largest acceleration occurred after lap 3 and the largest deceleration was after lap 11.
12. $v = 10.85$ m/s
13. $R = 7.81$ m, $h = 0.91$ m
14. $R = 17.81$ m
15.

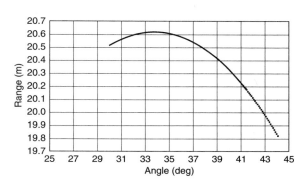

The range maximizes at an angle of approximately 34°.

16. (a) Horizontal velocity = 13 m/s
    Vertical velocity = 7.5 m/s
    (b) Horizontal velocity = 13 m/s
    (c) Time at maximum height = 0.765 s
    (d) d_v = 2.866 m, d_h = 9.945 m
    The ball will travel 22.466 m.

17. (a) corresponds to uniform acceleration. (b) is constant velocity; this is uniform acceleration in the special case of $a = 0$. (c) represents nonuniform acceleration (i.e., the acceleration is present but is not constant). Equations (1) to (4) would apply to (a) and (b).

Chapter 4

1. Moments are (a) 20 N × 0.65 m = 13 Nm and (b) 20 N × 0.65 m × cos(30) = 11.26 Nm

2. Take moments about bottom lefthand corner, for example. The resultant force is 1390 N acting at a distance of 51.9 cm from this point.

3. The volume is $\pi r^2 L = 4.71 \times 10^{-3} m^3$, and the mass is 5.18 kg. The center of mass lies on the axis of the cylinder at a distance 0.3 m from one end. The moment of the arm would be 5.18 × 9.8 × 0.3 = 15.25 Nm.

4. Couple = 2 × 50 × 2.5 = 250 Nm. The glider will rotate clockwise.

5. R_n = 800 cos(35) = 655.3 N; R_p = 800 sin(35) = 458.9 N. This can happen if a friction force is present to prevent a slide down the incline. In the absence of any friction, the skier would accelerate down the incline, but he is possibly on a section with no snow, or he has dug his skis into the surface.

6. 350 N tension in each rope

7. 355.4 N in each rope

8. M = 25 N × 0.25 m = 6.25 Nm and M = 30N × 0.2 m = 6 Nm

9.

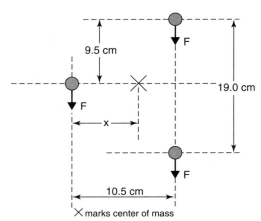

3F × x = F × 0.105 + F × 0.105 so that x = 0.07m. The object could be suspended from a number of its corners and cm found from point of intersection of verticals.

10. The center of mass is at 3.3, 5.0.

11. Moment of couple = 2 × 40 N × 0.05 m = 4 Nm

12. Moment = 100 N × 0.5 m = 50 Nm

Chapter 5

1. (a) 2 m/s, (b) 2 m/s, (c) 2 m/s
    Rolling friction will reduce velocity progressively in a real case. Also, air resistance.

2. $F = G\dfrac{m_1 m_2}{r^2} = \dfrac{6.67 \times 10^{-11} \times 80 \times 5.98 \times 10^{24}}{(6.38 \times 10^6)^2}$

    $= 783.92$ N

    Repeat the calculation using $r = 6.385 \times 10^6$ gives $F = 782.69$ N, a difference of 1.23 N.

3. Acceleration $= 10/1.5 = 6.66$ m/s^2
    Force $= ma = 65 \times 6.66 = 433.3$ N

4. Acceleration $= 20/0.01 = 2000$ m/s^2
    Force $= 0.2 \times 2000 = 400$ N assuming the acceleration is uniform and constant over the 0.01-s time interval.

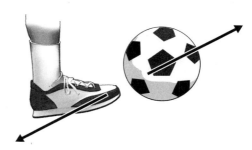

5. $W = 25 \times 9.81 = 245.25$ N

6. Normal reaction force $= 500$ N
    Static friction force $= \mu R = 0.18 \times 500 = 90$ N
    Dynamic friction force $= \mu R = 0.15 \times 500 = 75$ N

7. (a) $W = 686.7$N; $F = 0.65 \times 686.7 = 446.355$ N
    (b) $F = 0.62 \times 686.7 = 425.754$ N

8. $F = ma = 150 \times 3 = 450$ N
    Friction force $= 0.3 \times 150 \times 9.81 = 441.45$ N
    Total force $= 891.45$ N

9. Accelerating force $= 20 \times 4 = 80$ N
    Friction $= 20$ N
    Coefficient of dynamic friction $= 20$ N$/196.2$ N $= 0.102$

10. $v_{\max} = \sqrt{\dfrac{7.5 \times 9.81 \times (\sin 20 + 0.65 \cos 20)}{(\cos 20 - 0.65 \sin 20)}} = \sqrt{97.72} = 9.885\, m/s$

11. Friction force $= \mu R = 0.002 \times 0.046 \times 9.81 = 0.0009$ N
    Deceleration $=$ Force/mass $= 0.0009/0.046 = 0.0196$ m/s^2
    Distance rolled, $v^2 = u^2 + 2as$
    Initial velocity $= u$; final velocity $= v = 0$
    So that:
    $u = 2.5$ m/s
    $s = (2.5)^2/(2 \times 0.0196) = 159.438$ m
    and for $u = 5$ m/s
    $s = 637.75$ m

12. Momentum $= mv = 70 \times 9 = 630$ kg.m.s^{-1}

13. $1\text{mph} = \dfrac{1.6 \times 10^3}{3600}\dfrac{m}{s} = 0.444$ m/s

Velocity change $= 205 \times 0.444 = 91.1$ m/s

Change in momentum of ball $= 9.11\text{kg.m.s}^{-1}$

so that:

Average force $=$ Momentum change/Time $= 9.11/0.005 = 1822\text{N}$

14. The ranges of the football, calculated from a spreadsheet, are as follows: 2.35 m, 7.75 m, 13.77 m, 19.32 m, and 24.14 m for initial velocities of 5, 10, 15, 20, and 25 m/s, respectively.

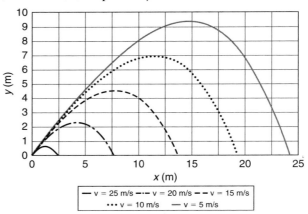

Chapter 6

1. $W = (2.8 \text{ m}) \times (560 \text{ N}) = 1568 \text{ J}$

2. Work done $= (4575) \times (15) \times \cos(10°) = 67582 \text{ J}$

3. Dividing the horizontal axis up into 8 equal sections

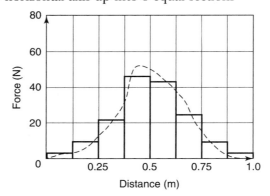

The approximate average forces over the eight intervals are 3.4, 9.3, 21.0, 44.9, 41.5, 24.4, 9.3, and 3.4 N, respectively (estimated by measuring the heights of the bars and converting to forces).

$W = (F_1 + F_2 + \dots\dots\dots\dots + F_8) \times (\Delta x)$

where $\Delta x = (x_f - x_i)/8$ is the width of each interval on the x axis.

In this case, $\Delta x = 0.125$ m and:

$W = (3.4 + 9.3 + 21 + 44.9 + 41.5 + 24.4 + 9.3 + 3.4) \times 0.125 = 157.2 \times 0.125 = 19.65 \text{ J}$

4. $e = 5/6.3 = 0.794$

5. Relative velocity before $= 55$ m/s; Relative velocity after $= 20$m/s; $e = 20/55 = 0.364$

6. $e_{min} = \sqrt{\dfrac{135}{254}} = 0.729$, $e_{max} = \sqrt{\dfrac{147}{254}} = 0.761$

7. $0.9 = \sqrt{\dfrac{h}{2}}$, $\dfrac{h}{2} = 0.81$, h $= 1.62$ m

8. Bounce 1 $= 1.24 - 0.25 = 0.99$ m; Bounce 2 $= 1.37 - 0.25 = 1.12$ m

   (measured to the bottom of the ball); $e_{min} = \sqrt{\dfrac{0.99}{1.83}} = 0.735$;

   $e_{max} = \sqrt{\dfrac{1.12}{1.83}} = 0.782$

9. Velocity of kicking foot, coefficient of restitution between boot and ball, mass of foot, mass of ball, angle of kick, ball struck head on or off center

10. $e = 4/6.3 = 0.635$, $s = \dfrac{u^2}{2a} = \dfrac{16}{2 \times 9.81} = 0.815 m$

11. $e = -v_v/u_v$, $u_h = v_h$ if no friction, but friction will reduce v_h. The angle of incidence will not be equal to the angle of reflection.

12. The downward vertical velocity is the same for both. The ball with topspin has greater horizontal velocity after impact with the court. The ball with no spin has a greater angle of reflection with respect to the horizontal.

13. PE $= mgh = 70 \times 9.81 \times 10 = 6867$ J

14. KE $= \frac{1}{2}mv^2 = \frac{1}{2}(75)(11)^2 = 4537$ J

15. Initial PE $= mgh = mg\,(10)$

    Final KE $= \frac{1}{2}mv^2$

    Therefore: $\frac{1}{2}mv^2 = mg\,(10)$

    $v^2 = 20g$

    $v = 14$ m/s

16. Force moved $= 981$ N. (This assumes that no additional force is required to accelerate the bar upward.) Work done $= 981 \times 0.7 = 686.7$ J; Power $= 686.7/0.6 = 1144.5$ W

17. Impulse $=$ Force $\times$ Time $= 1250 \times 0.003 = 3.75$ Ns. Velocity change $= 3.75/0.12 = 31.25$ m/s. Velocity of rebound $= 16.25$ m/s.

18. Frequency of oscillations and friction coefficient can be found from positions and amplitude of maxima. Maxima are to be found at, for example, $t = 0.016$ s, amp $= 2.97$; $t = 0.078$ s, amp $= 2.86$; $t = 0.141$ s, amp $= 2.75$; $t = 0.204$ s, amp $= 2.65$. Periodic time is $T = \frac{1}{3}(0.204 - 0.016) = 0.062 s$, so that frequency $= f = 1/T = 15.96$ Hz, angular frequency $= 2\pi f = 100.3$ rad/s. Friction coefficient, b, is:

    $\log_e\left(\dfrac{A_n}{A_1}\right) = \dfrac{-bt}{2m}$ so that $\log_e\left(\dfrac{2.65}{2.97}\right) = \dfrac{-b(0.204 - 0.016)}{2m}$

    $b/m = 1.213$

Chapter 7

1. (a) Absolute angles measured with respect to the horizontal are 54.7, 60.3, 69.3, 77.9, 91.4°

   (b) Angular velocities at frames 2, 3, and 4 are 291, 352, and 443°/s, respectively

   (c) Angular acceleration 3038°/s² or 53 rad/s²

2. Angular acceleration $= \dfrac{(30 - 10)}{1.2} = \dfrac{20}{1.2} = 16.66$ rad/s²

Angle turned $= \dfrac{(30^2 - 10^2)}{2 \times 16.66} = 24$ rad or $1376°$

3. Angular velocity $= \dfrac{(120 - 10)}{0.71 - 0.5} = \dfrac{110}{0.21} = 523.8°/s$ or 9.14 rad/s

4. (a) Angular velocity $= \omega = \alpha t = 2.5 \times 0.8 = 2.0$ rad/s
   (b) $114°/s$

5. Linear velocity $= v = \omega r = 20 \times 0.5 = 10$ m/s

6. (a) $\omega^2 = 2 \times 24 \times 250 \times \pi/180 = 209.43$
   $\omega = 14.47$ rad/s
   (b) $v = 14.47 \times 0.8 = 11.57$ m/s

7. Angular acceleration $= \alpha = \dfrac{1.5 - 1}{0.47 - 0.35} = \dfrac{0.5}{0.12} = 4.17$ rad/s^2

8. Velocity $= \omega r = \dfrac{2000 \times \pi \times 0.75}{180} = 26.18$ m/s

9. $a_T = \dfrac{2.5}{3} = 0.833$ m/s^2

   $a_r = \dfrac{v^2}{r} = \dfrac{(12.5)^2}{20} = 7.812$ m/s^2

   $a = \sqrt{a_r^2 + a_T^2} = 7.857$ m/s^2

10. Tangential acceleration $= \alpha r = 15 \times 1.7 = 25.5$ m/s^2

    Centripetal acceleration $= \dfrac{v^2}{r} = \omega^2 r = (14.7)^2 \times 1.7 = 367.4$ m/s^2

    Overall acceleration $= \sqrt{a_r^2 + a_T^2} = 368.3$ m/s^2

11. $a = \dfrac{v^2}{r} = \dfrac{100}{30} = 3.33$ m/s^2

12. $a_T = \dfrac{8 - 10}{4} = -0.5$ m/s^2

    $a_r = \dfrac{v^2}{r} = \dfrac{8^2}{20} = \dfrac{64}{20} = 3.2$ m/s^2

13. Average angular velocity over first 0.22 s $= 7.49$ rad/s

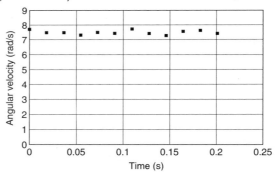

Chapter 8

1. $205(N) \times x(m) = 130(N) \times 0.55(m), x = 130 \times 0.55/205 = 0.349$ m
2. $250(N) \times 0.4(m) = F(N) \times 0.25(m), F = 250 \times 0.4/0.25, F = 400$ N
3. (a) The force exerted by the biceps is:
   $F \times (0.04$ m$) = 95 \times (0.35$ m$), F = 95 \times 0.35/0.04 = 831.25$N
   (b) The force exerted by the humerus on the ulna is:
   $G - F + 95 = 0, G = 831.25 - 95 = 736.25$ N
   (c) Mechanical advantage $= 4/35 = 0.114$

4. Moment = 110 N × 0.3 m = 33 Nm

5. 110 N × 0.34 m = 185 N × x, x = 110 × 0.34/185 = 0.202 m

6. Angular acceleration = α = (6 × 2 × π)/0.05 = 753.98 rad/s², Torque

$$= I\alpha = \tfrac{2}{5} \times 0.156 \times \frac{(7.19 \times 10^{-2})^2}{4} \times 753.98 = 0.201 \text{ Nm}$$

7. ω = 25 rad/s, $v_y = \tfrac{2}{3}\omega r$, r = 0.11 m

Therefore:

v_y = 0.666 × 25 × 0.11 = 1.83 ms^{-1}

8. m = 85 kg, h = 1.28m, T = 2.4 s

About the bar, the moment of inertia is:

$$I_{bar} = \frac{mghT^2}{4\pi^2} = 155.73 kg.m^2$$

About the center of mass:

$I_{cm} = I - mh^2 = 155.73 - 85 \times (1.28)^2 = 155.73 - 139.26 = 16.46 kg.m^2$

9. α = −1/5.2 = −0.192 rad/s^{-1}, torque = $\tau = I\alpha$ = 0.318 × −0.192
= −0.061 Nm

10. $v = \sqrt{\tfrac{10}{7}gh} = \sqrt{\dfrac{10 \times 9.81 \times \sqrt 2}{7}} = 4.451 ms^{-1}$

KE = $\tfrac{1}{2}mv^2$ = 2.972 J

Rotational energy = $\tfrac{1}{2}I\omega^2 = \tfrac{1}{2}I\dfrac{v^2}{r^2} = \tfrac{1}{2}\tfrac{2}{5}mr^2\dfrac{v^2}{r^2}$ = 0.4 × KE = 1.189 J

11. m = 75 kg, M_{up} = 0.682 × 75 = 51.15 kg, M_{low} = 0.318 × 75 = 23.85 kg

Coordinate of head = 63,153; hip = 105,87; foot 160,147 (approximate cm)

Length of upper segment = $\sqrt{(63-105)^2 + (153-87)^2}$ = 78.23 cm

Length of lower segment = $\sqrt{(105-160)^2 + (87-147)^2}$ = 81.39 cm

COM_{up} = 0.5 × (63 + 105), 0.5 × (153 + 87) = 84,120

COM_{low} = 0.5 × (105 + 160), 0.5 × (147 + 87) = 132.5, 117

Combined COM = 0.682 × 84 + 0.318 × 132.5, 0.682 × 120 + 0.318 × 117 = 99.42, 119.0

Moment of inertia about center of mass = 7.7659 kg.m² (apply parallel axis theorem as shown in text)

12. Assume arm adducts an angle of 180° or π rad. If we assume angular momentum is conserved, the center of mass of the combined body will remain unmoved during the arm adduction. The torque experienced by the arm (1) will be equal and opposite to the torque experienced by the rest of the body (2). Therefore:

$\tau = I_1\omega_1 = I_2\omega_2$ and $I_1\int\omega_1 dt = I_2\int\omega_2 dt$

Therefore:

$I_1\theta_1 = I_2\theta_2$ where θ_1 and θ_2 are the angles turned by the arm and the rest of the body, respectively.

We need to assume something about the lengths of the two rods. Let us take the arm as being 0.6 m long and the rest of the body as 1.9 m long. For simplicity, we can assume that the center of mass of the body remains at the center of the rest of the body. Therefore:

$I_2 = \tfrac{1}{12}M_2L^2 = \tfrac{1}{12} \times 0.95M \times (1.9)^2 = 0.95M \times 0.3008$

and an average value for I_1 would be:

$$I_1 = \frac{1}{12}M_1 l^2 + M_1 r^2 = \frac{1}{12}0.05M(0.6)^2 + 0.05M \times (0.992)^2 = 0.05M$$

$\times 0.4098$ assuming an arm angle of 90°.

So, the angle of tilt will be approximately:

$$\theta_2 = \frac{I_1\theta_1}{I_2} = \frac{0.05M \times 0.4098}{0.95M \times 0.3008} \times 180 = 12.9°$$

Notice that the mass, M, cancels out of this last equation for the angle of tilt.

Chapter 9

1. (a) 3.598 ms^{-1}
   (b) 55.58 ms^{-2}
2. (a) Backswing between 1.025 and 1.892 s (duration, 0.867 s). The swing is between 1.892 and 2.758 s (duration, 0.866 s).
   (b) Maximum velocity on backswing = 11.14 m/s; on swing = 36.31 m/s
   (c) Acceleration 256.7 m/s^2 at 2.183 s. (Answers Ch9Q2Ans)
3.

		Falling	Rising
Smoothed	Slope =	−1.7496	4.6648
Unsmoothed	Slope =	−1.7509	4.6692

Noise varies with position on the graph but is reduced by a factor of approximately 2 on the smoothed angular velocity graph. Perhaps more importantly, the noise is of lower frequency in the sense that sharp edges are rounded off. (Answers Ch9Q3Ans)

4. Look at R^2 values for 2nd and 3rd order polynomials (Answers: Ch9Q4Ans)
5. The coordinates of the three missing points are:

Field	t (s)	Interpolated Values, x	Interpolated Values, y	Interpolated Values, z
164	1.3583	−205.73	−351.05	733.56
165	1.3667	−223.26	−369.02	720.78
166	1.375	−243.30	−390.94	709.84

(Answers: Ch9Q5Ans)

Chapter 10

1. See Ch10Q1Ans chart *mass height*
2. See Ch10Q1Ans chart *angular velocity*
3. $h = -39.876t^2 + 124.69t + 955.59 \qquad R^2 = 1$
4. $\omega = 0.9618t - 1.4952 \qquad R^2 = 0.9993$
   $\omega = -0.0738t + 5.2731 \qquad R^2 = 0.9659$
5. downward acceleration of mass = 2(39.876) = 79.752 mm/s^2
   Peak velocity of wrist = 7706 mm/s filtered, 7690 mm/s unfiltered
   Peak velocity of punch bag = 760 mm/s filtered, 1130 mm/s unfiltered
   Acceleration of punch bag = 23200 mm/s^2 or 23.2 m/s^2

Chapter 11

1. (a) $N_{rots} = 0.241$
   (b) Deflection = 15.9 mm
   (c) $C_s = 2.13$
   (d) $C_L = 0.216$
   (Answers Ch11Q1Ans)

UNITS OF MEASUREMENT AND MATHEMATICAL METHODS

1. The SI system of Units

The fundamental mechanical units for length, mass, and time in the International System of Units (SI) system are:

The meter (m)

The kilogram (kg)

The second (s)

Prefixes can be used in conjunction with SI units so that the prefixed units are related to one another by powers of 10. These prefixes are presented in Table A1(a).

In addition to mass, length, and time, there are SI base units for temperature, electric current, amount of substance, and luminous intensity. These base units are presented in Table A1(b).

Prefixed units are commonly used in order to get working units of a convenient size. For example, it is easier to write "1 mm" than to use 0.001 m or even 1×10^{-3} m. However, the kilogram unit is an oddity in the sense that, for historical reasons, it already has the "kilo" prefix already present in the base unit; this means that kg is almost never prefixed for obvious reasons. Some derived units useful in mechanics are shown in Table A1(c).

2. Trigonometry

    (i) The Pythagorean Theorem

In any right-angled triangle:

$$c^2 = a^2 + b^2$$

Table A.1 (a) Prefixes used in the metric system

Multiple	Prefix	Abbreviation
10^9	giga	G
10^6	mega	M
10^3	kilo	k
10^{-1}	deci	d
10^{-2}	centi	c
10^{-3}	milli	m
10^{-6}	micro	μ
10^{-9}	nano	n

Table A.1 (b) Base units in the SI system

Dimension	Unit	Symbol
Mass	Kilogram	kg
Length	Meter	m
Time	Second	s
Temperature	Degree Kelvin	K
Electrical current	Ampere	A
Amount of substance	Mole	mol
Luminous intensity	Candela	cd

Table A.1 (c) Derived units

Dimension	Unit	Symbol
Acceleration	Meters per second squared	m/s^2 or $m.s^{-2}$
Angle	Radian	rad
Area	Meter squared	m^2
Concentration	Moles per meter cubed	mol/m^3 or $mol.m^{-3}$
Density	Kilograms per meter cubed	kg/m^3 or $kg.m^{-3}$
Energy	Joule (or Nm)	J
Impulse	Newton seconds	Ns
Moment of inertia	Kilogram meters squared	$kg.m^2$
Momentum	Kilograms meters per second	$kg.m/s$ or $kg.m.s^{-1}$
Power	Watts (or Nm/s)	W
Pressure	Pascal (N/m^2)	Pa
Speed	Meters per second	m/s or $m.s^{-1}$
Torque	Newton meters	Nm
Velocity	Meters per second	m/s or $m.s^{-1}$
Volume	Meters cubed	m^3
Work	Joules or Newton meters	J or Nm

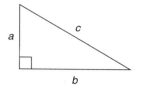

(ii) Sine, Cosine, and Tangent

In a right-angled triangle, the angles can be evaluated with sin, cos, or tan.

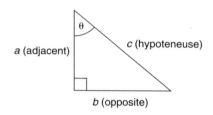

$$\sin \theta = \frac{b}{c}$$

$$\cos \theta = \frac{a}{c}$$

$$\tan \theta = \frac{b}{a}$$

Angles can be calculated from lengths by using the inverse relationships. For example, the angle θ could be written as:

$$\theta = \sin^{-1}\left(\frac{b}{c}\right)$$

or arcsin (b/c) or asin (b/c). On a calculator (or within a software package), the angle may be expressed in radians or degrees depending on how it is set up. Degrees can be converted to radians by remembering that 360° is 2π rad (1 rad is 57.3°).

(iii) Sine Rule

In any triangle (whether right-angled or not), the angles and lengths of the sides are related by the sine rule. Labeling the angles:

A: Opposite side of length a
B: Opposite side of length b
C: Opposite side of length c

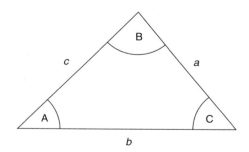

then we have:

$$\frac{a}{\sin A} = \frac{b}{\sin B} = \frac{c}{\sin C}$$

(iv) Cosine Rule

In any triangle:

$$c^2 = a^2 + b^2 - 2ab \cos C$$
$$b^2 = a^2 + c^2 - 2ac \cos B$$
$$a^2 = b^2 + c^2 - 2bc \cos A$$

These three equations can be used singly or together, depending on what information is known in the triangle.

3. Vector Analysis

(i) Adding and Subtracting Vectors by the Head-and-Tail Method

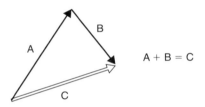

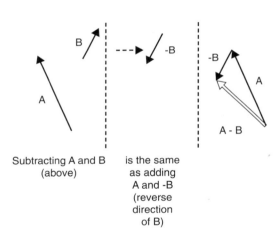

Subtracting A and B (above) is the same as adding A and -B (reverse direction of B)

(ii) Coordinate Axes And Unit Vectors

A righthanded set of coordinate axes x, y, z is always used for vector analysis. The unit vectors i, j, and k, are vectors of unit length pointing along the x, y, and z directions, respectively.

Any vector, A, can then be written in terms of its components along the coordinate axes:

A_x = Component along the x axis

A_y = Component along the y axis

A_z = Component along the z axis

Thus:

$$A = A_x i + A_y j + A_z k$$

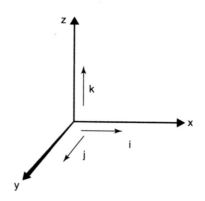

(iii) Adding or Subtracting Two or More Vectors Using Their Components

To add two vectors, **A** and **B**:

$$A + B = (A_x + B_x)i + (A_y + B_y)j + (A_z + B_z)k$$

To subtract two vectors, **A** and **B**:

$$A - B = (A_x - B_x)i + (A_y - B_y)j + (A_z - B_z)k$$

(iv) Components of a Two-dimensional Vector

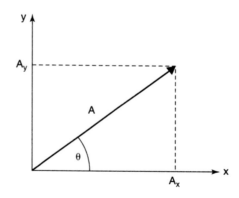

If **A** makes an angle θ with the x axis, then:

$$A_x = A \cos \theta$$
$$A_y = A \sin \theta$$

Also, the magnitude of the vector **A** is:

$$|A| = \sqrt{A_x^2 + A_y^2 + A_z^2}$$

(v) Components of a Three-dimensional Vector

If:

α = angle of vector with the x axis

β = angle of vector with the y axis

γ = angle of vector with the z axis

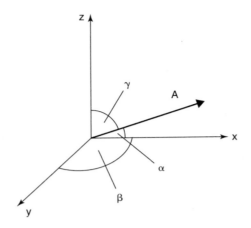

Then:

$$\cos \alpha = \frac{A_x}{|A|}$$

$$\cos \beta = \frac{A_y}{|A|}$$

$$\cos \gamma = \frac{A_z}{|A|}$$

where $|A|$ is the magnitude or length of vector **A**.

(vi) The Scalar (Dot) Product of Two Vectors, **A** and **B**

This is written as **A.B**, and the result is a scalar quantity.
If the angle between the two vectors **A** and **B** is θ, then:

$$\textbf{A.B} = |A|.|B|.\cos\theta$$

In terms of the vector components:

$$\textbf{A.B} = (A_xB_x + A_yB_y + A_zB_z)$$

(vii) The vector (cross) product of two vectors **A** and **B**.

The vector product is written as:

$$\textbf{A} \times \textbf{B}$$

and is itself a vector. If the angle measured between **A** and **B** is θ, then the vector product is of magnitude:

$$|\textbf{A} \times \textbf{B}| = |A|.|B|.\sin\theta$$

and in a direction perpendicular to the plane containing **A** and **B**. **A** $\times$ **B** is in the direction given by a simple righthand rule: if your fingers curl around from **A** to

B, then your thumb points in the direction of the crossproduct. (For more information on vector analysis, refer to Spiegel, 1959.)

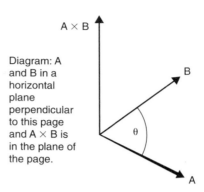

Diagram: A and B in a horizontal plane perpendicular to this page and A × B is in the plane of the page.

In terms of vector components, the crossproduct is:

$$A \times B = \begin{vmatrix} i & j & k \\ A_x & A_y & A_z \\ B_x & B_y & B_z \end{vmatrix} = i(A_yB_z - A_zB_y) + j(A_zB_x - A_xB_z) + k(A_xB_y - A_yB_x)$$

4. Errors in Data and Their Treatment

Experimentally measured quantities (e.g., distance, velocity) have uncertainties (errors) because of limitations in the measurement process. These uncertainties can be classified either as:

(i) *Systematic uncertainties* (errors), in which the quantity is measured consistently too big or too small. For example, a measuring ruler or tape might be the wrong length because of being stretched or because of temperature or humidity variations.

(ii) *Random uncertainties* (errors), in which the uncertainty can be positive or negative. For example, the height of a person measured over and over again will not be recorded exactly the same each time; the person doing the measuring will make small mistakes on each attempt.

Effect of Uncertainties on Calculated Quantities

Assume a quantity, c, is being calculated according to the equation:

$$c = a \times b$$

where a and b are measured quantities susceptible to uncertainties. We can then ask: What is the uncertainty in c? Let us assume that the measurement of a and b gives a range of possible values:

$$a \pm \Delta a \text{ and } b \pm \Delta b, \text{ respectively}$$

where Δa and Δb are the uncertainties in a and b, respectively. Taking natural logarithms:

$$\ln c = \ln(ab) = \ln a + \ln b$$

Differentiating:

$$\frac{dc}{c} = \frac{da}{a} + \frac{db}{b}$$

Therefore:

Fractional uncertainty in c = Fractional uncertainty in a + Fractional uncertainty in b

Multiplying by 100, we find

$$\frac{dc}{c} \times 100 = \frac{da}{a} \times 100 + \frac{db}{b} \times 100$$

% Uncertainty in c = % Uncertainty in a + % Uncertainty in b

5. Mean of N Observations

If a fixed quantity, X, is measured repeatedly N times, the mean (or average) of all the observations is:

$$X_{av} = \frac{1}{N} (X_1 + X_2 + X_3 + \,..........\, + X_N) \text{ (sometimes written as } \overline{X})$$

This mean is likely to be a better estimate of X than the individual observations X_i (i is used as a subscript standing for the numbers 1 to N). The mean is sometimes written as:

$$X_{av} = \frac{1}{N} \sum_{i=1}^{N} X_i$$

where the Σ stands for "summation."

Standard deviation of N observations: For a measure of the spread of the observations about a mean, the standard deviation is:

$$\sqrt{\frac{1}{N-1} \sum (X_i - X_{av})^2}$$

Table A.1 (d) Summary of other functions of a and b*	
Functions of a, b	**Method of Calculating Uncertainty in c**
$c = a + b$	Uncertainty in c is $\Delta c = 2(\Delta a + \Delta b)$ Work out percentage uncertainty by dividing this by c and $\times$ 100%
$c = a - b$	Uncertainty in c is $\Delta c = 2(\Delta a + \Delta b)$ Work out percentage uncertainty by dividing this by c and $\times$ 100%
$c = a \times b$	Percent uncertainty in c = Sum of percentage uncertainties in a and b
$c = a \div b$	Percent uncertainty in c = Sum of percentage uncertainties in a and b

*For more information on uncertainties and their treatment, refer to Topping J: *Errors of Observation and Their Treatment*, edn. 4. London: Chapman and Hall; 1972.

This is the "unbiased" version of the standard deviation; for details of the biased version and more on statistics, see Vincent (2005).

6. Graphs

Graphs are often used to display data points of the form (x, y) and to investigate any possible relationship between y and x. The following points should be observed when drawing graphs of x, y data:

- Examine the data and choose the axes and associated scales so that the data points occupy a substantial fraction of the available area.
- Choose the scale increments on the axes using convenient values.
- Label the axes with the quantity being plotted and the units of measurement.

Here are some axes, three done incorrectly and the fourth correctly:

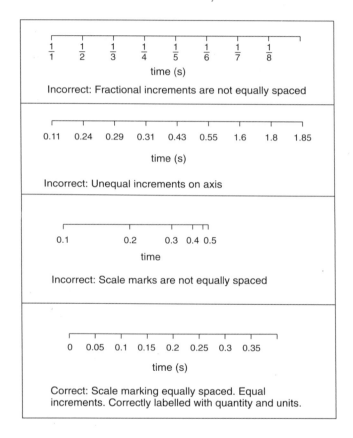

To further illustrate the use of graphs, we will consider some arbitrary velocity–time data shown in Table A1(e).

A graph of the data follows the table on pp. 322.

By inspection of the graph on the top, it appears that it shows a linear relationship between velocity and time. In the graph on the bottom, a straight line has been drawn on the graph by eye through the data points. This is the way it would have to be done if graph paper were being used. The slope of this line can be estimated by taking measurements with a ruler and estimating the sides of the triangle drawn on the graph with the data line as hypoteneuse. This would give:

$$\text{Slope} = 9.76/2.79 = 3.50 \text{m/s}^2$$

The intercept is the point where the drawn line crosses the velocity axis at $t = 0$. This value appears to be close to 1.5 m/s.

Table A.1 (e)	Illustrative velocity–time data
Time	**Velocity (m/s)**
0	1.5
0.3	2.8
0.6	3.8
0.9	4.2
1.2	5.6
1.5	6.3
1.8	7.8
2.1	8.9
2.4	9.4
2.7	10.3
3	11.7
3.3	12.5

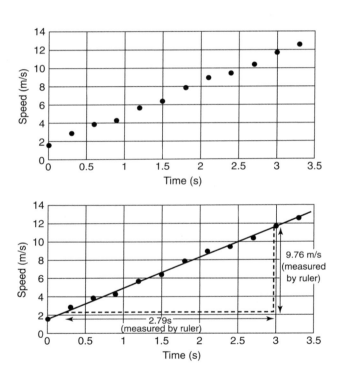

Least-squares Regression Line

In the example above, whereas the *y* data (dependent variable) is subject to some uncertainty, the *x* data (independent variable) can be considered exact. The objective is to find the coefficients *a* and *b* in the expression:

$$y = a + bx$$

such that the sum of the vertical deviations squared of the data points from the line is minimized. The resulting line is called the least-squares line of best fit or linear regression line. The formulas used are:

$$b = \frac{N\Sigma xy - \Sigma x \Sigma y}{N\Sigma x^2 - (\Sigma x)^2}$$

$$a = \frac{\Sigma y - b\Sigma x}{N}$$

It is now necessary to calculate the sum of the y's, the sum of the x^2's, and the sum of the x's times the y's. Putting the data into Table A1(f) and calculating these sums:

The numbers in the bottom row of the table are the sums of the columns. Hence:

$$\Sigma x = 19.8, \; \Sigma y = 84.8, \; \Sigma x^2 = 45.54 \text{ and } \Sigma xy = 182.52$$

Therefore, the coefficients a and b in the regression line are:

$$b = \frac{12 \times (182.52) - (19.8) \times (84.8)}{12 \times (45.54) - (19.8)^2} = \frac{-511.2}{-154.44} = 3.31$$

$$a = \frac{84.8 - 3.31 \times 19.8}{12} = 1.605$$

In the next graph, two things have been added: (1) a series of error bars on the data points representing ± 1 standard deviation above and below the data and (2) the least-squares regression line giving the straight line of best fit to the data. The conclusion from this is:

(i) The best-fit, least-squares regression line goes through the envelope created by the upper and lower standard deviation lines. This gives us confidence that we are really are dealing with a linear relationship between the variables.

(ii) The slope and intercept values generated from the regression are 3.31 and 1.605, respectively. Clearly, comparing this with the results obtained by visual fitting of a straight line (3.5 and 1.5), the benefits of using the regression method are obvious.

Fortunately, most spreadsheet packages and statistical programs include least square regression for linear and curve fitting. The value of the regression coefficient

Table A.1 (f)   A step in calculating the regression coefficients a and b

x	y	x²	x × y
0	1.5	0	0
0.3	2.8	0.09	0.84
0.6	3.8	0.36	2.28
0.9	4.2	0.81	3.78
1.2	5.6	1.44	6.72
1.5	6.3	2.25	9.45
1.8	7.8	3.24	14.04
2.1	8.9	4.41	18.69
2.4	9.4	5.76	22.56
2.7	10.3	7.29	27.81
3	11.7	9.00	35.1
3.3	12.5	10.89	41.25
19.8	**84.8**	**45.54**	**182.52**

R^2 is 0.9958. This indicates an extremely good fit to a straight line because it is very close to 1. For more information on regression, see Vincent (2005).

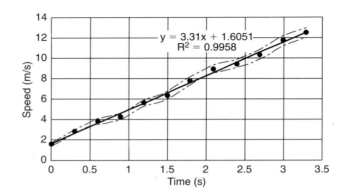

7. Elementary Ideas of Calculus

(i) Differentiation

The fundamental idea of differentiation is to find the slope of a tangent drawn to a curve at a point. For example, in the following example, the tangent is drawn to the curve at three particular values of x.

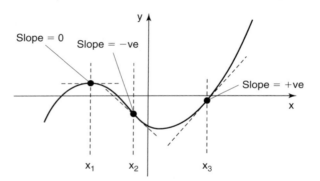

The idea of differentiation is to evaluate the slope at a point by taking it as:

$$\frac{\Delta y}{\Delta x}$$

That is, dividing a small increment in y by a small increment in x. In differentiation, this process is taken to the limit as Δx approaches 0, and the result is written as:

$$\frac{dy}{dx}$$

the derivative of y with respect to x. The process can be repeated to produce the second derivative, $\frac{d^2y}{dx^2}$. If y is known as an explicit function of x, then dy/dx can often be evaluated using a range of analytical methods. If y is not known as an explicit function of x, then numerical techniques can be used to approximate the derivative dy/dx and higher derivatives. Table A1 (g) gives some common functions and their first derivatives.

Table A.I (g)	Some functions and their derivatives
Function y	**Derivative dy/dx**
x	1
x^2	$2x$
x^3	$3x^2$
$\sin x$	$\cos x$
$\sin \omega x$	$\omega \cos \omega x$
$\cos x$	$-\sin x$
$\cos \omega x$	$-\omega \sin \omega x$
e^x	e^x
e^{-x}	$-e^{-x}$
$\log_e x$	$1/x$
e^{kx}	ke^{kx}

(ii) Integration

The essential idea of integration is to find the area bounded by a curve or function. Consider the graph of y versus x:

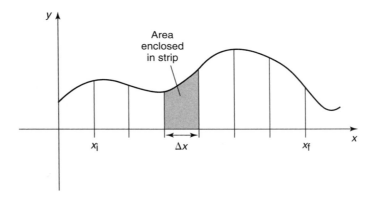

The area under the curve of y against x can be approximated as the sum of the areas of a number of strips each Δx wide and stretching from the initial x-value x_i to the final x value, x_f. Each strip has an area given by Δx multiplied by a y value indicative of the height of the strip. In integration, the area of these strips is added together:

$$\Sigma y \times \Delta x$$

Δx in such a way that the number of strips is allowed to increase to infinity and the width of the strips Δx becomes infinitesimally small. Then, the area under the curve between the limits x_i and x_f is written as the *integral* of y with respect to x:

$$\int_{x_i}^{x_f} y dx$$

If y is known as an explicit function of x, then the integral can often be written down or derived using a number of standard methods. The integrals of some common functions are given in Table A1(h).

Table A.I (h)	Some functions and their integrals
Function y	**Integral $\int ydx$**
1	x
x	$1/2x^2$
x^2	$x^3/3$
$\cos x$	$-\sin x$
$\cos \omega x$	$-\omega (\sin \omega x)/\omega$
$\sin x$	$-\cos x$
$\sin \omega x$	$-\omega (\cos \omega x)/\omega$
e^x	e^x
e^{-x}	$-e^{-x}$
$\log_e x$	$1/x$
e^{kx}	ke^{kx}/k

If y is not known as an explicit function of x, then approximate numerical methods of integration must be used. Two major forms of numerical integration are in common use: Euler's method and Runge-Kutta methods. For more information on calculus and numerical integration, refer to Smith and Minton (2002).

References

Smith RT, Minton RB: *Calculus*, edn. 2. New York: McGraw-Hill; 2002.

Spiegel MR: *Schaum's Outline of Vector Analysis*. Schaum Publishing; 1959.

Topping J: *Errors of Observation and Their Treatment*, edn. 4. London: Chapman and Hall; 1972.

Vincent WJ: *Statistics in Kinesiology*, ed. 3. Champaign, IL: Human Kinetics; 2005.

ANATOMY AND MOVEMENT OF THE ANKLE AND FOOT

The proximal joint of the foot is the talocrural, or ankle, joint (Fig. A2-1). It is a uniaxial hinge joint formed by the tibia and fibula (tibiofibular joint) and the tibia and talus (tibiotalar joint). The axis of rotation for the ankle joint is a line between the two malleoli running oblique to the tibia and not in line with the body. The movement of dorsiflexion (plantarflexion) occurs at the ankle joint as the foot moves toward (away from) the leg (Fig. A2-2). The average range of motion is 50° plantarflexion and 20° dorsiflexion.

Moving distally from the talocrural joint is the subtalar or talocalcaneal joint consisting of the articulation between the talus and the calcaneus, referred to as the hindfoot. All of the joints in the foot, including the subtalar joint, are shown in Figure A2-3.

The axis of rotation for the subtalar joint runs from the posterior, lateral plantar to the anterior, dorsal medial surface of the talus (Fig. A2-4).

Tri-plane movement is allowed to occur about the subtalar's single axis because of simultaneous actions in the sagittal, frontal, and transverse planes because the axis is oblique running through all of the planes. These tri-plane movements at the subtalar joint are called *supination* and *pronation*. Figure A2-5 shows the differences in subtalar movements between open- and closed-chain positioning. In the weight-bearing closed kinetic system, the movement of pronation consists of calcaneal eversion, talar adduction, and plantarflexion; the talus moves on the calcaneus. Eversion is the movement in the frontal plane in which the lateral border of the foot moves toward the leg in non–weight-bearing or the leg moves toward the foot in weight bearing as the calcaneus lies on its medial surface.

The transverse plane motion is abduction with the toes pointing out, and it occurs with external rotation of the foot on the leg and lateral movement of the calcaneus in the non–weight-bearing position, or internal rotation of the leg with

Figure A2.1 The talocrural joint, commonly called the ankle joint, refers to the articulations between the tibia and the talus (tibiotalar joint) and the tibia and the fibula (tibiofibular joint). The tibia and fibula create a mortise, making the joint very stable unless the mortise is altered through injury. *(Modified with permission from Hamill J, Knutzen KM: Biomechanical Basis of Human Movement. Philadelphia: Williams and Wilkins; 1995.)*

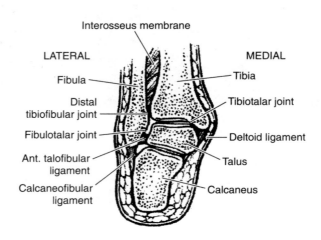

respect to the calcaneus and medial movement of the talus in weight bearing. The movement of supination is just the opposite.

Motion of the foot during running is shown in Figure A2-6 for one leg cycle.

Of the remaining articulations in the foot, the mid-tarsal or transverse tarsal joint has the most functional significance. It actually consists of two joints, the calcaneocuboid on the lateral side and the talonavicular on the medial side of the foot. In combination, they form an S-shaped joint with two axes, oblique and longitudinal. Movement at the midtarsal joint is dependent on the subtalar position.

Figure A2.2
Plantarflexion and dorsiflexion occur around a mediolateral axis running through the ankle joint. The range of motion for plantarflexion and dorsiflexion is approximately 50° and 20°, respectively. Plantarflexion and dorsiflexion can be produced with the foot moving on a fixed tibia or with the tibia moving on a fixed foot. *(Modified with permission from Hamill J, Knutzen KM: Biomechanical Basis of Human Movement. Philadelphia: Williams and Wilkins; 1995.)*

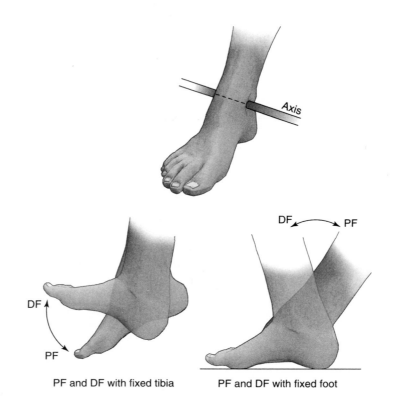

PF and DF with fixed tibia   PF and DF with fixed foot

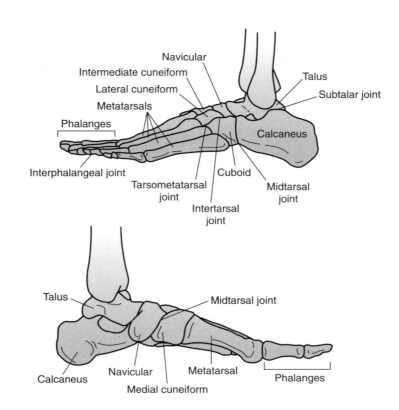

Figure A2.3   Thirty different joints in the foot work in combination to produce the movements of the rearfoot, midfoot, and forefoot. The subtalar and midtarsal joints contribute to the movements of pronation and supination. The intertarsal, tarsometatarsal, metatarsophalangeal, and interphalangeal joints contribute to movement of the forefoot and toes. *(Modified with permission from Hamill J, Knutzen KM: Biomechanical Basis of Human Movement.* Philadelphia: Williams and Wilkins; 1995.)

When the subtalar joint is in pronation, the two axes of the midtarsal joint are parallel, which unlocks the joint, creating hypermobility in the foot. Figure A2-7 shows these two axes for two cases.

During supination of the subtalar joint, the two axes running through the midtarsal joint converge and are no longer parallel. This locks the joint in creating a rigidity in the foot necessary for efficient force application during later stages of stance.

Figure A2.4   The axis of rotation for the subtalar joint runs diagonally from the posterior, lateral, plantar surface to the anterior, medial, dorsal surface. The axis is situated approximately 42° in the sagittal plane and 16° in the transverse plane. *(Modified with permission from Hamill J, Knutzen KM: Biomechanical Basis of Human Movement.* Philadelphia: Williams and Wilkins; 1995.)

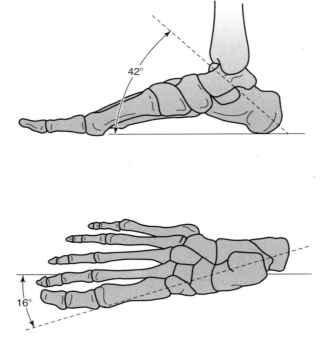

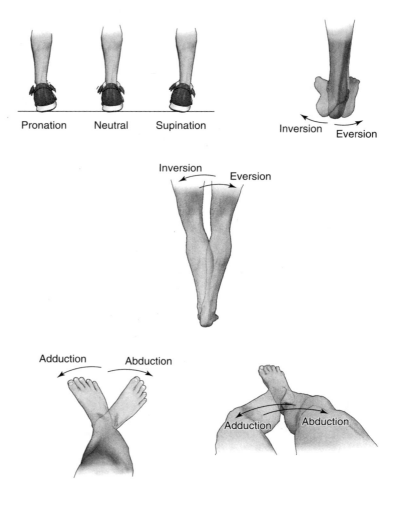

Figure A2.5 Movements at the subtalar joint are termed *pronation* and *supination*. With the foot off the ground, the foot moves on a fixed tibia and the subtalar movement of pronation is produced by eversion, abduction, and dorsiflexion. Supination in the open chain is produced by inversion, abduction, and plantarflexion. In a closed kinetic chain, with the foot fixed on the ground, much of the pronation and supination is produced by the weight of the body acting on the talus. In this weight-bearing position, the tibia moves on the talus to produce the movements of pronation and supination. *(Modified with permission from Hamill J, Knutzen KM: Biomechanical Basis of Human Movement. Philadelphia: Williams and Wilkins; 1995.)*

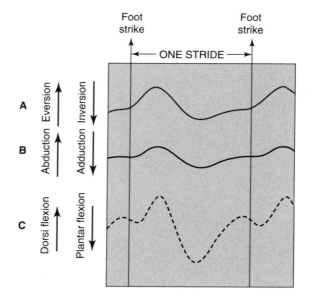

Figure A2.6 The pattern of motion of the foot during one running stride is presented. The foot (A) everts and inverts, (B) abducts and adducts, and (C) plantar flexes and dorsiflexes in the running stride. *(Modified with permission from Hamill J, Knutzen KM: Biomechanical Basis of Human Movement. Philadelphia: Williams and Wilkins; 1995.)*

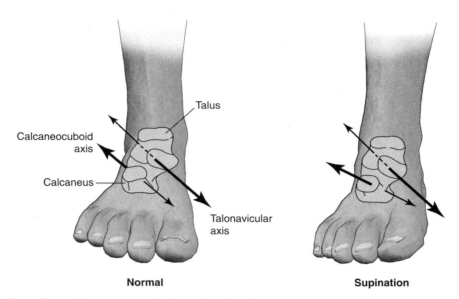

Normal   **Supination**

Figure A2.7   The midtarsal joints consist of the articulations between the calcaneus and the cuboid (calcaneocuboid joint) and the talus and the navicular (talonavicular joint). Each joint has an axis of rotation that runs obliquely across the joint. When the two axes are parallel to each other, the foot is flexible and can freely move. If the axes do not run parallel to each other, the foot is locked in a rigid position. This occurs with the supination movement. *(Modified with permission from Hamill J, Knutzen KM: Biomechanical Basis of Human Movement. Philadelphia: Williams and Wilkins; 1995.)*

Figure A2.8   The metatarsal head should be oriented in a plane that is perpendicular to the heel in a normal alignment in the foot. There are many variations in this alignment, including forefoot valgus (in which the medial side of the forefoot drops below the neutral plane), forefoot varus (in which the medial side lifts), rearfoot valgus (in which the calcaneus is everted), and rearfoot varus (in which the calcaneus is inverted). There can also be tibial and subtalar varum or valgus, in which the tibia or talus moves laterally or bmedially, respectively. *(Modified with permission from Hamill J, Knutzen KM: Biomechanical Basis of Human Movement. Philadelphia: Williams and Wilkins; 1995.)*

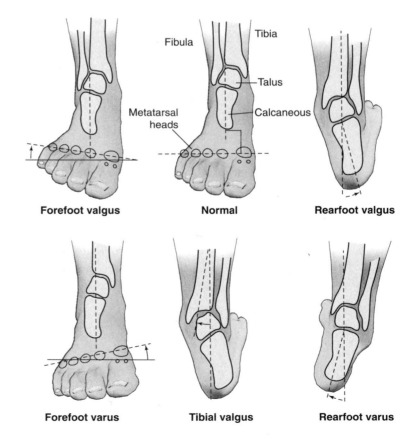

The forefoot is composed of the metatarsals and the phalanges and the respective joints between them. The function of the forefoot is to maintain the transverse metatarsal arch, the medial longitudinal arch, and the flexibility in the first metatarsal. The plane of the forefoot at the metatarsal head, formed by the second, third, and fourth metatarsals, should be oriented perpendicular to the vertical axis of the heel in normal forefoot alignment. This is the neutral position for the forefoot (Fig. A2-8). If the plane is tilted so that the medial side lifts, it is termed *forefoot supination* or *varus*. If the medial side drops below the neutral plane, it is termed *forefoot pronation* or *valgus*. Figure A2-8.

REFERENCE

Hamill J, Knutzen KM: *Biomechanical Basis of Human Movement.* Philadelphia: Williams and Wilkins; 1995.

INDEX